Neuromuscular Disease: A Case-Based Approach

Neuromuscular Disease

A Case-Based Approach

Second Edition

Jessica E. Hoogendijk
University Medical Center Utrecht

Marianne de Visser
Amsterdam University Medical Center

Pieter A. van Doorn
Erasmus MC, University Medical Center Rotterdam

Erik H. Niks
Leiden University Medical Center

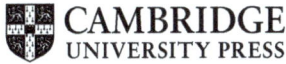

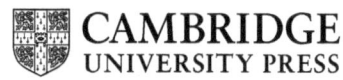

Shaftesbury Road, Cambridge CB2 8EA, United Kingdom

One Liberty Plaza, 20th Floor, New York, NY 10006, USA

477 Williamstown Road, Port Melbourne, VIC 3207, Australia

314–321, 3rd Floor, Plot 3, Splendor Forum, Jasola District Centre, New Delhi – 110025, India

103 Penang Road, #05–06/07, Visioncrest Commercial, Singapore 238467

Cambridge University Press is part of Cambridge University Press & Assessment, a department of the University of Cambridge.

We share the University's mission to contribute to society through the pursuit of education, learning and research at the highest international levels of excellence.

www.cambridge.org
Information on this title: www.cambridge.org/9781108744188

DOI: 10.1017/9781108881593

© Jessica E. Hoogendijk, Marianne de Visser, Pieter A. van Doorn, and Erik H. Niks 2025

This publication is in copyright. Subject to statutory exception and to the provisions of relevant collective licensing agreements, no reproduction of any part may take place without the written permission of Cambridge University Press & Assessment.

When citing this work, please include a reference to the DOI 10.1017/9781108881593

First published 2013
Second Edition 2025

A catalogue record for this publication is available from the British Library.

Library of Congress Cataloging-in-Publication Data
Names: Hoogendijk, Jessica E., 1957– author. | Visser, Marianne de, author.| Doorn, Pieter A. van, author. | Niks, Erik H., author.
Title: Neuromuscular disease : a case-based approach / Jessica E. Hoogendijk, University Medical Center Utrecht, Marianne de Visser, Amsterdam University Medical Center, Pieter A. van Doorn, Erasmus MC, University Medical Center Rotterdam, Erik H. Niks, Leiden University Medical Center.
Description: 2nd edition. | Cambridge, United Kingdom ; New York, NY : Cambridge University Press, 2024. | Revised edition of: Neuromuscular disease / John H.J. Wokke [et al.]. 2013. | Includes bibliographical references and index.
Identifiers: LCCN 2024017717 | ISBN 9781108744188 (paperback) | ISBN 9781108881593 (ebook)
Subjects: LCSH: Neuromuscular diseases – Case studies. | Musculoskeletal system – Diseases – Case studies. | Diagnosis, Differential – Case studies.
Classification: LCC RC925.55 .H66 2024 | DDC 616.7/44–dc23/eng/20240509
LC record available at https://lccn.loc.gov/2024017717

ISBN 978-1-108-74418-8 Paperback
ISBN 978-1-108-88159-3 Cambridge Core

Cambridge University Press & Assessment has no responsibility for the persistence or accuracy of URLs for external or third-party internet websites referred to in this publication and does not guarantee that any content on such websites is, or will remain, accurate or appropriate.

Every effort has been made in preparing this book to provide accurate and up-to-date information that is in accord with accepted standards and practice at the time of publication. Although case histories are drawn from actual cases, every effort has been made to disguise the identities of the individuals involved. Nevertheless, the authors, editors, and publishers can make no warranties that the information contained herein is totally free from error, not least because clinical standards are constantly changing through research and regulation. The authors, editors, and publishers therefore disclaim all liability for direct or consequential damages resulting from the use of material contained in this book. Readers are strongly advised to pay careful attention to information provided by the manufacturer of any drugs or equipment that they plan to use.

Contents

List of Contributors vii
Foreword by Benedikt Schoser ix
Preface to 2nd Edition xi

Part I Evaluation and Treatment of Patients with a Neuromuscular Disorder

1. Neuromuscular Diseases: Anterior Horn Cell Disorders, Peripheral Neuropathies, Neuromuscular Junction Disorders, Myopathies 1
2. History Taking and Clinical Examination 5
3. Differential Diagnoses by Presenting or Prominent Clinical Feature 15
4. Electrodiagnostic Studies *Stephan Goedee* 35
5. Imaging *Stephan Goedee* 42
6. Muscle and Nerve Pathology 47
7. Genetic Testing *Wouter van Rheenen* 52
8. Management 57

Part II Neuromuscular Cases

Disorders of the Anterior Horn Cell

1. Amyotrophic Lateral Sclerosis (ALS) 71
2. Primary Lateral Sclerosis (PLS) 77
3. Progressive Muscular Atrophy (PMA) 79
4. Segmental Spinal Muscular Atrophy 82
5. Spinal and Bulbar Muscular Atrophy (SBMA; Kennedy Disease) 84
6. Spinal Muscular Atrophy (SMA) Type 1 85
7. Spinal Muscular Atrophy (SMA) Type 3 *Renske Wadman* 88
8. Postpolio Syndrome (PPS); Poliomyelitis Anterior Acuta, West Nile Virus Poliomyelitis, Acute Flaccid Weakness in Children 91

Peripheral Neuropathies

9. Guillain–Barré Syndrome (GBS) and Miller–Fisher Syndrome (MFS) 94
10. Chronic Inflammatory Demyelinating Polyneuropathy (CIDP) 97
11. IgM Anti-MAG Polyneuropathy 99
12. Polyneuropathy, Organomegaly, Endocrine Manifestations, Monoclonal Protein, and Skin Changes (POEMS) Syndrome 104
13. Vasculitic Neuropathy 107
14. Small-Fibre Neuropathy (SFN) 110
15. Sensory Neuronopathy (SNN, Ganglionopathy) 114
16. Wartenberg Migrant Sensory Neuropathy 116
17. Multifocal Motor Neuropathy (MMN) 118
18. Peripheral Nerve Hyperexcitability Syndromes: Morvan Syndrome 122
19. Idiopathic Brachial Plexus Neuropathy, Neuralgic Amyotrophy (NA) 124
20. Diabetic Neuropathy 127
21. Alcoholic Polyneuropathy 130
22. Chronic Idiopathic Axonal Polyneuropathy (CIAP) 131
23. Critical Illness Polyneuropathy and Myopathy (CIPM) 135
24. Drug-Induced Polyneuropathies: Amiodarone Polyneuropathy 137
25. Lyme Radiculopathy 139
26. Leprosy 142
27. Charcot–Marie–Tooth Disease (CMT) Type 1A/Hereditary Neuropathy with Liability for Pressure Palsies (HNPP) 144
28. Charcot–Marie–Tooth Disease (CMT) Type 2A and Type 2B 149
29. Hereditary Sensory and Autonomic Neuropathy (HSAN) Type 4 151
30. Hereditary Transthyretin (TTR) Amyloidosis 154

Disorders of the Neuromuscular Junction

31 Myasthenia Gravis with Acetylcholine Receptor Antibodies (AChR MG) 157
32 Myasthenia Gravis with Muscle-Specific Kinase Antibodies (MuSK MG) 161
33 Drug-Induced Myasthenia Gravis: Immune Checkpoint Inhibitor (ICI)-Related 163
34 Lambert–Eaton Myasthenic Syndrome (LEMS) 165
35 Congenital Myasthenic Syndromes (CMS): Dok7 168

Myopathies

36 Duchenne Muscular Dystrophy (DMD) 173
37 Becker Muscular Dystrophy (BMD) 176
38 Facioscapulohumeral Muscular Dystrophy (FSHD) 180
39 Myotonic Dystrophy Type 1 (DM1) 182
40 Myotonic Dystrophy Type 2 (DM2) 185
41 Limb Girdle Muscular Dystrophy (LGMD) R1, Calpain-Related 187
42 Limb Girdle Muscular Dystrophy (LGMD) R9, FKRP-Related 191
43 Bethlem Myopathy, a Collagen VI-Related Myopathy (LGMDD5); Ullrich Congenital Muscular Dystrophy 193
44 Oculopharyngeal Muscular Dystrophy (OPMD) 196
45 Emery–Dreifuss Muscular Dystrophy (EDMD) 198
46 Caveolinopathy, Rippling Muscle Disease 200
47 Distal Myopathies: Miyoshi Myopathy, Dysferlinopathy; Anoctaminopathy 202
48 Distal Myopathies: GNE Myopathy 206
49 Myofibrillar Myopathies: Desminopathy 209
50 Skeletal Muscle Channelopathies: Non-Dystrophic Myotonia; Myotonia Congenita (Becker) 212
51 Skeletal Muscle Channelopathies: Hypokalaemic Periodic Paralysis 216
52 Pompe Disease (Glycogen Storage Disease (GSD) Type II; α-Glucosidase Deficiency) 218
53 McArdle Disease (Glycogen Storage Disease (GSD) Type V); Myophosphorylase Deficiency, Rhabdomyolysis 224
54 Carnitine Palmitoyltransferase-II (CPT2) Deficiency 227
55 Mitochondrial Myopathies: Chronic Progressive External Ophthalmoplegia (CPEO) 230
56 Ryanodine Receptor 1 (RYR1)-Related Disorders 234
57 Congenital Myopathies: X-Linked Myotubular Myopathy 238
58 Congenital Myopathies: Nemaline Myopathy 240
59 Juvenile Dermatomyositis (JDM) 243
60 Dermatomyositis (DM) 247
61 Immune-Mediated Necrotizing Myopathy (IMNM) 252
62 Inclusion Body Myositis (IBM) 256
63 Endocrine Myopathy: Hypothyroid Myopathy; Hyperthyroid Myopathy 260
64 Drug-Induced Myopathies: Hydroxychloroquine Myopathy 262
65 A- or Paucisymptomatic HyperCKaemia 266
66 Exertional Rhabdomyolysis 269

Video legends 271
Index 274

Supplementary videos are available at www.cambridge.org/neuromuscular

Contributors

Pieter van Doorn
Department of Neurology
Erasmus MC, University Medical Center
Rotterdam, The Netherlands

Stephan Goedee
Department of Neurology
University Medical Center Utrecht
Utrecht, The Netherlands

Jessica Hoogendijk
Department of Neurology
University Medical Center Utrecht
Utrecht, The Netherlands

Erik Niks
Department of Neurology
Leiden University Medical Center
Leiden, The Netherlands

Wouter van Rheenen
Department of Neurology
University Medical Center Utrecht
Utrecht, The Netherlands

Marianne de Visser
Department of Neurology
Amsterdam University Medical Center
Amsterdam, The Netherlands

Renske Wadman
Department of Neurology
University Medical Center Utrecht
Utrecht, The Netherlands

Foreword

During the past three decades, interest in neuromuscular medicine has increased exponentially.

This neurology section turned from a descriptive diagnostic setting into a molecular diagnostic and currently gene therapeutic subject.

However, the base of all this development remains the deep phenotyping or, more holistically, the Gestalt approach to neuromuscular disorders.

In this book, four 'icons' of the neuromuscular world, Marianne de Visser, Jessica Hoogendijk, Erik Niks, and Pieter van Doorn, jointly describe emblematic clinical case reports of the whole spectrum of these acquired and inherited more than 800 distinct disorders.

In this book, all sections of the nervous system, from motor neurons via the spinal cord and peripheral nerve through the neuromuscular endplate into the skeletal muscle, are reflected in case presentation to raise awareness, interest, knowledge, and clues for beginners, professionals, and to esteemed experts of the field.

A state-of-the-art summary supports these case reports for evaluating people with neuromuscular disorders using neuromuscular-specific ancillary investigations such as electrophysiology, imaging, and genetic testing by Stephan Goedee and Wouter van Rheenen.

This book, written in the beautiful Dutch tradition of clinical perception of medicine, will help set the framework for teaching and learning about patients living with neuromuscular disorders.

Taking up this ongoing novel 'therapy area' of neuromuscular disorders, this book is in high demand, as treating rare diseases is re-learning rare diseases.

Benedikt Schoser

Preface to 2nd Edition

Neuromuscular diseases (NMD) are classified as rare diseases affecting less than 5 individuals in 10,000, but collectively NMD are quite common. Diagnosis of NMD can be difficult, but due to advancements in particular in genetic testing, some adult patients may receive a better-defined or alternative diagnosis to the one established during childhood.

This book contains 66 neuromuscular cases across the spectrum of NMD that aim to familiarize the reader with the wide spectrum of clinical features in NMD, the diagnostic strategies, and therapeutic possibilities. Asking about symptoms and problems in daily life, the family history, and careful neurological examination often largely help to make an appropriate clinical and differential diagnosis. In the second edition of this book, 23 tables of differential diagnoses are included that assist in the diagnostic process. Additional laboratory investigations are often helpful and include at least assessment of serum creatine kinase (CK) activity in patients suspected to have a myopathy, anti-acetylcholine receptor, and other antibodies in patients with fluctuating weakness, and a range of laboratory tests to identify risk factors for polyneuropathy in patients with a neuropathy. The basics of electromyography (EMG) and nerve ultrasound (NUS) are described and illustrated. EMG examination is important in the diagnosis of motor neuron disease, helpful to diagnose polyneuropathy, and essential to dissect polyneuropathy into axonal and demyelinating subgroups. If a hereditary disease is suspected, up-to-date DNA analysis is often the diagnostic approach of choice. The basics of genetic diagnostic tests, including suggestions when and how to use them, are described. In inflammatory diseases of muscle, myositis blots to detect myositis-specific antibodies can be used to search for specific comorbidities. Advanced imaging techniques, especially MRI and muscle ultrasound, can be helpful to make the diagnosis or to guide the location of a muscle biopsy. An appropriate sequence of examinations usually allows for making an accurate diagnosis. However, despite advanced and targeted investigations, offering a precise diagnosis may remain a challenge.

Once a diagnosis has been made, other medical disciplines sometimes have to be consulted, for example a medical geneticist in case of a hereditary disease. Some patients with a hereditary myopathy, but also those with, for example, amyloidosis, require consultation of a cardiologist. Targeted treatment for hereditary neuromuscular disorders is currently limited to only a few diseases, but it is hoped that gene therapy will become more widely applicable in the near future. Most patients with immune-mediated diseases, especially those with immune-mediated polyneuropathy, and patients with myasthenia gravis or myositis can nowadays be treated successfully, but there is still a need for more effective drugs with fewer side effects, and new drugs are currently under investigation.

Management of patients with an NMD often also involves rehabilitation care in all its aspects, and there are current standards of care for anaesthesia, pregnancy, the transition of paediatric care to adulthood care, and palliation. Therefore, this book is relevant for a wide range of medical professionals, care givers, students, and others interested in patients with an NMD.

We are indebted to the late Professor John Wokke for his eminent contribution to the first version of this book, which was published in 2013. This second edition is fully revised and updated, now containing also paediatric cases and many new cases, new figures, and videos. To assist in the diagnostic process, we added 23 tables of differential diagnoses of a wide range of clinical problems (e.g., axial weakness, bulbar weakness, or pure motor distal weakness). However, we did not aim at completeness and this book is not intended to be a comprehensive textbook.

We thank Drs Stephan Goedee (Chapters 4 and 5), Wouter van Rheenen (Chapter 7), and Renske Wadman (Case 7) for their contributions, Professor

Preface to 2nd Edition

Eleonora Aronica and Dr Wim van Hecke for their help with the muscle pathology, Professor Peter Barth and Dr Anneke van der Kooi for providing Cases 58 and 64 Dr Janneke Hoeijmakers and Professor Jan Verschuuren for providing Figures 14.3 and 32.1, Professor Karin Faber and Dr Henk-Jan Westeneng for providing Videos 39.2-3 and 62.1, and Dr Merel van Maerle for her recommendations regarding genetic counseling in Chapter 8.

We foremost thank our patients, who form the basis of this book. They agreed to have their disease, or their child's disease, pictured in a photograph or video, trusting this will help in educating medical professionals and thus contribute to the treatment and care for patients with a neuromuscular disease.

Jessica E. Hoogendijk
Marianne de Visser
Pieter A. van Doorn
Erik H. Niks

Part I Evaluation and Treatment of Patients with a Neuromuscular Disorder

Chapter 1

Neuromuscular Diseases: Anterior Horn Cell Disorders, Peripheral Neuropathies, Neuromuscular Junction Disorders, Myopathies

Currently, there is a rapid, ongoing increase in our understanding of genetic neuromuscular disorders at the molecular level: many causative genes have been found, giving hope for targeted genetic treatments, already proven effective in some diseases. In immune-mediated neuromuscular disorders, pathogenetic mechanisms are better understood, and this enables the development of more precise immunotherapies. Increased knowledge has led to a refinement of classifications and has added numerous subtypes to the already hundreds of possible neuromuscular diagnoses. Patients can only benefit from future targeted therapies if an accurate diagnosis is made. Moreover, a diagnosis needs not only to be precise; the diagnostic trajectory needs to be swift, as current and future treatments will be aimed at the prevention or the restriction of irreversible damage.

The best way to diagnose a neuromuscular disease at this point is probably to recognize the phenotypical pattern, to know its differential diagnosis, and to proceed from there. The classic categorization of neuromuscular disorders in diseases of the anterior horn cell, peripheral nerves, neuromuscular junction, and skeletal muscle is not always sufficiently helpful as a starting point in the diagnostic process. For example, inclusion body myositis may mimic an anterior horn cell disease. Kennedy disease, an anterior horn cell disease, affects muscle too, and may present with a myopathy – suggesting CK elevation. In distal weakness, it might be cumbersome to differentiate between neurogenic and myopathic disease, and some drugs can cause both a neuropathy and a myopathy, or a combination of a myopathy and a neuromuscular junction disorder. Yet, from a practical point of view it is useful to keep to this anatomical–functional division: it provides a basic insight in functions, in understanding disease mechanisms, and in applying diagnostic and therapeutic tools. Therefore, we give a brief clinical characterization of the four categories of neuromuscular disorders. Details on physiology and pathophysiology are not discussed here.

Anterior Horn Cell Disorders

Anterior horn cell diseases, except for those caused by the polio virus and some other viruses, are progressive degenerative diseases of the motor neurons in the spinal cord and brainstem. These disorders may be hereditary, such as spinal muscular atrophy (SMA) types 1 to 3 in children and SMA 4 in adults, familial amyotrophic lateral sclerosis (ALS), Kennedy disease, and distal hereditary motor neuropathies (HMN; distal SMA). ALS, progressive muscular atrophy (PMA), primary lateral sclerosis (PLS), and segmental SMA are commonly sporadic. The clinical hallmarks of anterior horn cell disease are the lower motor neuron signs of weakness, wasting (atrophy), fasciculations, and reduced or absent tendon reflexes. In ALS, the upper motor neuron is also involved and in PLS this is the sole manifestation, characterized by hypertonia (spasticity), pseudobulbar symptoms, hyperreflexia, and abnormal plantar response. ALS, PMA, and PLS are collectively classified as *motor neuron diseases*.

Clinical assessment, that is, history taking and neurological examination, and exclusion of mimics usually suffice to establish a diagnosis of ALS or postpolio syndrome (PPS). Electrodiagnostic assessment (nerve conduction studies and needle electromyography) is a crucial step in the diagnostic process of PMA, segmental SMA, and distal HMN. Hereditary diseases (SMA, Kennedy disease) require genetic testing as first-tier ancillary investigation.

Infectious diseases affecting the anterior horn cells such as poliomyelitis anterior acuta are diagnosed by virus isolation from stool or pharyngeal swabs and the polio-like disease caused by West Nile virus (WNV) by testing of serum or cerebrospinal fluid to detect WNV-specific IgM antibodies.

Therapy is mostly supportive in distal HMN and segmental SMA, including physiotherapy, orthotics, occupational therapy, and pain and fatigue management. In motor neuron diseases, multidisciplinary treatment is required (i.e., a rehabilitation physician for preservation of motor abilities, a gastroenterologist for instalment of a percutaneous endoscopic or radiologic gastrostomy, a pulmonologist for (noninvasive) ventilation, a palliative care specialist, and others).

Significant advances in basic and clinical research paved the way for approved therapies in SMA with a focus on strategies aiming at increased survival motor neuron (SMN) protein expression, either via antisense oligonucleotides, small molecules, or viral gene transfer. These strategies have led to dramatic improvement of survival and motor function.

Peripheral Neuropathies

Disorders of nerve roots, plexus, or peripheral nerves are the most frequent neuromuscular diseases. Conditions caused by compression of one nerve root or nerve are usually handled by the general practitioner or neurologist based in a community hospital. Polyneuropathies are readily distinguishable from disorders of the anterior horn cell, neuromuscular junction, and skeletal muscle by the presence of sensory disturbances, but these may be mild and pure motor neuropathies do exist. Neuropathies can also be purely sensory. Neuronopathies, localized in the dorsal root ganglion, are associated with specific conditions, such as cancer. Typical pain patterns can point to a localization in nerve roots, plexus, or peripheral nerves. Neuropathic pain can be severe and should be treated appropriately.

Polyneuropathies can have many causes. Distinction between subacute and chronic disease course, onset in childhood or adulthood, symmetric and asymmetric symptomatology, length-dependent and non-length-dependent, and axonal and demyelinating pathogenesis is a useful approach for making a differential diagnosis. Nerve conduction studies complemented by ultrasound examination can establish a demyelinating pathogenesis. These are often immune-mediated. Recognition of these disorders has become increasingly important because of the increasing treatment options. Most polyneuropathies are chronic, symmetric, distal, and axonal. The most frequent causes are metabolic. Diabetic polyneuropathy, monoradiculopathy, and plexopathy can occur without a known prior history of type 2 diabetes. Evidence-based guidelines are useful in the diagnostic work-up of polyneuropathies.

Hereditary polyneuropathies can be axonal or demyelinating, as established with nerve conduction studies. In particular, axonal hereditary polyneuropathies can sometimes have their onset in adulthood, and these patients need not have typical deformities such as hollow feet. This is also the case in young children in whom often a pes planus is seen. Weakness can also present more proximal with difficulty rising from the floor and running. Many genes have now been identified, and these disorders can be increasingly diagnosed at the gene level, which is important for genetic counselling. Gene therapies for hereditary polyneuropathies have not been developed yet. Treatment is mainly supportive, including physiotherapy, orthotics, occupational therapy, pain and fatigue management, and – when indicated – orthopaedic surgery.

Neuromuscular Junction Disorders

Myasthenia gravis (MG) is the most common autoimmune disease affecting the neuromuscular junction. If the disease manifests with the typically fluctuating, variable, and fatigable ptosis and diplopia, the diagnosis can be readily made, but ancillary investigations are always indicated. MG can be distinguished into an ocular and generalized phenotype. MG is caused by antibodies directed at the acetylcholine receptor (AChR) situated on the postsynaptic membrane, or, much more rarely, at muscle-specific kinase (MuSK), which is needed for maintenance and clustering of the AChR. In particular, in ocular myasthenia, and rarely in generalized myasthenia, antibodies are absent or not detectable with current methods (e.g., seronegative MG). The diagnosis then rests upon the clinical phenotype, response to symptomatic treatment, and typical electrophysiological findings. The thymus plays a role in the pathogenesis of AChR MG showing hyperplasia or thymoma. Therapeutic strategies range from cholinesterase inhibitors, immunosuppressive or immunomodulatory treatment to immunotherapies that more specifically address distinct targets of the main immunological players in MG pathogenesis. If bulbar or respiratory muscles are affected, an emergency condition may occur, warranting adequate treatment and close monitoring in an intensive care unit (ICU). A myasthenic crisis is life-threatening, but if recognized early it is generally well manageable, with a good prognosis.

Lambert Eaton myasthenic syndrome (LEMS) is caused by antibodies directed at the voltage-gated calcium^{2+} channel in the presynaptic nerve ending. The influx of calcium is needed for the release of acetylcholine in the synaptic cleft. The clinical features are different from MG (namely, proximal weakness, autonomic dysfunction, and areflexia), and fluctuating weakness is less obvious as compared with MG. Apart from antibody testing, the diagnosis can be made by specific electrophysiological abnormalities. LEMS is strongly associated with small cell lung cancer, which should be screened for.

Congenital myasthenic syndromes (CMS) are extremely rare and heterogeneous genetic diseases with variable phenotypes. Most CMS are treatable. Some agents that benefit one type of CMS can be ineffective or harmful in another type, and therefore an accurate molecular diagnosis prior to symptomatic treatment is paramount.

The neuromuscular junction may be targeted by various drugs and toxins. Botulinum toxin (as drug or foodborne) and snake venoms such as β-bungarotoxin (cobra, mamba) block the ACh release at the presynaptic nerve terminal, which is resistant to anti-venoms. Organophosphates, present in pesticides such as parathion and used as poison (e.g., Novichok), inhibit acetylcholinesterase, which causes an excess of acetylcholine and may result in a possibly fatal cholinergic crisis including paralysis. Curare, snake venoms such as α-bungarotoxin, and muscle-relaxant drugs such as pancuronium competitively block the AChR prohibiting depolarization. Suxamethonium chloride (succinylcholine) is a muscle relaxant that binds to the AChR, causing depolarization, but not allowing for repolarization and subsequent depolarization, because it is broken down slowly. Tetrodotoxin, found in the liver of puffer fish, blocks the voltage-gated Na$^+$ channel. Diaphragm paralysis can follow very quickly.

Myopathies

Myopathies – diseases of the skeletal muscles – can be acquired or hereditary. The distinction, important because of the differences in diagnostic work-up and treatment options, rests initially upon careful history taking focused on age of onset and rate of progression. Acquired myopathies are commonly immune-mediated, and weakness progresses in weeks or a few months. A more protracted course can, however, occur, and these immune-mediated myopathies may lack inflammatory changes in a muscle biopsy, which may add to the difficulties in differentiating this group of diseases from a muscular dystrophy. An increasing number of autoantibodies is linked to the pathogenesis, and some forms are associated with cancer, which requires screening.

Hereditary myopathies are caused by DNA variants causing dysfunction or absence of proteins involved in, for example, the extracellular matrix, sarcolemmal structure and function, the nuclear envelope, metabolic pathways and mitochondria, the contractile apparatus, and ion channels. In particular, if the sarcolemma is affected, there is leakage of intracellular substances such as CK. A serum CK elevation of more than 10 times the upper limit of normal is commonly consistent with a myopathy. In many myopathies, however, CK activity is only mildly increased and may even be normal.

Many hereditary myopathies have specific complaints or abnormalities on clinical examination, needle electromyography (EMG), or muscle biopsy. Muscle biopsies should best be performed in a neuromuscular centre, in order to allow for appropriate processing. The final diagnosis, however, is made by genetic investigation, and EMG and muscle biopsy are often not indicated in the diagnostic work-up. The possibilities to diagnose a myopathy at the genetic level are expanding very rapidly, albeit a fair proportion is still awaiting a definite molecular diagnosis. Neuromuscular multidisciplinary teams therefore should include, among others, clinical and molecular geneticists, who can help interpret the results of genetic analyses and offer genetic counselling to patients and their families.

Causal treatment of hereditary myopathies is currently mostly restricted to enzyme replacement therapy, which is effective in Pompe disease, in which gene transfer therapy is now also in development. Rehabilitation treatment includes optimizing physical functioning and engagement in social life. In many progressive myopathies, there is an imminent danger of insufficient swallowing and respiratory function. Cardiac involvement can occur in various myopathies, leading to cardiomyopathy, dysrhythmias, or conduction abnormalities with the risk of sudden death. These complications require close monitoring to ensure timely interventions such as percutaneous endoscopic gastrostomy, noninvasive ventilation at home, or prevention or treatment of cardiac failure or instalment of devices (pacemakers, defibrillators).

Chapter 2

History Taking and Clinical Examination

History Taking

The main aim of a first consultation will concentrate on establishing a diagnosis. However, there are two other major aims: capturing the expectations of the patient and appreciating the impact of the complaints on daily life.

Purpose of the Visit and Expectations

If a patient presents with rapidly progressive weakness, fast-track diagnosing and effective and immediate treatment, if possible, are obviously required. For patients with a chronic disease, however, the purpose of their visit may vary. Some people are concerned about transmitting their disease to their children. Most of the patients are keen on obtaining an accurate diagnosis even if there is no causative treatment. This is particularly important in genetic conditions that will have an impact on family planning. Still others seek relief of symptoms, regardless of the precise nature of their illness. Many patients ask for a consultation in the hope that a severe disease diagnosis can be excluded. These considerations steer the diagnostic and therapeutic trajectory.

Diagnosis

Patients often present their symptoms related to functional tasks, which may provide important diagnostic clues. Examples include having heavy objects slip from the fingers (e.g., in inclusion body myositis), inability to turn a key (e.g., in amyotrophic lateral sclerosis (ALS) or in multifocal motor neuropathy), cannot run or does not shake hands (myotonia), a feeling of a 'folded sock' (sensory abnormality in polyneuropathy), neck pain (weakness of neck extensors). The patient's own words cannot be replaced by structured questions or questionnaires. It is also important to have a child formulate complaints as much as possible before asking the parents.

Notwithstanding the importance of the patient's own words, direct and specific questions should always be raised to pinpoint the onset of the disease, and to assess the rate of progression and the nature and extent of the problems. Relatives may also give valuable additional information.

Time Course and Duration of the Disease

Information about the onset of the disease and rate of progression as precisely as possible is paramount in the diagnostic process. First, if symptoms and signs worsen every day, week, or month, or fluctuate over time, an acquired disorder (usually with autoimmune or acquired metabolic or toxic pathogenesis) is likely. If the disease worsens little over years or decades, a genetic pathogenesis is much more likely. Careful history taking may be needed to determine the onset of the disease and its rate of progression. One should also consider that if patients, for example, lose the ability to walk, they may perceive this as an acute deterioration, whereas, in fact, the muscle weakness in the legs has progressed gradually. Second, assessing the rate of progression also determines therapeutic policies. A patient in whom symptoms and signs of weakness of respiratory muscles occur within a short time frame and increase every hour will need immediate action to safeguard respiration.

The following questions can be helpful in assessing the disease onset and time course: Are motor milestones reached, like rolling over, crawling, and independent walking? Is the patient keeping up with peers at school? At sports? What was the age at first symptoms? Are there fluctuations throughout the day? Do the complaints worsen over time? Over a period: days, weeks, months, years? Over decades? When did the patient start to use a walking aid? When could the patient still do things that are impossible now, such as getting out of a car, rising up from a chair, walking up/down stairs?

Information from the History That Can Point to Specific Clinical Features

- *External ophthalmoplegia and ptosis:*

  Double vision? Does double vision disappear at closing one eye? Drooping eyelid(s)? Fixed or fluctuating, on one or both sides? Symmetric?

- *Facial weakness:*

  Inability to whistle? Inability to drink through a straw? Inability to blow up a balloon? Difficulty to 'bury one's eyelashes' (squeeze eyes tight shut)? Dry eyes at awakening? Little facial expression when crying?

- *Bulbar weakness:*

  Difficulty speaking clearly? Hoarse voice? Nasal speech? Having to swallow repeatedly? A sensation of food getting stuck in the throat? Food or fluids coming through the nose? Coughing or gagging when swallowing? Weight loss? Infants: Weak crying? Poor sucking?

- *Respiratory muscle weakness:*

  Exercise-induced shortness of breath? Dyspnoea or feeling uncomfortable lying flat? Sleeping with how many cushions/pillows? Vivid dreams? Morning headache? Morning drowsiness? Daytime sleepiness? These symptoms of hypoventilation during the night are usually not admitted voluntarily and should be specifically asked for.

- *Axial weakness:*

  Difficulty holding one's head in an upright position? Difficulty rising from supine to sitting position? Difficulty holding one's head up while swimming or driving a car? Infants: Head lag? Difficulty remaining in an upright position while walking?

- *Weakness and wasting of arm or leg muscles:*

  Have arms or legs become thinner? Myalgia? Difficulty lifting objects above the head? Difficulty handling small objects? Difficulty opening a jar? Difficulty rising from a chair? Difficulty walking up or down the stairs? Moving off the stairs to the floor? Tipping over? Falls? Needing walking aid? Wheelchair? Weakness non-fluctuating? Fluctuating? Intermittent? In attacks? Provoking factors (cold, carbohydrates)? Children: Jumping, hopping? Complaints bilateral? Symmetric?

- *Sensory impairments:*

  Pins and needles in the feet? In the hands? Pain on slight touch? Numb feeling? Perception of walking on cotton wool or on a folded sock? Burning pain? Symmetric? Insecure walking in the dark?

- *Autonomic dysfunction:*

  Dizziness on standing up? Palpitations? Feeling of fullness after a small quantity of food? Changes in micturition? Obstipation or diarrhoea? Problems achieving or maintaining an erection? Abnormal sweating?

- *Fasciculations, myokymia, cramp, myotonia, rippling, contracture, pain:*

  A complaint of stiffness may be related to myotonia or muscle contracture, non-neuromuscular neurological signs (rigidity, dystonia, spasticity), or rheumatological conditions. Pain is the main symptom of cramp. Helpful questions include: Are there muscle twitches? Painful, involuntary, and unprovoked, accompanied by abnormal foot or hand posture, lasting up to minutes and shortened by stretching (cramp)? Confined to calves? Symmetric? Only at night-time? Cramp-like stiffness with or without pain provoked by activity? Sustained contraction with delayed relaxation when, for example, making a fist, closing the eyes (myotonia)? Plexopathy: lancinating pain in upper or lower limb? Radiculopathy: irradiating pain? Polyneuropathy: cramp? Pins and needles, pain at light touch (e.g., a bed sheet), burning pain? Myopathy: muscle pain? Stiffness? During exertion? Following exertion? Symmetric and proximal? Focal?

- *Rhabdomyolysis:*

  Episodes with dark brown (Coca-Cola-like) urine? Elicited by strenuous exercise, such as running? Accompanied by myalgia?

- *Skin changes:*

  Rash? Itching? Photosensitive? Ulceration? Excessive scars? Laxity?

- *Cardiac involvement:*

  Palpitations? Unexplained fainting? Swollen feet? Dyspnoea?

Family History

If there is a suspicion of hereditary disease, the family history should be taken systematically (preferably by drawing a family tree). How large is the family? Are there family members with similar complaints? Are the parents related? Does the family belong to an isolated community? Are the parents and siblings alive? At which age did they die? From what cause? Sometimes, specific information concerning family members should be specifically asked for (e.g., cataract in the father at a relatively young age – myotonic dystrophy type 1). Sudden death (myotonic dystrophy type 1 or 2 and other muscular dystrophies with cardiac involvement)? Features of mitochondrial disease such as epilepsy, migraine, deafness, diabetes mellitus? Cognitive deficit (Duchenne muscular dystrophy (DMD)) or decline, or behavioural changes (e.g., ALS)?

Previous Medical History

The onset of neuromuscular complaints can be preceded by conditions or signs of systematic disease in many neuromuscular disorders (e.g., a syncope preceding a diagnosis of a myopathy with cardiac involvement, epilepsy in a patient later diagnosed with *LAMA2*-related congenital muscular dystrophy). Unrelated conditions in the past may explain present symptoms or signs. A herniated lumbar disc at some time earlier, for example, can explain atrophy or hypertrophy and fasciculations in the ipsilateral calf.

Ask about use of medications, alcohol, and/or drugs. Is there a temporal relation to onset of symptoms?

Impact on Daily Life

For the purpose of offering appropriate treatment options and advice on supportive measures, it is important to obtain information about the home situation and the impact of complaints on daily activities and social life (see also Chapter 8, Management). The possibilities of rehabilitation medicine may be under- or overestimated by patients. Patients may also differ in their perception of the burden of their complaints and impairments. This influences the extent of the diagnostic investigations and the weighing of intended effects of treatments against the possible adverse effects. Obviously, this requires careful shared decision making.

Clinical Examination

Neuromuscular Examination in Infants and Toddlers: Some Points of Attention

Neuromuscular examination in infants and toddlers is best done with improvisation and observation. It is important to gain trust, not to rush, and to allow the child to play while in the meantime checking the various muscles for spontaneous anti-gravity movement in a random order. Examining a child who is shy can start while the child sits on the parent's lap and work from the feet upward. It may also help not to undress the child immediately, but first study some of the larger muscle groups in this position, for example by having the child reach for objects overhead and making a contest or game out of holding them. This also allows examination of the external eye muscles and facial expression while the child follows the object of interest. Tendon reflexes can also be tested in this sitting position. Axial and proximal leg muscles can be examined when the child lies on the floor and is encouraged to stand and walk towards the parents or an interesting toy. When possible, a next step would be to have the child run towards or alongside one of the caregivers. Proper running requires a moment in which both feet are above the floor and is normally achieved anywhere between two and four years of age. Before this, a child is usually able to jump or make a small hop on one leg. Preschool children are generally also able to walk on their toes and heels if given a clear example. More detailed examination of cranial nerves including mouth and tongue in young children is often best saved for last.

Neuromuscular Examination in Children and Adults

The neuromuscular examination can be best done in a structured manner. See Table 2.1 for an example. The examiner decides which parts of the examination need to be performed extensively, and which do not.

Cognition and Behaviour

Mental retardation, among other features of central nervous system involvement, is a hallmark of some congenital muscular dystrophies, in particular α-dystroglycanopathies. In DMD, and in children and adults with myotonic dystrophy type 1, there is an increased prevalence of various cognitive disabilities on neuropsychological testing, and psychiatric co-diagnoses such as attention-deficit/hyperactivity disorder and autism spectrum disorder. At presentation, patients with myotonic dystrophy, in particular type 1, typically may appear dull and apathetic, which increases the level of the diagnostic suspicion. In about 10% of patients with ALS there is frank frontotemporal dementia, and in about 30–50% there are cognitive

Table 2.1 Example of a structured neuromuscular examination

- General impression, cognition, language and speech, pseudobulbar affect
- Posture and walking pattern (scoliosis, hyperlordosis, waddling gait, bent spine, dropped head, walking on heels and on tiptoes), atrophy, hypertrophy, joint contractures in the legs, rigid spine, Gowers sign, Trendelenburg sign, Romberg sign
- Inspection with patient lying down or sitting: skin abnormalities, fasciculations, atrophy in the hands, myotonia, cramp (during muscle strength testing), joint contractures in the arms, range of motion abnormalities (frozen shoulder), hypermobility, foot or hand deformities, scars
- Cranial nerves, test for fatigability as indicated; forced cough
- Muscle strength testing: neck, arms, hands, trunk (rising from supine to sitting position), legs, feet
- Sensory testing as indicated
- Arms outstretched (tremor? pseudo-athetosis?)
- Coordination (finger-to-nose, heel-to-shin, tandem walking)
- Tendon reflexes

and or behavioural impairments. This information can be obtained from relatives (if asked specifically), or requires observation of language, social cognition, and behaviour (apathy or inhibition), or by using a screening tool such as the Edinburgh Cognitive and Behavioural ALS Screen (ECAS). Behaviour can also be altered in Morvan syndrome. Importantly, a lack of facial expression due to facial weakness should not be mistaken for a sign of cognitive impairment or a psychiatric condition.

Posture, Walking Pattern, Skin

Many physicians prefer starting the neurological examination by observing posture and gait. Observation of the patient in a standing position can reveal focal atrophy and hypertrophy, dropped head, bent spine, winging of the scapula, and abnormal curvature of the spine (scoliosis). Walking with hyperlordosis indicates weakness of the gluteal musculature, walking with locked knees (genu recurvatum) indicates quadriceps weakness, waddling gait indicates weakness of hip abductors. Walking on heels (foot dorsal flexors) and on tiptoe (foot plantar flexors) and testing for Gowers sign (gluteus maximus and quadriceps muscles) and Trendelenburg sign (hip abductors) are more sensitive means for detecting weakness than examination on the bench. Inspection of the whole body allows for detection of fasciculations and skin abnormalities. The latter comprise rashes and scaling (myositis), ulceration (myositis, sensory neuropathies), excessive scars (keloids), and nail dystrophy (amyloidosis), among many others. Amputated toes can be a complication of sensory neuropathies.

Fasciculations, Myokymia, Cramp, Myotonia, Rippling, Contracture, Hypermobility (Laxity), and Deformities

- Fasciculations are non-rhythmic, spontaneous, simultaneous contractions of all muscle fibres belonging to a single motor unit. Fasciculations are visible during the physical examination as twitches, and with ultrasound. They do not result in coordinated movement of a muscle. Electromyography (EMG) shows fasciculation potentials. They occur in neurogenic disorders, and in healthy people.
- Myokymia is a spontaneous, rhythmic or semi-rhythmic, uniform, continuous muscle contraction. Myokymia occurs periodically and is self-limiting in seconds to hours. The lower eyelid is affected commonly in healthy people. In disease, myokymia results from hyperexcitability of peripheral nerve motor axons. The EMG shows myokymic and neuromyotonic discharges.
- Cramp is an involuntary painful contraction of a muscle or muscle group that may result in an abnormal position of the limb. A cramp lasts seconds to minutes and can be shortened by stretching. Cramps may be provoked by exercise, for example during the neurological examination, but occur also in rest. Needle EMG shows continuous motor unit action potential activity. Their origin is in the lower motor neuron (anterior horn cell or nerve), but cramp also occurs in non-neuromuscular neurological diseases (Parkinson disease), non-neurological conditions, and in healthy people.
- In myotonia, as in muscle contracture (see below), there is stiffness following voluntary contraction due to delayed relaxation. This may be painless or painful. Myotonia can occur in any skeletal muscle. It can be elicited by percussion of the thenar, or by asking the patient to squeeze the hands or close the eyes for several seconds, and then suddenly release the grasp or open the eyes. In some diseases, myotonia

decreases after repeated contraction (warming-up effect); in other diseases, it can worsen. EMG shows typical myotonic discharges and complex repetitive discharges.
- Rippling muscle is composed of involuntary rolling skeletal muscle contractions that are mechanically induced by muscle stretching or percussion. Usually, this is accompanied by transitory local muscle mounding and percussion-induced rapid contractions. Needle EMG shows no motor unit action potential activity (EMG is 'silent'), indicating that these contractions originate in the contractile apparatus, and are not induced by depolarization of the muscle fibre membrane.
- Muscle contractures manifest with stiffness due to the inability of the muscle to relax normally in some myopathies. This may be either very painful (McArdle disease) or painless (Brody disease). In severe cases of McArdle disease, patients refrain from any activity out of fear of provoking a painful contracture. Stretching is not helpful. These contractures last for several minutes. As in rippling muscle disease, these muscle contractions are electrically silent on EMG.
- Joint contractures (arthrofibrosis, or rigid contracture of an articular joint) are caused by prolonged immobility of a joint. Joint contractures occur in particular in myopathies that affect the extracellular matrix (e.g., collagen VI-related myopathies) or in other myopathies, such as Emery–Dreifuss muscular dystrophy or *LAMA2*-related congenital muscular dystrophy.
- Joint contractures may result in deformities (scoliosis, hollow feet, hammer toes, claw hands). Hollow foot is best examined when the patient is lying down or in sitting position with the feet dangling. Deformities can also be caused by other conditions, for example Charcot foot in diabetes mellitus.
- Hypermobility (hyperlaxity) is an abnormally increased range of motion in a joint. Hypermobility is a feature of some, mostly congenital, myopathies. Often it is confined to distal joints, but hypermobility can also be generalized. Various criteria sets are in use to assess hypermobility. The simplest is the Beighton score, in which both proximal and distal joints are tested in a predefined way; see Table 2.2.

Table 2.2 Beighton scale for hypermobility

1. Passive dorsiflexion and hyperextension of the fifth MCP joint beyond 90°
2. Passive apposition of the thumb to the flexor aspect of the forearm
3. Passive hyperextension of the elbow beyond 10°
4. Passive hyperextension of the knee beyond 10°
5. Active forward flexion of the trunk with the knees fully extended so that the palms of the hands rest flat on the floor

Scoring: 1–4 are tested bilaterally. Maximum score 9. Abnormal: > 4/9 in adults, >5/9 in children.

External Ophthalmoplegia and Ptosis

External ophthalmoplegia may manifest with diplopia. Monocular diplopia is not due to external ophthalmoplegia. In acquired disorders, ophthalmoplegia is accompanied by diplopia, which is fatigable in myasthenia gravis (see Table 2.5 later in the chapter). Usually, chronic progressive external ophthalmoplegia (CPEO) remains unnoticed by the patient, since there is no diplopia. Ptosis is present when the upper eyelid is lower than its normal anatomical position, typically 1–2 mm below the superior corneoscleral limbus. The levator palpebrae muscle is affected in neuromuscular causes of ptosis. Ptosis due to weakness of the tarsalis superior muscle (Horner syndrome) is never complete. Many healthy people have an asymmetric palpebral fissure. However, asymmetric ptosis with or without diplopia should be examined for fatigability (see below). In disorders of the neuromuscular junction, and in particular myasthenia gravis, ptosis is usually unilateral or asymmetric. Ptosis, unilateral or bilateral, should be differentiated from blepharospasm, in which there is contraction of the orbicularis oculi muscle and no compensatory contraction of the frontalis muscle, as seen in ptosis.

Facial Weakness

Facial weakness is best examined by asking the patient to firmly close the eyes (orbicularis oculi muscle) and whistle or firmly pout the lips. Asymmetric closure of the mouth as in facioscapulohumeral dystrophy can be very subtle. Bilateral facial involvement may also present as reduced facial expression.

Bulbar Weakness

It is notoriously difficult to distinguish the various forms of dysarthria from one another. Bulbar dysarthria is often flaccid and nasal with softening of the consonants, especially P, T, and K. The speech can be soft and hoarse. Inspiratory stridor and laryngospasm may result from predominance of vocal cord adduction in cases of vocal cord abduction paresis. Dysphagia is diagnosed based on the history. If there is dysphagia, the patient in general will be referred to the ear, nose, throat (ENT) specialist for further characterization by fibre-optic endoscopic evaluation of swallowing (FEES) or videofluoroscopic swallow studies (VFSS). Inspection of the tongue for enlargement (DMD, amyloidosis, Pompe disease, hypothyroidism), atrophy, and fasciculation is best done with the tongue relaxed on the floor of the mouth. Slow and sluggish mobility of the tongue indicates involvement of the central nervous system. Upper motor neuron signs further include a 'pseudobulbar affect' (inappropriate laughing, crying, or yawning), and the less specific pseudobulbar reflexes.

Respiratory Muscle Weakness

Acute (or acute-on-chronic) respiratory failure leads to restlessness, tachycardia, tachypnoea, use of sternocleidomastoid or scalene muscles, or failure to string more than a few words together in a sentence. Counting in one breath can be used for monitoring. In chronic neuromuscular disorders, the clinical signs of respiratory failure may be very subtle. When there is emerging hypercapnia, the patient may easily fall asleep. Weakness of respiratory muscles may be shown by weak coughing (the patient attempts to cough with maximal force after deep inhalation). However, also in the absence of abnormalities on physical examination, if the history reveals complaints that indicate hypoventilation during the night, this should be investigated further during the patient's first visit. Forced vital capacity (usually expressed as percentage of that expected based on age and height) is easily done. A postural drop of more than 20 percentage points in supine as compared with sitting position indicates diaphragm weakness. A capillary blood gas analysis can be used to reveal hypercapnia, respiratory acidosis, or normal pH with compensatory increase of bicarbonate and base excess.

Axial Weakness

Weakness of neck flexors (dropped head) and neck extensors is best examined in supine and prone positions, respectively. If there is a bent spine (camptocormia) that is appearing in standing position, increasing during walking, and abating in supine position (making orthopaedic causes less likely) and no signs of a movement disorder, weakness of paraspinal muscles is likely. If there is no bent spine, the strength of the erector spinae muscles may be difficult to examine, and involvement of these muscles sometimes is shown only on MRI imaging. Weakness of abdominal muscles may be apparent on rising from supine to sitting position. Beevor sign is the upward movement (towards the head) of the umbilicus on lifting the head in supine position, caused by weakness of lower, but not upper, abdominal muscles.

Winging of Scapula

Symmetric winging is normal in young children. In older children and adults, scapula(e) alata(e) points to a dysfunction of nerve or muscle. Medial winging (inferior angle of scapula rotates medially and scapula translates superiorly) is most prominent on push-up and pushing against a wall. It is caused by dysfunction of the long thoracic nerve or the serratus anterior muscle. Lateral winging (shoulder droops with inferior translation of the scapula and the inferior angle rotates laterally) is more prominent by abduction of the arm and external rotation against resistance. This is caused by dysfunction of the spinal accessory nerve or dorsal scapular nerve, or by weakness of the muscles they innervate: the trapezius and rhomboid muscles, respectively. In healthy children, the scapula translates horizontally, without rotation of the inferior angle. Of note, strength of the deltoid muscle cannot be examined in the usual way if there is ipsilateral scapula alata, because most fibres arise from the scapula. To test the strength of the deltoid muscle in these cases, the scapula must be fixated by manual force on the thorax.

Wasting and Weakness of Arms and Legs

Muscle atrophy and hypertrophy can be difficult to assess, in particular in elderly people, if not focal and asymmetric. The tonus of diseased muscle is different from healthy muscle, but appreciation of this requires some experience. Muscle MRI can be helpful. Muscle strength is examined by manual muscle testing (MMT), which allows for testing many muscles in a short amount of time. It is necessary to test many muscles, as wasting and weakness of different muscles occur in different diseases. Using MMT, muscle strength is universally quantified by means of the 6-point Medical Research Council (MRC) scale; see Table 2.3. Some examiners prefer a subclassification of grade 4 weakness into 4−, 4, and 4+, or prefer using a 0–10 scale, but this adds to the inter- and intraobserver variability, especially in patients with mild or moderate weakness. MMT requires that the patient is able to give maximum strength (hampered by, e.g., pain and psychological factors), that the tested limb is in the right position (e.g., not locked), that the impact of the examiner's force is on the right place relative to the joint, that the patient is explicitly encouraged throughout the test until the muscle 'breaks', and that the examiner interprets the result relative to the patient's age and own muscle strength. The same holds for quantitative muscle testing (QMT), for example, measuring grip strength using a Vigorimeter, in which the result is expressed on a linear scale. QMT is mainly used in research settings. For a list of muscles, their actions, and innervation, see Table 2.4.

Fatigability

In suspected myasthenia gravis, several tests can be used to assess fatigability of muscle strength; see Table 2.5. A neostigmine test can also be useful in

Table 2.3 Medical Research Council scale for assessment of muscle strength

Grade	
Grade 0	No contraction
Grade 1	Flicker or trace of contraction
Grade 2	Active movement, with gravity eliminated
Grade 3	Active movement against gravity
Grade 4	Active movement against gravity and some resistance
Grade 5	Normal strength: active movement against full resistance

Table 2.4 Main action and innervation of the most important muscles

Action Test all muscles against resistance	Muscle	Nerve	Spinal segmental
Shoulder and arm			
Elevation of shoulder	Trapezius	Spinal accessory	C1, C2, C3, C4
Elevation and abduction of arm (arm sideways)	Trapezius	Spinal accessory	C1, C2, C3,
Pushing arm forward above the horizontal level: fixation of scapula	Serratus anterior	Long thoracic	C5, C6, C7
Pushing arm forward up to the horizontal level (activities such as bench pressing and push-ups)	Pectoralis major, clavicular head	Lateral pectoral	C5, C6
Adduction of arm (pull arm across the front of the body, as in hugging)	Pectoralis major, sternocostal head	Pectoral	C6, C7
Adduction of arm (palpable when coughing; downstroke when swimming, rowing and climbing, hammering)	Latissimus dorsi	Thoracodorsal	C6, C7, C8
Abduction of upper arm	Supraspinatus 0°–30° Deltoid[a] 30°–180°	Suprascapular Axillary	C5, C6
External rotation of arm, elbow fixed against trunk (playing tennis, cello)	Infraspinatus	Suprascapular	C5, C6
Flexion of forearm	Forearm supinated: biceps brachii, brachialis Forearm halfway brachioradialis	Musculocutaneus Radial	C5, C6
Extension of forearm	Triceps brachii	Radial	C6, C7
Supination of forearm	Supinator	Radial	C6, C7
Pronation of forearm; also flexion of forearm	Pronator	Median	C6, C7
Extension and abduction of hand (on radial side)	Extensor carpi radialis longus	Radial	C5, C6
Extension and adduction of hand (on ulnar side)	Extensor carpi ulnaris	Radial (posterior interosseus)	C7, C8

Table 2.4 (cont.)

Action Test all muscles against resistance	Muscle	Nerve	Spinal segmental
Flexion and abduction of hand (on radial side)	Flexor carpi radialis longus	Median	C6, C7
Flexion and adduction of hand (on ulnar side)	Flexor carpi ulnaris	Ulnar	C7, C8, T1
Extension of fingers at metacarpophalangeal joints	Extensor digitorum Thumb: extensor pollicis brevis	Radial (posterior interosseus)	C7, C8
Flexion of fingers at proximal and distal interphalangeal joints, respectively[b]	Flexor digitorum superficialis and profundus	Median	C7, C8, T1
Flexion of distal phalanx of thumb	Flexor pollicus longus	Median	C7, C8
Abduction (upward movement) of thumb with back of hand on flat surface	Abductor pollicis brevis	Median	C8, T1
Opposition of thumb (towards little finger)	Opponens	Median	C8, T1
Abduction of little finger with back of the hand on flat surface	Abductor digiti minimi	Ulnar	C8, T1
Abduction of index finger with palm of hand on flat surface	First dorsal interosseus	Ulnar	C8, T1
Hip and leg			
Patient prone: heel to buttock	Hamstrings[c]	Sciatic	L5, S1, S2
Patient prone: extend flexed leg; alternative (patient supine): extend the leg with the limb flexed in hip and knee	Quadriceps femoris	Femoral	L2, L3, L4
Patient supine: flexion of thigh (advances limb during walking)	Iliopsoas Aided by tensor fasciae latae	Femoral Superior gluteal	L2-4, L4, L5, S1
Patient supine: adduction of thigh	Adductors	Obturator	L2, L3, L4
Patient supine: abduction of thigh	Gluteus medius and minimus, tensor fasciae latae	Superior gluteal	L4, L5, S1
Patient supine: extension of thigh (movement towards bench)[d]	Gluteus maximus Hamstrings[c]	Inferior gluteal Sciatic	L5, S1, S2
Patient supine: dorsiflexion[e] of the foot	Anterior tibial	Deep peroneal or fibular	L4, L5
Patient supine: inversion of the foot (inward dorsiflexion)	Posterior tibial	Tibial	L4, L5
Patient supine: eversion of the foot (outward dorsiflexion)	Peroneus longus and brevis	Superficial peroneal or fibular	L5, S1
Patient supine: dorsiflexion of the distal phalanx of the big toe/toes	Extensor hallucis/digitorum longus	Deep peroneal or fibular	L5, S1
Patient supine: dorsiflexion of the toes	Flexor hallucis/digitorum longus	Tibial	L5, S1, S2
Patient supine: extension and plantar flexion of foot	Gastrocnemius	Tibial	S1, S2
Patient supine with knee and hip flexed: plantarflexion of the foot	Soleus	Tibial	S1, S2

[a] Deltoid muscle: elevation and retraction of abducted arm; function hampered if supraspinatus muscle is paralysed.
[b] Flexor digitorum profundus II and III muscles: flexion of distal phalanx of index and middle fingers with proximal phalanx fixed (median nerve, C7, C8). Flexor digitorum IV and V muscles have the same function for ring and little fingers (ulnar nerve, C7, C8).
[c] Hamstrings: biceps femoris, semitendinosus, and semimembranosus muscles.
[d] The gluteus maximus muscles and hamstrings act together when walking, running, and climbing; the gluteus regulates flexion of hip when sitting down.
[e] Dorsiflexion of foot is synonymous with extension.

the evaluation of neuromuscular transmission disorder (Table 2.6).

Sensory Impairments

See Table 2.7 for the main modalities of sensation. The examiner decides to what extent the sensory system needs to be evaluated. It is best to start with examination of tactile sense over various areas of the body using a wisp of cotton. Pain sense can best be evaluated comparing the feet with more proximal areas. If normal, a generalized neuropathy with involvement of small myelinated sensory fibres is unlikely. If small fibre neuropathy is suspected, detailed sensory testing is appropriate, and includes, among others, the assessment of negative signs (hypoaesthesia) and positive signs (allodynia, hyperalgaesia, aftersensation, diminished pinprick). Making a diagnosis of small fibre neuropathy can also include quantitative sensory testing (QST) and intraepidermal nerve fibre density (IENFD). The proprioceptive system can best be evaluated starting with the Rydell–Seiffer 128 Hz tuning fork at the tip of the hallux. If vibration is not perceived, or only for a split second, the examination must be extended to more proximal areas (base of hallux, midfoot, ankle, mid-tibia, knee, anterior superior process of the pelvic bone). If the patient feels the vibrations at the hallux for five seconds or longer, a generalized neuropathy with involvement of large myelinated sensory fibres is unlikely. Vibration sense (and the APR) diminishes in healthy old age. If vibration sense is normal, evaluation of joint position and movement sense will add little diagnostic value. If proprioception is severely impaired, there can be sensory ataxia of the limbs, pseudoathetosis, and a positive Romberg sign. Coordination testing of arms and legs can be severely impaired with eyes closed, which can give a false impression of weakness. In particular in elderly people, who often have a feeling of imbalance and a fear of falling from various causes, a Romberg sign can be easily false-positive if the patient is not reassured and gently distracted from the task.

Tendon Reflexes

Hypo- or areflexia in an early stage of disease points to a disorder of the anterior horn cells or of the peripheral nerves, in particular demyelinating neuropathy. In axonal polyneuropathies, which are much more frequent than demyelinating polyneuropathies, only the ankle jerk may be absent, with preserved knee jerk and tendon reflexes in the arms. In disorders of the neuromuscular junction, muscle tendon reflexes remain preserved until late in

Table 2.5 Tests for fatigability in suspected myasthenia gravis

- Observe increasing dysarthria while taking a history, or counting in one breath.
- Sustained upward and sideways gaze for 2 minutes, or re-examine following blinking repeated 20 times.
- Lifting the head in supine and prone position for 1 minute.
- Holding the arms outstretched for 3 minutes or re-examine deltoid muscle strength following contraction against resistance repeated 20 times.
- Ten deep squats.

Table 2.6 Neostigmine test

1. Inform the patient about the test and the possible side effects.
2. Start with 0.5 mg atropine SC or IM (to prevent side effects of neostigmine).
3. After 5 minutes: specific neurological examination/tests (see below). This part of the test can also be used to assess a possible placebo effect.
4. After the examination: administer 1.5 mg neostigmine SC or IM.
5. After 5 and 10 minutes and when no improvement is observed, repeat after 15, 20, and 30 minutes: specific neurological examination/tests.
6. Observe the patient for at least 30 minutes after neostigmine administration for possible side effects. (abundant fasciculations, decreased heart rate, gastrointestinal complaints like diarrhoea).

Neostigmine test is positive:
If there is no improvement of the functional tests after atropine and when there is a clear increase in muscle force after neostigmine administration.

Specific neurological examination depending on localization of weakness to assess the result of a neostigmine test:
Test for diplopia, ptosis, dysarthria: seconds that arms can be held in sitting position, or straight leg test in supine position, number of times able to stand from squatting, or number of words counting aloud in one breath).

Table 2.7 Evaluation of the somatosensory system

	Nerve fibres	Qualities	Symptoms	Examination
Exteroceptive system (vital sensation)	Small myelinated or unmyelinated: slow conducting	Crude touch Pain Temperature	Pain An/hypalgesia Hyperalgesia Loss of temperature sense*	Pinprick
Proprioceptive system (gnostic sensation)	Large myelinated fibres with thick myelin sheaths: fast conducting	Tactile sense Vibration sense Position sense	Numbness Tremor Uncoordinated movements Postural instability	Wisp of cotton. Rydel–Seiffer tuning fork (128 Hz) Fingertip–nose test, eyes closed Romberg test

Neuropathic pain can be burning, aching, or lancinating.
*Assessment of temperature sense is usually cumbersome in the consultation room.
Hyperesthesia is increased sensitivity to a stimulus and dysesthesia is distorted sensitivity to a stimulus. Allodynia is abnormal pain due to a stimulus that does not normally provoke pain.
Paraesthesias are abnormal spontaneous sensations (prickling, tingling, numbness, itching).
Romberg test: Standing becomes insecure when the eyes are closed as compared with eyes open.
Observe if the patient remains stable when turning around rapidly.

the disease course. A normal or brisk tendon reflex in an atrophic and weak limb suggests involvement of the upper motor neuron, as can be found in ALS. It is not always easy to establish if a tendon reflex is low or absent. The patient should be relaxed, the limb should be in the right position, the examiner should apply the right technique, and the hammer should be sufficiently heavy.

Autonomic Dysfunction

Assessment of orthostatic hypotension is an easy-to-perform test for autonomic dysfunction. It is defined as a decrease in systolic blood pressure of ≥ 20 mmHg and/or a decrease in diastolic pressure of ≥ 10 mmHg, three minutes after rising from a supine position. Additional autonomic function tests include measurement of how heart rate and blood pressure respond during exercises such as deep breathing and forcefully breathing out (Valsalva manoeuver).

Functional Neurological Symptom Disorder (FND)

It is important to diagnose an FND at an early stage, preferably at the first consultation. Refraining from ancillary investigations will prevent the finding of unrelated or difficult-to-interpret findings, which in turn may lead to more, sometimes invasive, investigations. A timely diagnosis may be beneficial for adequate treatment and recovery. Findings that indicate an FND are, for example, co-contraction of agonists and antagonists, intermittent contraction, sudden loss of contraction, a walking pattern showing extreme endorotation or exorotation, and an over-expression of effort. The Hoover sign is positive if seemingly present weakness of hip extension returns to normal with contralateral hip flexion against resistance.

Of note, impaired use of arms and legs due to pain or orthopaedic conditions, such as give way or sudden loss of muscle strength at examination should not be mistaken for an FND.

Chapter 3

Differential Diagnoses by Presenting or Prominent Clinical Feature

Differential Diagnoses

- 3.1 External ophthalmoparesis and/or ptosis
- 3.2 Facial weakness
- 3.3 Bulbar weakness
- 3.4 Respiratory insufficiency as an early sign
- 3.5 Axial weakness: dropped head, bent spine
- 3.6 Scapular winging
- 3.7 Proximal weakness, (near-)normal sensation
- 3.8 Distal weakness, normal sensation, subacute, or progressive in a few years
- 3.9 Distal weakness, usually symmetric, normal sensation, very slowly progressive
- 3.10 Sensory or sensorimotor distal symmetric impairment: (predominantly) sensory polyneuropathies
- 3.11 Sensory or sensorimotor multifocal or asymmetric impairment: (radiculo)neuropathies or mutifocal neuropathies
- 3.12 Sensory or sensorimotor proximal asymmetric or unilateral impairment brachial or lumbosacral plexopathy; radiculopathy
- 3.13 Dysautonomia
- 3.14 Ataxia in neuromuscular disorders
- 3.15 Postural tremor in neuromuscular diseases
- 3.16 Abnormal muscle fibre activity: fasciculations, myokymia, cramp, muscle contracture, myotonia, and rippling
- 3.17 Pain and stiffness
- 3.18 Muscle hypertrophy
- 3.19 Joint contractures, hypermobility (hyperlaxity), and deformities in neuromuscular disorders
- 3.20 Neonatal hypotonia: neuromuscular causes
- 3.21 Cardiac involvement in neuromuscular disorders
- 3.22 Asymptomatic/paucisymptomatic hyperCKaemia
- 3.23 Rhabdomyolysis

Note that these listings are not exhaustive. Abbreviations: AD: autosomal dominant; AR: Autosomal recessive; genes in italic.

Useful Database

Neuromuscular Home Page (wustl.edu)

Box 3.1 External ophthalmoplegia and/or ptosis (supranuclear and internuclear causes excluded)

Ophthalmoparesis is defined by dysfunction of the extraocular muscles (EOM). Localization supranuclear, nuclear/nerve (CN III, IV, and VI), neuromuscular junction, or muscle. External ophthalmoparesis is not accompanied by pupillary abnormalities and may manifest with diplopia. Chronic progressive external ophthalmoplegia (CPEO) usually remains unnoticed by the patient, since there is no diplopia. Ptosis is present when the upper eyelid is lower than its normal anatomical position, typically 1–2 mm below the superior corneoscleral limbus. Ptosis can be unilateral or bilateral and acquired or congenital.

Usually present at birth

Nucleus/nerve
- Congenital cranial dysinnervation disorders (CCDDs), resulting from developmental errors in innervation of one or more cranial nerves/nuclei. CCDDs include Moebius syndrome (VI, VII), Duane syndrome (VI), congenital fibrosis of the extraocular muscles (CFEOM) (III), Marcus Gunn ptosis (V, VII), and others.

Neuromuscular junction
- Transient neonatal myasthenia gravis due to placental transfer of maternal antibodies against acetylcholine receptor; ptosis may be unilateral, external ophthalmoplegia is uncommon.
- Congenital (hereditary) myasthenic syndromes. Usually mild, asymmetric. Sometimes only ptosis. Onset at birth or in first decade. **Case 35**

Muscle
- Congenital myopathies: Multi/minicore myopathy (AR *RYR1*, AR *SELENON/SEPN1*, ophthalmoparesis and mild ptosis in severe cases); XR myotubular myopathy (*MTM1*, mostly ptosis, sometimes limited eye movements); centronuclear myopathy (AD *DNM2*, AR or AD *BIN1*); severe nemaline myopathy (AR *LMOD3*, AR *KLHL40* – rare). **Cases 57, 58**
- Congenital ptosis (levator muscle dysgenesis) mostly unilateral

Childhood or adult onset – unilateral

Nucleus/nerve
- Ischaemic 3rd or 6th nerve palsy (mostly elderly patients), associated with cardiovascular risk factors. Acute-onset ptosis and ophthalmoplegia (3rd nerve palsy without pupillary involvement).
- Compression of oculomotor nerves outside the orbita; 3rd nerve compression associated with mydriasis (meningeoma, aneurysm, in particular of communicans posterior artery, sinus cavernosus thrombosis, tentorial herniation).
- Intraorbital pathology including tumor, trauma, surgery, vascular, inflammatory, and infectious aetiologies (tuberculosis and cysticercosis). May involve 3rd, 4th, or 6th nerve; usually associated with pain and sometimes proptosis.
- Painful ophthalmoplegic neuropathy due to unspecified inflammation of sinus cavernosus (Tolosa–Hunt syndrome: unilateral orbital pain, ipsilateral oculomotor paralysis, rapid response to steroids).
- Horner syndrome: miosis, tarsalis muscle weakness, anhydrosis (ipsilateral sympathetic pathway).

Childhood or adult onset – Bilateral, symmetric, or asymmetric

Nucleus/nerve
- Riboflavin transporter deficiency (RTD, Fazio–Londe, Brown–Violetta–Van Laere syndromes): childhood onset, AR *SLC52A2* and *SLC52A3*; progressive cranial neuronopathy (sensorineural deafness, optic atrophy; occasionally ptosis and facial weakness), motor and sensory neuropathy. Treatment: start oral riboflavin supplementation immediately.
- Miller–Fisher syndrome, Guillain–Barré syndrome (severe cases). **Case 9**
- CANOMAD syndrome: chronic ataxic neuropathy, external ophthalmoplegia, M-protein, disialosyl antibodies.
- Wernicke encephalopathy due to thiamine deficiency: external ophthalmoplegia (6th and 3rd nerve palsy, may be asymmetric); nystagmus most common symptom; acute-onset cognitive changes and gait ataxia.

Neuromuscular junction
- Myasthenia gravis. Fluctuating, unilateral or asymmetric. **Cases 31, 32**
- Convergence spasm (intermittent episodes of convergence, miosis, and accommodation with disconjugate gaze). May mimic myasthenia gravis.
- Congenital myasthenic syndromes. Usually onset in first decade. **Case 35**
- Botulism. Rapidly progressive, associated with bulbar weakness, limb weakness, respiratory insufficiency, mydriasis, and nausea.

Muscle
- Myotonic dystrophy type 1, mostly ptosis and sometimes lateral gaze limitation AD *DMPK*. **Case 39**
- Oculopharyngeal muscular dystrophy, AD *PABPN1*; ptosis most prominent. **Case 44**
- Oculopharyngodistal myopathy: AD/AR *LRP12, GIPC1, NOTCH2NLC, RILP1* (repeat expansion in untranslated region). Ptosis first symptom in half of cases. Onset in late adolescence or early adulthood. Mostly Japanese and Chinese patients.
- Mitochondrial myopathy. CPEO, either isolated or as part of a multisystem disease, e.g., Kearns–Sayre syndrome due to *de novo* mitochondrial DNA (mtDNA) deletions. Other cases are caused by multiple mtDNA due to nDNA mutations, e.g., *TWNK, POLG, POLG2, TK2, MTTL1, RRM2B, SLC25A4, DNA1, MGM1, RNASEH1*, AD or AR. **Case 55**
- Recessive myosin myopathy (MyHC IIa): external ophthalmoplegia, ptosis, facial weakness, proximal weakness. AD/AR *MYH2*.
- VCP-related myopathy (ptosis and ophthalmoplegia, uncommon). AD *VCP*
- Pompe disease (unilateral or asymmetric ptosis) AR *GAA*. **Case 52**
- Thyroid-associated ophthalmopathy. Graves disease, hypothyroidism, or thyroid cancer. **Case 63**
- Acquired aponeurotic ptosis (e.g., due to hard or soft contact lenses) or involutional (older age): may be unilateral.

Box 3.2 Facial weakness

Facial weakness can be due to a defect in the motor nucleus, nerve root or trajectory of the facial nerve (neurogenic), neuromuscular junction, or as a myopathic feature. Unilateral or bilateral (myopathic face). If bilateral, may be asymmetric. Clinical characteristics: facial droop, absent forehead wrinkles, nasolabial or periorbital folds; lagophtalmos (incomplete eyelid closure); open mouth posture or tent-shaped upper lip; drooling; and inability to make facial expressions, wrinkle the forehead, whistle, and/or difficulties with articulation of labial consonants.

Usually present at birth

Nerve
- Moebius syndrome (MBS): mostly sporadic (*de novo* AD mutations in *PLXND1* and *REV3 L* found to be associated with MBS), congenital, nonprogressive condition: facial palsy (often bilateral) and additional involvement (usually bilateral) of CN VI. Dysfunction of other CNs (V, X, XI, and XII) often present. Absence of the pectoral muscle may occur. Caused by failure of development or degeneration of cranial nerves.
- Congenital facial weakness
  - Congenital fibrosis of extraocular muscles (ptosis and restricted vertical and horizontal gaze), with or without congenital facial palsy; AD *TUBB3*
  - Charge syndrome (coloboma, heart defects, choanal atresia, retarded growth and development, genital and ear abnormalities); AD *CHD7*; ~40% of patients have uni/bilateral facial nerve palsy.
  - Hereditary congenital facial paresis (HCFP); AR *HOXB1* – HCFP shares clinical features with Moebius syndrome, but these are different clinical entities with a different pathogenesis.

Neuromuscular junction
- Transient neonatal myasthenia gravis due to placental transfer of maternal antibodies against acetylcholine receptor; ptosis may be unilateral, external ophthalmoplegia uncommon.
- Congenital (hereditary) myasthenic syndromes. Usually mild, asymmetric. In some forms sparing of extraocular weakness or only ptosis. Onset at birth or in first decade. **Case 35**

Muscle
- Congenital myotonic dystrophy type 1: myopathic face and tent-shaped mouth, ptosis, dysphagia, weak cry/cough, respiratory failure, hypotonia and generalized weakness, clubfeet; sparing of extraocular muscles. **Case 39**
- Congenital myopathies, e.g., myotubular/centronuclear myopathy, nemaline myopathy, recessive *RYR1*-related multiminicore myopathy, associated with external ophthalmoplegia; onset in childhood or early adulthood (AR multiminicore myopathy, AD centronuclear myopathy). **Cases 56, 57, 58**

Childhood or adult onset

Nerve
- Idiopathic facial palsy (Bell palsy); 70% of facial palsies. Any age (also children < 10 years), most commonly > 65 years.
- Infections (HIV, herpes zoster, Lyme, leprosy, *Mycobacterium* tuberculosis). Facial nerve palsy is a common manifestation of Lyme neuroborreliosis, mostly in adults. About one-third bilateral, usually occurring consecutively.
- Sarcoidosis: cranial nerve involvement most common manifestation of neurosarcoidosis; CN II, VII, and VIII most frequently affected. Facial nerve palsy occurs in about 10%, may be the presenting sign. In about one-third, facial nerve palsy is bilateral, recurrent, or simultaneous. Can occur at any age, but often between the ages of 20 and 60 years; rare < 2 years.
- Immune-mediated: in Guillain–Barré syndrome cranial neuropathy in half of the patients, most commonly facial palsy (mostly bilateral), followed by bulbar and oculomotor palsy. **Case 9**
- Light chain (AL) amyloidosis: facial nerve palsy may be an isolated manifestation. Occurs mostly between 60 and 70 years.
- Traumatic, neoplastic, iatrogenic origin (e.g., most commonly occurs due to temporomandibular joint replacement, mastoidectomy, and parotidectomy).
- Melkersson–Rosenthal syndrome: granulomatous disorder of unknown cause: triad of recurrent facial palsy (mostly unilateral), orofacial swelling, and fissured tongue. Commonly an incomplete clinical pattern. Facial palsy mostly transient, recurrence in 10%. Frequently found in females in the 2nd or 3rd decade.

Neuromuscular junction
- Myasthenia gravis: fluctuating, often asymmetric weakness; present in most patients, extraocular and bulbar muscles are affected first, and subsequently weakness of facial muscles and limb muscles. **Case 31**

Muscle
- Facioscapulohumeral muscular dystrophy (FSHD) type 1 and type 2. Often subtle, unilateral; if bilateral often asymmetric; prominent in infantile onset FSHD. FSHD1: AD *DUX4* (repeat deletion); FSHD2: AD *SMCHD1*. **Case 38**
- Myotonic dystrophy type 1. Bilateral, myopathic face, ptosis. Facial weakness in myotonic dystrophy type 2 usually milder. **Cases 39, 40**
- Inclusion body myositis (IBM); facial weakness may be prominent in elderly women. **Case 62**
- Various other neuromuscular diseases: spinal and bulbar muscular atrophy (SBMA, Kennedy disease) **Case 5**, LGMDD2 (early-onset cases), LGMDR13, Danon disease, oculopharyngeal muscular dystrophy (OPMD) **Case 44**, oculopharyngodistal muscular dystrophy (OPDM), some mitochondrial myopathies **Case 55**

Box 3.3 Bulbar weakness

Bulbar weakness can be due to a defect in the motor nucleus, or trajectory of the lower cranial nerves (IX–XII) (neurogenic), neuromuscular junction, or as a myopathic feature. Clinical features are dysphagia, dysarthria, hoarseness, hypophonia, weakness of masticatory muscles and tongue. Not all features need to be present. For example, in amyotrophic lateral sclerosis, patients with dysphagia are also dysarthric, whereas in inclusion body myositis there is often dysphagia, but no dysarthria.

(Sub)acute onset

Nucleus/nerve
- Ischaemic lesion of lower brainstem. Also signs of CNS involvement.
- Infection or meningeal malignancy
- Immune-mediated: regional variant of GBS. **Case 9**

Neuromuscular junction
- Toxins. Dysfunction of neuromuscular junction, e.g., botulism. Also ptosis, diplopia, rapidly descending weakness, fixed dilated pupils, and other signs of nicotinic cholinergic blockade.

Fluctuating, progression in days–months

Neuromuscular junction
- Myasthenia gravis (MG), especially prominent in MuSK MG. **Cases 31, 32, 33**
- Congenital myasthenic syndromes, inherited disorders caused by genetic defects at presynaptic, synaptic or postsynaptic levels). Fatigable weakness involving ocular, bulbar, and limb muscles. Bulbar weakness may be presenting sign. Onset at or shortly after birth, or in first two years. Mostly AR, AD less common. Multiple genes involved. **Case 35**

Progression in months

Upper and lower motor neuron
- Bulbar-onset amyotrophic lateral sclerosis (ALS/MND). Upper and lower motor neuron involvement. Onset with dysarthria, followed by choking on liquids. Often accompanied by pseudobulbar affect (forced laughter, crying, yawning). Familial in ~10%. **Case 1**
- Villaret syndrome (unilateral palsy of CN IX–XII and the cervical sympathetic nerve, usually due to mass in the posterior retroparotid space.

Progression in years. Dysphagia, no dysarthria

Muscle
- Inclusion body myositis (IBM). Food gets stuck in the throat. Asymmetric deep finger flexor and quadriceps weakness. **Case 62**
- Oculopharyngeal muscular dystrophy (OPMD). Mostly AD *PABPN1*. **Case 44**
- Oculopharyngodistal myopathy (OPDM). AD *LRP12, GIPC1, NOTCH2NLC, RILP1*. Ptosis first symptom in most cases. Adult onset. Japanese and Chinese patients. Repeat expansion disease.

Progression in years. Dysphagia, dysarthria, tongue weakness, respiratory insufficiency

Upper motor neuron
- Pseudobulbar palsy/primary lateral sclerosis. Isolated upper motor neuron disorder. Dysarthria, pseudobulbar affect, dysphagia, bladder symptoms. May be stable for years and unlikely to convert to ALS, if EMG remains normal beyond the first 3–4 years. **Case 2**

Lower motor neuron (anterior horn cell, nerve)
- Spinal and bulbar muscular atrophy (SBMA, Kennedy disease). XR *Androgen Receptor* repeat expansion. **Case 5**
- Riboflavin transporter deficiency (RTD, Brown–Violetta–Van Laere syndrome, Fazio–Londe syndrome. Childhood onset. Rarely adult onset. Progressive cranial and peripheral neuronopathy. Hearing loss (first symptom), loss of vision, bulbar weakness, occasionally ptosis and facial weakness, respiratory weakness, sensory ataxia, AR *SLC52A2, SLC52A*. Treatment with oral riboflavin, start immediately after diagnosis.
- Facial-onset sensorimotor neuronopathy (FOSMN): characteristic phenotype with paresthesia and numbness within the trigeminal nerve region, which spreads to the scalp and subsequently descending to the face, upper trunk, upper extremities, and in some cases to the lower extremities. Later bulbar weakness, tongue atrophy, and fasciculations, and less frequent weakness in the extremities. Respiratory insufficiency rare. Progression in months–years. Rare.
- Charcot–Marie–Tooth disease (axonal) with vocal cord paralysis. AR *GDAP1*, AD*TRP4*

Muscle
- Vocal cord and pharyngeal weakness with distal myopathy (VCPDM). AD *MATR3*

Box 3.4 Respiratory insufficiency as an early sign

Respiratory insufficiency may be the presenting symptom in rapidly progressive neuromuscular disease. In chronic disease, its manifestation may be acute-on-chronic, caused by, e.g., upper airway infection. Sometimes in patients unaware of having a neuromuscular disease (e.g., in myotonic dystrophy type 1), when there is disproportionate weakness of the diaphragm (relative to bulbar, axial, or limb weakness), or because weakness of other muscles went unnoticed). Isolated respiratory insufficiency (no weakness of other muscles) is not a feature of neuromuscular disorders.

Patients may present at the emergency room or with difficulty weaning at the intensive care unit (ICU).

Anterior horn cell/nerve
- Bulbar-onset amyotrophic lateral sclerosis (ALS). **Case 1**
- Guillain–Barré syndrome (GBS). **Case 9**
- Brachial plexus neuropathy/neuralgic amyotrophy (NA) with phrenic nerve involvement. **Case 19**
- ICU-acquired weakness, critical illness neuropathy and myopathy (CIP, CIM). Symmetric proximal or generalized arm and leg weakness. No facial or oculomotor weakness. **Case 23**

Neuromuscular junction
- Myasthenia gravis, in particular in MuSK MG. **Cases 31, 32**
- Neurotoxins, e.g., food-borne botulism, associated with bulbar weakness and rapidly descending weakness, mydriasis, and other signs of nicotinic cholinergic blockade.
- Drug-induced, e.g., immune checkpoint inhibitor-related myasthenia-myositis-myocarditis. **Case 33**

Muscle
- Myotonic dystrophy type 1 (DM1) AD *DMPK*. **Case 39**
- Pompe disease AR *GAA*. **Case 52**
- Hereditary myopathy with early respiratory failure (HMERF). Adult onset. Also early distal weakness AD*TTN*, childhood-onset AR titinopathies

Box 3.5 Axial weakness: dropped head, bent spine (camptocormia)

Camptocormia is an excessive involuntary trunk flexion. It usually presents while standing, walking, or exercising and is alleviated while sitting, in recumbent position, standing against a wall, or using walking support. In neuromuscular disease, dropped head and bent spine are caused by weakness of neck extensors and/or paraspinal (erector spinae) muscles.

This table does not include diseases featured by scoliosis (mainly in early-onset disorders) or lumbar hyperlordosis as manifestations of axial weakness.

With bulbar weakness, with or without diaphragm weakness

Neuromuscular junction
- Myasthenia gravis, in particular MUSK MG. Dysphagia and dysarthria. Weakness of respiratory muscles. May be progressive in hours. **Cases 31, 32, 33**

Muscle
- Inclusion body myositis (IBM). **Case 62**
- Other subtypes of myositis. Dropped head may rarely be presenting symptom. **Cases 60, 61**
- Sporadic late-onset nemaline myopathy (SLONM) presents commonly with atrophy and weakness of proximal arm or leg muscles, sometimes with axial, bulbar, and respiratory weakness. Nemaline rods in muscle biopsy. Sometimes monoclonal gammopathy. Consider treatment when rapidly progressive.

With diaphragm weakness, (initially) without bulbar weakness

Anterior horn cell
- Amyotrophic lateral sclerosis (ALS). Thoracic onset, diaphragm weakness. Later spreading to other regions. **Case 1**
- Spinal muscular atrophy (SMA) types 2, 3. AR *SMN*. **Case 7**

Muscle
- Pompe disease. Often with weakness in erector spinae muscles, with local fatty changes on MRI. AR *GAA*. **Case 52**
- Multiminicore disease, selenoprotein deficiency. AR *SELENON/SEPN1*. Early onset. With rigid spine, scoliosis, facial weakness.
- VCP-myopathy. AD *VCP*, adult onset. Rimmed vacuoles in muscle biopsy. CK normal–mildly elevated. Associated with Paget disease of bone, frontotemporal dementia, ALS.

No bulbar or diaphragm weakness

Anterior horn cell
- Spinal muscular atrophy (SMA) types 2, 3. AR *SMN*. **Case 7**

Nerve
- Chronic inflammatory demyelinating polyneuropathy (CIDP). Rare. Signs of polyneuropathy also present. **Case 10**

Muscle
- Central core disease AD *RYR1*. Adult onset. **Case 56**
- Limb girdle muscular dystrophy 1 (LGMDR1), AD *CAPN3*

Box 3.5 (cont.)

- Post-radiation. Delayed complication of large-field (mantle) radiation, e.g., for Hodgkin lymphoma. In combination with more extensive myopathy, plexopathy, phrenic nerve involvement, myelopathy.
- Isolated neck extensor myopathy (INEM). Onset mostly > 40 years. Weakness may progress to shoulder girdle and proximal arm muscles. CK normal. Muscle biopsy to exclude other diagnoses. Most cases of isolated dropped head or bent spine remain unsolved, also after extensive ancillary investigations.

Non-neuromuscular disorders

- Neurodegenerative diseases with hypo/bradykinesia: (Parkinson disease, multisystem atrophy).
- Cervical dystonia: repetitive/ patterned head or neck movements or postures.
- Orthopaedic conditions: not redressable in supine position.

Box 3.6 Scapular winging

Medial winging (inferior angle of scapula rotates medially and scapula translates superiorly) is most prominent on push-up and motion against the wall. Caused by dysfunction of the long thoracic nerve or to serratus anterior muscle involvement.

Lateral winging (shoulder droops with inferior translation of the scapula and the inferior angle rotates laterally is accentuated by abduction of the arm and external rotation against resistance). Caused by dysfunction of the spinal accessory nerve or dorsal scapular nerve, or by weakness of the muscles they innervate: the trapezius and rhomboid muscles, respectively.

Acute, unilateral

Nerve
- Surgical damage (cervical mass excision, lymph node biopsy, thyroidectomy, carotid surgery).
- Other injury of the posterior cervical area (traction injuries, and motor vehicle accidents damaging the plexus brachialis or individual nerves, or detachment of muscle from scapula).

Evolving in days–weeks

Nerve
- Neuralgic amyotrophy (idiopathic or hereditary plexus brachialis neuropathy). Long thoracic nerve involvement in about two-thirds of the cases. Usually preceded by severe pain. Bilateral in one quarter of patients. **Case 19**
- Repetitive compression or stretch injuries to the long thoracic nerve causing medial winging (e.g., due to carrying a backpack).

Slowly progressive

Nerve
- Scapuloperoneal spinal muscular atrophy (SPSMA). Also vocal cord paresis, hearing loss, kyphoscoliosis. Onset at any age, also congenital. Slowly progressive. AD *TRPV4*

Muscle
- Facioscapulohumeral dystrophy types 1 and 2 (FSHD). Typically asymmetric. AD *DUX4/SMCHD1*. **Case 38**
- Dystrophinopathies (DMD, BMD, DMD/BMD carriers (can be asymmetric) XR *DMD*. **Cases 36, 37**
- AD Limb girdle muscular dystrophies (LGMDs): LGMDD1 F (*TNPO3*); LGMDD1 G (*HNRNPDL*).
- AR LGMDs: LGMDR1 (*CAPN3*) **Case 41**; LGMDR3/4 α/β-Sarcoglycan-related; LGMDR9 (*FKRP*) **Case 42**; LGMDR14 (*POMT2*); LGMDR18 (*TRAPPC11*); LGMDR21 (*POGLUT1*).
- Emery–Dreifuss muscular dystrophy. Scapuloperoneal weakness. Early contractures, cardiac involvement. XR *FHL1*; AD *LMNA*. **Case 45**
- Pompe disease. Limb girdle and axial weakness AR *GAA*. **Case 52**
- Myofibrillar myopathies, AD, e.g., *DES*. **Case 49**
- Multisystem proteinopathy (MSP) AD *VCP*.
- Myotonic dystrophy type 1. Often asymmetric, occurs in all subtypes. AD *DMPK*. **Case 39**
- Congenital myopathies. Centronuclear myopathy (e.g., *MYF6*); Nemaline myopathy (e.g., *ACTA1*). **Case 58**
- Reducing body myopathy (*FHL1*). Pathology: characteristic cytoplasmic bodies. Also myofibrillar abnormalities. Many clinical phenotypes. May be asymmetric. May be rapidly progressive.

Box 3.7 Proximal weakness, (near-)normal sensation

Proximal weakness pertains to weakness of muscles that move the shoulder and hip and proximal muscles that move the elbow and knee. Specifically, one muscle group may be involved, e.g., in spinal muscular atrophy (SMA) type III, the iliopsoas muscle is early affected, whereas this muscle is spared until later in the disease course in Becker muscular dystrophy (BMD).

CK elevation > 10 × ULN indicates myopathy, and makes pure neurogenic diseases unlikely. However, in many acquired and hereditary myopathies CK is normal or only mildly to moderately increased. Autosomal dominant muscular dystrophies in general present with lower CK than X-linked and autosomal recessive muscular dystrophies.

Unilateral or asymmetric

Anterior horn cell
- Progressive muscular atrophy (PMA), usually presenting with asymmetric muscle weakness, fasciculations, progression may be variable, but usually resembling that of ALS. **Case 3**
- Poliomyelitis anterior acuta and other neurotropic viruses, postpolio syndrome. **Case 8**
- Segmental spinal muscular atrophy in proximal or distal arms or legs. Asymmetric, very slow progression or stable. Rarely, progression to ALS. **Case 4**

Nerve
- (Mono)radiculopathy, plexopathy, mononeuropathy. Pain and atrophy, often also sensory involvement. Causes: diabetes, compression, tumor ingrowth, inflammation, post-radiation.

Usually symmetric, progression in weeks–months

Nerve
- Guillain–Barré syndrome (GBS). Rapidly progressive (days–weeks). 30–70% has no sensory involvement. CK normal. **Case 9**
- Chronic inflammatory demyelinating polyneuropathy (CIDP). Areflexia. CK normal. **Case 10**

Neuromuscular junction
- Rarely, AChR myasthenia gravis presents with a limb girdle distribution of weakness. **Case 31**
- Lambert–Eaton myasthenic syndrome (LEMS) can be progressive in months. **Case 34**

Muscle
- Myositis. Deltoid and iliopsoas most severely affected. Myalgia.
  - Immune-mediated necrotizing myopathy (IMNM) CK markedly elevated. **Case 61**
  - (Juvenile) dermatomyositis (J)DM). Typical skin features, CK often elevated, may be normal. **Cases 59, 60**
  - Overlap myositis (with connective tissue disease (CTD)). CK usually mildly elevated.
  - Anti-synthetase syndrome. With arthralgias and interstitial lung disease (ILD). CK usually mildly elevated.
- Immune checkpoint inhibitor-related myasthenia-myositis-myocarditis. **Case 35**
- Other drugs. **Case 64**
- Amyloid myopathy, mostly AL-amyloidosis.
- Sarcoid myopathy. Myalgia, also with slow progression. Sometimes also polyneuropathy.
- Endocrine, notably hypothyroidic myopathy. CK may be elevated > 10 ×; **Case 63**. Hypovitaminosis D, if severely deficient. Cushing myopathy: muscle atrophy, low CK.
- Intensive care unit-acquired weakness (critical illness polyneuropathy and myopathy, CIPM). Weakness generalized, sparing facial and ocular muscles. **Case 32**

Usually symmetric, progression in years

Anterior horn cell (hypo-areflexia)
- Spinal muscular atrophy (SMA), AR *SMN*. **Cases 6, 7**
- Flail arm (proximal, man-in-the-barrel) variant of motor neuron disease (MND). May be asymmetric. Predominantly lower motor neuron signs. Progression slower than in ALS; **flail leg** (see flail arm).
- Bulbospinal muscular atrophy (BSMA, Kennedy disease). CK often elevated due to muscle involvement, XR *Androgen receptor* repeat expansion. **Case 5**

Nerve (hypo-areflexia)
- Motor chronic inflammatory demyelinating polyneuropathy (CIDP), often also proximal weakness. Progressive in months–years. **Case 10**

Neuromuscular junction
- Lambert–Eaton myasthenic syndrome (LEMS). Proximal–distal spread of (fluctuating) weakness in months–years. Also autonomic dysfunction (dry mouth, erectile dysfunction) and decreased to absent reflexes. **Case 34**
- Congenital myasthenic syndromes, mostly *DOK7* and *GFPT1*. **Case 35**

Box 3.7 (cont.)

Muscle
- AD Limb girdle muscular dystrophies (LGMDs): *DNAJB6, TNP03, HNRNPDL, CAPN, COL6A1-3*. **Case 43**
- AR LGMDs: *CAPN, DYSF, SGCA, SGCB, SGCG, SGCD, TCAP, TRIM32, FKRP, TTN, POMT1, ANO5, FKTN, COL6A1-3, OMO2, LAMA2*, and other. **Cases 41, 42**
- Duchenne muscular dystrophy and Becker muscular dystrophy (DMD, BMD) Carriers can have asymmetric weakness. XR *DMD*, often deletion or duplication. **Cases 36, 37**
- Emery–Dreifuss muscular dystrophy (EDMD), contractures, humeroperoneal weakness. AD, AR *LMNA*; XR *EMD* **Case 45**; *SYNE1, SYNE2* reported as EDMD types.
- SNUPN-related myopathy. Childhood-onset, Severe. Proximal more than distal weakness. Respiratory insufficiency. Contractures. Dystophic and myofibrillar features in muscle biopsy. AR *SNUPN*
- Caveolinopathy, rippling muscle disease, may rarely cause distal weakness. AD *CAV3*. **Case 46**
- Pompe disease (glycogen storage disease (GSD) II). AR *GAA*. **Case 52**
- McArdle disease (glycogen storage disease (GSD) V). Elderly patients may have fixed weakness. AR *PYGM* **Case 53**
- Mitochondrial myopathy. Physical activity intolerance. Nuclear and mitochondrial DNA variants. **Case 55** Rarely without any other features of mitochondrial disease: AR *TK2*: mostly very early onset generalized weakness with rapid progression.
- Myotonic dystrophy type 2 (DM2). Myalgia. AD *CNBP* repeat expansion. **Case 40**
- VCP-related myopathy. AD *VCP* adult onset. Rimmed vacuoles in muscle biopsy.
- Congenital myopathies. Often with contractures, joint hypermobility, sometimes also CNS involvement. AR and AD, many genes, e.g., *RYR1, SELENON/SEPN1, NEB*. May present in adulthood. AD *RYR1, DNM2, BIN1, KBTBD13*. **Cases 56, 57, 58**

Episodic weakness

Muscle
- Periodic paralysis. Attacks of weakness lasting minutes–days. Onset in teens. Weakness focal or generalized. Often provoked by triggers. Associated with hypo- or hyperkalaemia. Sometimes development of fixed proximal weakness. Muscle channelopathies. Several types. AD *CACNA1S, SCN4A, KCNJ2, KCNJ18, KCNE3*. **Case 51**

Box 3.8 Distal weakness, normal sensation, subacute, or progressive in a few years

Progression in days–weeks

Anterior horn cell
- Poliomyelitis anterior acuta. Usually asymmetric, legs > arms. **Case 8**

Nerve
- Mononeuropathy, monoradiculopathy, plexopathy by compression, trauma, inflammation, ischaemia, e.g., diabetic plexopathy, vasculitic neuropathy (multifocal, axonal), Lyme disease, sometimes predominantly motor signs.
- Guillain–Barré syndrome (GBS). Symmetric. Usually also proximal weakness. **Case 9**
- Acute hepatic porphyric neuropathy. Wrist extensor and ankle dorsal flexor weakness. Usually symmetric. Proximal muscles often affected. Rapid progression to quadriparesis. Respiratory involvement. Fatal if untreated. Abdominal pain. Psychiatric and central nervous system symptoms. Dark urine. Especially in women of childbearing age.

Progression in weeks–months

Nerve
- Pure or predominant motor chronic inflammatory demyelinating polyneuropathy (CIDP). Proximal and distal, symmetric or multifocal. Areflexia. Demyelinating features with nerve conduction studies. **Case 10**
- Lead toxicity. Motor neuropathy. Wrist and finger extensors. Usually symmetric. Also gastrointestinal and cognitive disturbances, and anaemia.

Progression in months–years

Anterior horn cell
- Amyotrophic lateral sclerosis (ALS). Normal reflexes or hyperreflexia in atrophic limb. Onset often in hands or lower legs, asymmetric or unilateral. CK up to 10 × ULN. Familial in ~10%. **Case 1**
- Progressive muscular atrophy (PMA), often evolves to ALS, usually somewhat slower progression than ALS. **Case 3**
- Hirayama disease (or juvenile muscular atrophy of distal upper extremity or segmental/focal spinal muscular atrophy or monomelic amyotrophy). Unilateral weakness and atrophy in muscles of the hand and forearm without sensory loss.

Box 3.8 (cont.)

Usually in young men, often of Asian descent. Progression in months up to 8 years. In about one-third of patients less pronounced contralateral weakness of the hand and forearm. MRI (atrophy cervical spinal cord). **Case 4**
- Monomelic amyotrophy of lower limb or 'wasted leg syndrome': atrophy and muscle weakness restricted to one leg, distal or proximal. Initially slowly progressive disease course of 1–2 years followed by a stationary period lasting decades. Predominantly in males.
- Flail leg (distal) variant of MND. Asymmetric. Lower motor neuron signs. Progression slower than in ALS; sometimes initially difficult to distinguish from ALS.
- Postpolio syndrome. New or increased weakness and atrophy in patient with sequelae of polio, fatigue. **Case 8**

Nerve
- Multifocal motor neuropathy (MMN). Onset in finger and wrist extensor muscles, sometimes in ankle dorsal flexors. Asymmetric. Mild atrophy of muscles, cramps and fasciculations. No bulbar or respiratory muscle weakness. Motor conduction blocks. MRI and ultrasound proximal nerve thickening. Anti-GM1 IgM antibodies
- Asymmetric wasting of calf muscles due to tethered cord (i.e., abnormal tension on the spinal cord) or other damage to the (epi)conus/cauda due to spinal dysraphism, trauma, infection, or neoplasm (e.g., ependymoma). Sensory and bladder signs may be absent. CNS signs and clubfeet if congenital.

Muscle
- Inclusion body myositis (IBM). Asymmetric deep finger flexor weakness (flexors of distal phalanx), quadriceps muscle weakness, dysphagia. Muscle biopsy shows endomysial cell infiltrates. Anti-cN1A antibodies. Weakness of deep finger flexors can also be prominent in myotonic dystrophy **Case 62**

Box 3.9 Distal weakness, usually symmetric, normal sensation, very slowly progressive

Especially in the absence of sensory disturbances, it can be difficult to make a distinction between neurogenic and myopathic disease. In general, patients with a distal neurogenic disease more often have deformities (pes cavus, hammer toes, claw hands) and pronounced atrophy, especially with early childhood onset, compared with patients with a distal myopathy. In many distal myopathies, CK is only slightly increased (except in *DYSF* and *ANO5* distal myopathies).

Note that this list contains some genes known to cause both distal hereditary motor neuropathy (HMN/dSMA) and Charcot–Marie–Tooth disease (CMT/HMSN). About 100 genes are known to cause CMT, in which sensory abnormalities can be very mild or absent (e.g., *SORD*, *TRPV4*). Distal HMN/dSMA can also be accompanied by upper motor neuron signs. The clinical spectrum associated with a specific gene or gene variant is expanding, and genes also have been found to be associated with both AD and AR transmitted disease.

Onset in ankle dorsiflexors (these are examples, list is not exhaustive!)

Distal hereditary motor neuropathies/distal spinal muscular atrophy
- *HSPB1* (AD, AR); *HSPB3* and *HSPB8* (AD); *BICD2* {AD}; *BSCL2* (also called neuromyopathies, sometimes with pyramidal features, AD); *SORD* (AR) and *AARS1* (AD), sometimes with sensory abnormalities (CMT2); *SYT2*, features of NMJ disease; spinal muscular atrophy with lower extremity predominance (SMA-LED)/CMT 2O/dHMN *DYNC1H1* (congenital or early onset, also proximal leg weakness, AD)

Hereditary distal myopathies
- *MYH3* (AD); *MYH8* (AD). Onset in infancy with distal arthrogryposis, or childhood. *MYH7* (Laing) (AD), hanging big toe, later finger extensors, neck flexors. Childhood onset. In severe cases, loss of ambulation and diaphragm weakness. Sometimes cardiomyopathy. Pathology: nonspecific.
- *ACTA1* (AD); *NEB* (AR); *KLHL9* (AR). Onset in infancy or childhood. Pathology: nemaline rods.
- GNE-myopathy (Nonaka distal myopathy) – *GNE* (AR), quadriceps sparing, **Case 48**; HSPB1 (AD); *ADSSL1* (AR); *HNRNPA1* *HNRNPA2/B1* (AD); *TTN* (AD, AR); *VCP* (AD, myopathy and peripheral neuropathy), *SMPX* (XR); PLIN4 (AD). Mostly adult onset. Pathology: all may show rimmed vacuoles, some show necrosis and others dystrophy-like changes. AD titinopathy can be caused by copy number variants (deletions).
- *DES*, **Case 49**; *LDB3*; *MYO*; *FLNC*; *HSPB8*; *BAG3*; *CRYAB*; *DNAJB6*; *ACTN2*, mostly AD. Cardiomyopathy and diaphragmatic weakness. Sometimes neurogenic features (*HSPB8*). Mostly adult onset. Pathology: myofibrillar, vacuoles, cores.
- *CAV3* (AD), **Case 46**. Pathology: nonspecific. Immunostaining with CAV3 can be helpful: AD *DNM2*. Ptosis, contractures Achilles tendons and finger extensors.
- Adult-onset glycogen storage disease type III (GSDIII) (glycogen debrancher enzyme deficiency). Hypertrophic cardiomyopathy. AR *AGL*.

Box 3.9 (cont.)

Onset in ankle plantar flexors

Distal hereditary motor neuropathies (dHMN)/distal spinal muscular atrophy (dSMA))

- *VRK1* (AR); also myopathic features. Adult onset.

Hereditary distal myopathies

- *ANO5* (AR); *DYSF* (AR), **Case 47**; often asymmetric calf atrophy, CK ↑↑.
- *DNAJB6* (AD); *MYOT* (AD); *FLNC* (AD). Pathology: rimmed vacuoles, myofibrillar.

Onset in hands

Distal hereditary motor neuropathies (dHMN)/distal spinal muscular atrophy (dSMA))

- *GARS* (AD), cramp on exposure to cold.
- *BSCL2* (AD), sometimes with pyramidal signs in legs (Silver syndrome), also onset in legs.

Hereditary distal myopathies

- Welander distal myopathy – *TIA1* (AD, AR); *SMPX* (XR) finger extensor weakness. *SQSTM1*+ *TIA1*; digenic, finger extensor and respiratory muscles weakness; *FLNC* (AD) thenar, calf; *MATR3* (AD), vocal cord and pharyngeal muscles, extensor muscles; *DNAJB4* (AD) finger flexors. Pathology: rimmed vacuoles, myofibrillar.
- *POLG* (AD, AR). Rare presentation of POLG-related disease. Adult onset. Progresses to involve extraocular, bulbar, axial, proximal, and distal leg muscles. Pathology: mitochondrial.

Rarely, distal muscle weakness is a presenting sign in other myopathies.

- Consider, e.g., DM1, **Case 39**; FSHD, **Case 38**; OPDM, GSD III (debranching enzyme deficiency), Emery–Dreifuss muscular dystrophy, **Case 45**; central core disease (*RYR1*), **Case 56**. Caveats: DM1, FSHD, and OPDM are repeat disorders and cannot be detected in an NGS gene panel.

Box 3.10 Sensory or sensorimotor distal symmetric impairment: (predominantly) sensory polyneuropathies

Metabolic

- Diabetes mellitus (32–53% of all chronic axonal neuropathies), **Case 20**; chronic kidney disease, chronic liver disease, critical illness polyneuropathy (CIP), **Case 23**.

Nutritional deficiencies

- Vitamins B1, B6, B12 (sometimes also pyramidal tract involvement), vitamin E; copper. Progression can be rapid in severe Vit B1 deficiency.

Toxic

- Alcohol, often in combination with Vit B1 deficiency; frequent cause of chronic polyneuropathy. **Case 21**
- Chemotherapy, especially: vincristine, cisplatin (sensory ganglionopathy), oxaliplatin (acute, cold-induced paraesthesias), docetaxel, paclitaxel, bortezomib (more frequently induces polyneuropathy in Black patients with multiple myeloma), cytarabine (may mimic GBS). Symptoms may appear after stopping the drug, and may progress for months ('coasting' effect), in particular platinum-based chemotherapies, such as cisplatin; may be severe especially in patients already known to have polyneuropathy due to another cause (e.g., vincristine in patients with underlying CMT).
- Anti-infective drugs: chloramphenicol, dapsone, isoniazide, ethambutol, metronidazole, nitrofurantoin, quinolones, dideoxycytidine, thalidomide, other nucleoside analogs (often painful), linezolid, tedizolid, podophyllin (topical).
- Anti-inflammatory drugs: (hydroxy)chloroquine, colchicine (in both also myopathy), tacrolimus (typical polyneuropathy, but sometimes also GBS-like), anti-TNFα (may mimic CIDP).
- Cardiovascular drugs: amiodarone. May mimic CIDP. Neuromyopathy. **Case 24**, dronedarone, hydralazine, propafenone, perhexiline.
- Psychiatric medication: disulfiram, lithium.
- Other medications: pyridoxine (vitamin B6 intoxication may induce polyneuropathy), phenytoin, disulfiram, thalidomide (also coasting effect).
- Environmental toxins: arsenic, lead, mercury, thallium, organophosphate (may mimic Guillain–Barré syndrome, may be rapidly progressive), carbon disulfide, acrylamide, nitrous oxide (myeloneuropathy).

Box 3.10 (cont.)

Idiopathic

- Chronic idiopathic axonal polyneuropathy (CIAP) 24–27% of all neuropathies in hospital studies, and 37% of all chronic neuropathies in population-based studies. **Case 22**
- Idiopathic small fibre neuropathy (I-SFN). **Case 14**

Genetic

- Charcot–Marie–Tooth (CMT) disease/hereditary motor and sensory neuropathy (HMSN), atrophy distal legs and hands, claw hands and pes cavus, many subtypes, > 100 causative genes, AD, AR, XD. **Cases 27, 28**
- Hereditary sensory (and autonomic) neuropathy (HS(A)N) AD/AR SPTLC1/2 (HSAN1/2) and many other genes. **Case 29**
- Hereditary transthyretin (TTR) amyloidosis. AD, *TTR*. Relatively fast progression of polyneuropathy. Frequently misdiagnosed as CIDP or lumbar radiculopathy. **Case 30**
- Mutations in COL6A5 and genes for voltage-gated sodium channels such as SCN9A causing small-fibre neuropathy.
- Tangier disease, *ABCA1* (AR) demyelinating polyneuropathy, deficiency/absence of HDL, multisystem disease, orange- or yellow-coloured tonsils.
- Fabry disease, alpha-galactosidase deficiency, *GLA* (XR), usually onset in childhood.
- Mitochondrial disease.

Occurring in autoimmune disease

- Rheumatoid arthritis, SLE, Sjögren syndrome, sarcoidosis, thyroid dysfunction, cryoglobulinemia, vasculitis (often painful, mostly (multi)focal, can be systemic or nonsystemic). **Case 13**

Autoimmune inflammatory

- Sensory chronic inflammatory demyelinating polyneuropathy (CIDP), **Case 10**; chronic inflammatory sensory polyganglionopathy (CISP).
- Paraneoplastic sensory neuronopathy. **Case 15**

Infectious

- HIV, hepatitis B/C/E

Neoplastic

- Monoclonal gammopathy of undetermined significance (MGUS), IgM anti-myelin-associated glycoprotein (MAG) neuropathy, **Case 11**; multiple myeloma, osteosclerotic or solitary plasmacytoma, Waldenström macroglobulinemia, AL amyloidosis, POEMS (polyneuropathy, organomegaly, endocrinopathy, monoclonal gammopathy, skin changes). **Case 12**
- Paraneoplastic sensory neuronopathy (ganglionopathy). **Case 15**

Box 3.11 Sensory or sensorimotor multifocal or asymmetric impairment: (Radiculo)neuropathies or multifocal neuropathies

- Vasculitis, nonsystemic or secondary to, e.g., connective tissue disorders), progression in days–weeks. **Case 13**
- Diabetes mellitus (usually symmetric distal). **Case 20**
- Sarcoidosis
- Cryoglobulinaemia
- Paraneoplastic sensory neuronopathy (ganglionopathy). **Case 15**
- Multifocal chronic inflammatory demyelinating polyneuropathy (CIDP). **Case 10**
- Hereditary neuropathy with liability to pressure palsies (HNPP). **Case 27**
- Other entrapment neuropathies
- Neurofibromatosis
- Lyme (can be painful, can cause radiculitis). **Case 25**
- Leprosy (often in combination with loss of pain/painless wounds). **Case 26**
- Neoplastic invasion of nerves or roots (can be very painful).
- Lymphomatoid granulomatosis
- Wartenberg migrant sensory neuropathy. **Case 16**

Box 3.12 Sensory or sensorimotor proximal asymmetric or unilateral impairment: brachial or lumbosacral plexopathy; radiculopathy

- Diabetes mellitus. **Case 20**
- Inflammatory: autoimmune or infectious (e.g., CMV)
- Malignant infiltration
- (Hereditary) neuralgic amyotrophy (NA). **Case 19**
- Post-radiation. Symptoms and signs can appear up to 15 years after radiotherapy
- Post-injury
- Thoracic outlet syndrome
- Facial-onset sensorimotor neuronopathy (FOSMN): see Table 3.3.

Box 3.13 Dysautonomia

- Diabetes mellitus **Case 19**
- Guillain–Barré syndrome (GBS) (subacute onset, combination with weakness), Miller–Fisher syndrome. **Case 9**
- Amyloidosis (multisystem disease): e.g., AL amyloidosis, transthyretin (TTR) amyloidosis. **Case 30**
- Hereditary sensory and autonomic neuropathy (HSAN). **Case 29**
- Acute pandysautonomia
- Paraneoplastic sensory and autonomic polyganglionopathy. **Case 15**
- Lambert–Eaton myasthenic syndrome (LEMS). **Case 34**

Box 3.14 Ataxia in neuromuscular disorders

- Toxins and nutritional deficiencies
    - Pyridoxine (vitamin B6) intoxication. Ataxic sensory non-length neuropathy, Lhermitte sign. Likely after > 100–200 mg/day for several months.
    - Cisplatin toxicity. Ataxic sensory neuropathy, Lhermitte sign. Symptoms related to cumulative dose, usually after > 300 mg/m^2; may also develop after therapy has stopped ('coasting').
    - Vitamin B12 deficiency, nitrous oxide intoxication. Ataxic sensorimotor neuropathy. Pyramidal tract involvement.
- Cerebellar ataxia, neuropathy, and vestibular areflexia syndrome (CANVAS). Sensory large-fibre neuropathy; chronic cough may precede ataxia. Adult onset. AR *RFC1* (repeat expansion).
- Friedreich ataxia. Gait and limb ataxia, dysarthria, and loss of lower limb reflexes. Polyneuropathy may be present at onset. AR *FXN* (repeat expansion).
- Ataxia with vitamin E deficiency (AVED). Sensory neuropathy, ataxia, areflexia, extensor plantar response AR *TTPA*.
- Autosomal dominant spinocerebellar ataxias (SCAs) may also be associated with polyneuropathy. Often CAG repeat expansions.
- Charcot–Marie–Tooth disease with episodic ataxia, triggered by fever and heat. AD *NEFL*.
- Primary mitochondrial disorders, for example:
    - Kearns–Sayre syndrome (KSS): onset < 20 years, CPEO, retinitis pigmentosa, ataxia, cardiac conduction block. Sporadic mtDNA deletion.
    - Neuropathy, ataxia, and retinitis pigmentosa (NARP), myoclonus epilepsy with ragged red fibres (MERRF), (episodic) ataxia and polyneuropathy. Maternal inheritance, mtDNA variants.
    - Ataxia neuropathy spectrum (ANS), with, dysarthria, ophthalmoplegia (SANDO), myoclonic epilepsy, myopathy, sensory ataxia (MEMSA), and other combinations of clinical abnormalities AR *POLG, PEO1, TYMP*.
- Dysimmune sensory neuronopathies and neuropathies. Usually subacute, asymmetric, pseudoathetosis.
    - Paraneoplastic sensory neuronopathy and neuropathy (anti-Hu, anti-CRMP5, anti-amphiphysin). **Case 15**
    - Sjögren syndrome, SLE (anti-SSA, anti-SS, ANA, lupus anticoagulant).
    - Chronic ataxic neuropathy with ophthalmoplegia, M-protein (IgM), agglutination, and disialosyl antibodies (CANOMAD). Anti-GD1b, anti-GT1b, anti-GQ1b.
    - Miller–Fisher syndrome (MFS). Rapidly progressive: double vision, ataxia, areflexia (cranial nerve variant of GBS). **Case 9**
    - Autoimmune nodopathy. Often relatively young patients with ataxia, suspected to have GBS but continue to worsen, or to have CIDP and do not respond to IVIg or corticosteroids; these patients may have antibodies against neurofascin 155 (NF155), contactin1 (CNTN1) or Caspr1.
- Chronic inflammatory sensory polyganglionopathy (CISP)
- Chronic idiopathic ataxic neuropathy (CIAN)

Box 3.15 Postural tremor in neuromuscular diseases

- Spinal muscular atrophy (SMA) types 2 and 3. AR *SMN*. **Case 7**
- Spinal and bulbar muscular atrophy (SBMA, Kennedy disease) XR, *androgen receptor* repeat expansion. **Case 5**
- Charcot–Marie–Tooth disease, in particular demyelinating AD types *PMP22, MPZ, NEFL*. Disabling in children. **Case 27**
- Dysimmune neuropathies: IgM paraproteinaemic neuropathies, chronic inflammatory demyelinating polyneuropathy (CIDP), and multifocal motor neuropathy (MMN). **Cases 10, 11, 17**
- Myopathies associated with genes encoding sarcomere proteins *MYH2, MYH7, NEB, TNNT1, TPM3, MYL2, MYBPC1*. Postural, sometimes also action tremor, irregular, high-frequency, low-amplitude tremor, early-onset myopathy, joint contractures, and hypermobility.

Box 3.16 Abnormal muscle fibre activity: fasciculations, myokymia, cramp, muscle contracture, myotonia, and rippling

See Chapter 2 for a clinical description of these features. Clinically, these abnormalities may be difficult to distinguish from one another (e.g., fasciculations – myokymia; cramp – contracture). EMG can be helpful, but often fails to be diagnostic, as these features cannot always be provoked during the examination.

Twitches

Fasciculations
- All disorders of the lower motor neuron (anterior horn cell and peripheral nerves), in particular in ALS/MND/PMA, Kennedy syndrome (perioral), and the cramp-fasciculation syndrome. In SMA fasciculations mostly confined to the tongue. **Cases 1, 3, 4, 5, 6, 7, 8, 18**
- May be induced by treatment of myasthenia gravis with cholinesterase inhibitors (e.g., pyridostigmine), in particular in MuSK MG. **Cases 31, 32**
- 'Benign' fasciculations in healthy people, usually, but not always, restricted to the calves. At rest or after strenuous exercise. No wasting or weakness. No abnormalities on needle EMG, apart from fasciculation potentials.

Myokymia
- Peripheral nerve hyperexcitability syndromes (Morvan, Isaac). Stiffness. Autonomic dysfunction. Antibodies against CASPR2 and LGI1, which form part of the voltage-gated potassium channel complex. **Case 18**
- Autosomal dominant inherited syndromes involving episodic ataxia or neonatal epilepsy caused by defects in the potassium channels genes *KCNA1* and *KCNQ2*.
- Facial myokymia: due to a lesion of the nucleus of the facial nerve in the pons.
- Eyelid and other 'benign' myokymia, e.g., superior oblique myokymia (monocular; high-frequency oscillopsia). Nonprogressive.
- Post-radiation myokymia located in the face, tongue, limbs.

Physical activity-induced, short-duration cramp, cramp-like pain or stiffness

Anterior horn cell/nerve
- Cramp occurs in all disorders of the lower motor neuron (anterior horn cell and peripheral nerves), in particular in ALS/MND/PMA, Kennedy syndrome (including carriers), neuropathies, and the cramp-fasciculation syndrome. Very painful. **Cases 1, 3, 5, 18**
- Cramp in metabolic, endocrine, and electrolyte abnormalities (hypothyroidism, hypomagnesaemia, hypocalcaemia, renal or liver dysfunction, third trimester of pregnancy).
- Cramp provoked by strenuous exercise, and nocturnal cramp in the calves can occur in healthy people. Can be very painful.

Muscle
- Contracture in McArdle disease. Painful. Elevated CK. Abnormal non-ischaemic forearm test. AR *PYGM*. **Case 53**
- Contracture in Brody disease. Exercise induced and painless; exacerbated by cold. Elevated CK. AR *ATP2A1*.
- Contracture in carnitine palmitoyl transferase II (CPTII). Contractures occur during prolonged exercise. Normal CK. Rhabdomyolysis. AR *CPT2*. **Case 54**
- Cramp-like myalgia in Becker muscular dystrophy (XR *DMD*), myotonic dystrophy type 2 (AD *CNBP*), and hypothyroid myopathy. **Cases 37, 40, 63**
- Myotonia in myotonic dystrophy types 1 (AD *DMPK*) and 2 (AD *CNBP*). **Cases 39, 40**
- Myotonia in channelopathies: nondystrophic myotonic disorders and some periodic paralyses (AD *CLCN1; SCN4A*). **Case 50**
- Rippling muscle disease: rippling, mounding, percussion-induced rapid muscle contractions (PIRCS) due to *CAV3* mutation, without or with other features of *CAV3* mutations: myalgia, muscle hypertrophy, hyperCKaemia. May also be caused by AR *PTRF/CAVIN1* mutations. **Case 46**
- Rippling muscle disease due to autoimmune disorder with AChR and MURC/Cavin-4 antibodies. Associated with thymoma and myasthenia gravis.

Box 3.17 Pain and stiffness

Nerve root or plexus
- Sharp, lancinating, severe pain in the distribution of one or more dermatomes. Irradiating in nerve root involvement. Inflammation (e.g., Guillain–Barré syndrome, **Case 9**), infection (e.g., Lyme, **Case 25**), ischaemia (diabetes, **Case 20**), compression or ingrowth by malignancy.

Peripheral nerve
- Distal, continuous, symmetric burning pain, painful paraesthesia, allodynia: polyneuropathy with (isolated) involvement of small myelinated and unmyelinated nerve fibres. Small-fibre neuropathy (SFN), **Case 14**; and, e.g., diabetic polyneuropathy, **Case 20**
- Unilateral (sub)acute pain in the course of a distal peripheral nerve: vasculitic neuropathy. **Case 13**

Muscle
- Myotonia and muscle contracture are often described as painful stiffness. **Cases 50, 53**
- Myalgia: painful stiffness, mostly symmetric, proximal, aggravated by physical activity:
    ◦ Myositis (not IBM). **Cases 59, 60, 61**
    ◦ Sarcoidosis CK mildly elevated
    ◦ Vasculitic myopathy – muscular polyarteritis nodosa (M-PAN). Often with fever, no weakness. Normal CK. Usually systemic disease, but may be confined to muscle (PET/CT, muscle biopsy). Vasculitic myopathy occurs also in Behçet disease.
    ◦ (Eosinophilic) fasciitis (MRI, muscle biopsy).
    ◦ Some drug-induced myopathies. **Case 64**
    ◦ Polymyalgia rheumatica (ESR ↑, no weakness, CK normal).
    ◦ Hypothyroid myopathy, also weakness, fatigability, cramps; CK can be markedly elevated. **Case 63**
    ◦ Cramp-like myalgia in various muscular dystrophies, e.g., BMD, DM2, see Box 3.16.

Central nervous system
- Stiff person spectrum disorders (SPSD), rigidity and pain, thoracolumbar stiffness, triggered spasms, onset in back and legs, hyperlordosis, continuous motor unit activity in affected muscles, anti-GAD65 and other antibodies. Paraneoplastic in 5% of cases.

Box 3.18 Muscle hypertrophy

Tongue:
- Duchenne muscular dystrophy (DMD), Becker muscular dystrophy (BMD), amyloidosis, infantile-onset Pompe disease, hypothyroidism. **Cases 36, 37, 52, 63**

Calves (also pseudohypertrophy due to fatty replacement):
- DMD, BMD, DMD/BMD carriers, **Cases 36, 37.** Other muscular dystrophies: e.g., limb girdle muscular dystrophy (LGMD) R9, **Case 42**; Pompe disease, **Case 52**; myotonic dystrophy type 2, **Case 40**; core myopathies, **Case 56**; radiculopathy due to herniated disc (unilateral), Charcot–Marie–Tooth disease (CMT), **Cases 27, 28**

Generalized:
- Channelopathies (congenital myotonia, periodic paralysis), **Cases 50, 51**; rippling muscle disease, **Case 46**; peripheral nerve hyperexcitability syndromes, **Case 18**; RYR1–related conditions, **Case 56**

Box 3.19 Joint contractures, hypermobility (hyperlaxity), and deformities in neuromuscular disorders

Arthrogryposis (joint contractures in at least two areas, present at birth) – usually symmetric, distal more than proximal

- Amyoplasia
- Congenital AR spinal muscular atrophy (arthrogryposis of mainly the lower leg, usually not progressive), also known as spinal muscular atrophy lower extremity dominant (SMA-LED; AD *DYNC1H1*, *BICD2*).
- Congenital onset 5q-linked SMA (SMA type 0; AR *SMN*); X-linked infantile SMA (*UBA1*)
- Hereditary neuropathies (rare; e.g.,*TRP4* (AD))
- Congenital myasthenic syndromes, inherited disorders caused by genetic defects at presynaptic, synaptic or postsynaptic levels). Fatigable weakness involving ocular, bulbar, and limb muscles. Bulbar weakness may be presenting sign. Arthrogryposis. Onset at or shortly after birth, or in first two years. Mostly AR, AD less common. Multiple genes involved. **Case 35**

Box 3.19 (cont.)

- Recurrent arthrogryposis (maternal myasthenia gravis, usually untreated; transplacental transfer of AChR).
- Congenital myopathy (some forms of nemaline myopathy). **Case 58**
- Congenital muscular dystrophy (e.g., Fukuyama congenital muscular dystrophy (AR *FKTN*; **Case 47**), merosin-deficient congenital muscular dystrophy (AR *LAMA2*).
- *SNUPN*-related myopathy, titinopathy. AR

Hollow feet (pes cavus) or club feet

- Hereditary neuropathies with early onset. Pes cavus with hammer toes, later also claw hand. Also pes cavus in Friedreich ataxia, hereditary spastic paraplegia (HSP). **Cases 27, 28**
- Tethered cord syndrome, spina bifida (club feet)
- Caveolinopathy (*CAV3*), congenital myotonic dystrophy, congenital myopathies, titinopathies congenital-onset Bethlem myopathy (club feet usually disappear spontaneously), Ullrich congenital muscular dystrophy. **Cases 43, 46, 57, 58**

Proximal and distal contractures, joint hypermobility

- Collagen VI-related myopathy spectrum (*COL6A1*, *COL6A2*, *COL6A3*): Severe: Ullrich congenital muscular dystrophy (UCMD), mostly AR: Distal joint hypermobility, hip dislocation, prominent calcaneus, proximal, later also distal contractures, kyphoscoliosis, hypertrophic scars. Mild: Bethlem myopathy, mostly AD: Achilles tendon, long finger flexor, elbow, and spine, **Case 43.** *COL12* may be associated with similar phenotype.
- Emery–Dreifuss muscular dystrophy (EDMD). Contractures of neck and thoracolumbar extension (rigid spine), elbow flexion, and Achilles tendons. Humeroperoneal weakness and atrophy, cardiac arrhythmias and cardiomyopathy, XR, AR *EMD*, *LMNA*, *SYNE1*, *SYNE2*, *FHL1*, *TMEM43*. **Case 45**
- Limb girdle muscular dystrophy R1 (LGMDR1), AR *CAPN*. **Case 41**, titinopathies
- Joint contractures may develop in acquired myopathy. Contractures in juvenile dermatomyositis are associated with calcinosis.

Scoliosis

- Duchenne muscular dystrophy (DMD). XR *DMD*. **Case 36**
- Spinal muscular atrophy (SMA) type 2. AR *SMN*. **Case 7**
- Congenital myopathies. AD, AR *RYR1* (also hip dislocation, pes cavus), AR *SELENON/SEPN1*, AR/AD *NEB*, AR/AD *MYH2*, AR *MEGF10*, among others. RYR1 and SELENON mutations are also typically associated with rigid spine. **Case 56**

Deformities (Charcot arthropathy) and amputation

- Can result from sensory polyneuropathies, e.g., diabetes mellitus, **Case 20**; leprosy, **Case 26**; sensory and hereditary sensory autonomic neuropathy (HSAN), **Case 29**. Different pathogenetic mechanisms.

Box 3.20 Neonatal hypotonia: neuromuscular causes

A floppy infant is an infant with generalized hypotonia presenting at birth or in early life. Neonatal hypotonia is most often due to acquired or genetic disorders of the central motor neuron (60–80%). Clues to suspect a neuromuscular disease are a prenatal onset of symptoms, e.g., in case of polyhydramnios or joint contractures (arthrogryposis), and a positive family history. A combination of central and peripheral hypotonia can occur if respiratory insufficiency due to the neuromuscular condition induced asphyxia, in rare metabolic conditions and mitochondrial disease, or in congenital muscular dystrophy and congenital myotonic dystrophy.

Anterior horn cell

- Spinal muscular atrophy (SMA). Mutations in *SMN1* gene (AR). Requests specific DNA testing. Proximal weakness more than distal. No facial weakness. Normal eye movement. Intercostal muscle weakness with preserved diaphragm movement causes pronounced belly breathing. **Case 6**
- Spinal muscular atrophy with respiratory distress type 1 (SMARD1). Mutations in *IGHMBP2* gene (AR). Growth retardation. Distal weakness with foot deformity. Diaphragmatic weakness and weak cry.

Peripheral nerve

- Congenital hypomyelinating neuropathy. Mutations in several CMT genes (AD/AR). Clinical presentation similar to SMA with preserved ocular movements although more often with arthrogryposis.

Neuromuscular junction

- Transient neonatal myasthenia. Placental transfer of maternal anti-AChR or anti-MuSK antibodies. No correlation with maternal weakness, mothers may be minimally affected and undiagnosed. Good response to acetylcholinesterase inhibitors. Resolves spontaneously in 1 to 3 weeks.
- Congenital myasthenic syndromes (CMS). More than 30 genes involved in neuromuscular transmission, mainly AR. Generalized weakness including the facial muscles with ptosis. Arthrogryposis may be present. Episodic apneas. **Case 35**

Box 3.20 (cont.)

- Infantile botulism. Reduced acetylcholine release due to exotoxin of *Clostridium botulinum*. Transfer through contaminated environmental dust or honey. Feeding difficulties and constipation followed by bulbar and generalized weakness including ptosis and dilated pupils.

Muscle
- Congenital myopathies with neonatal onset. Multiple genes (AD/AR). Generalized weakness including the facial muscles. High arched palate. Some subtypes with external ophthalmoparesis, cardiomyopathy or early respiratory failure. Muscle biopsy may show typical abnormalities, but with substantial overlap between the genotypes and the histological classification:
    - Nemaline myopathy
    - Congenital fibre-type disproportion myopathy
    - Centronuclear myopathy. **Case 57**
    - Central core or multiminicore myopathy. **Case 56**
- Congenital muscular dystrophy (CMD). Classification as syndromic (with CNS involvement) or nonsyndromic.
- Secondary dystroglycanopathies. Genes involved in the glycosylation of α-dystroglycan (AR). Syndromic CMD with a variety of cerebral developmental abnormalities including polymicrogyria, lissencephaly, cerebellar involvement, corpus callosum dysgenesia, and hydrocephalus. Elevated CK.
- Laminin α2-related CMD. Mutations in *LAMA2* (AR) lead to merosin deficiency. Generalized weakness with respiratory failure and joint contractures. Elevated CK. Increased T2 signal of the cerebral white matter on MRI.
- CMD with collagen deficiency (Ullrich disease). Mutations in *COL6A1*, *COL6A2*, *COL6A3* (AD/AR). Combination of joint contractures and joint laxity. Early respiratory failure. CK normal or mildly elevated
- CMD with rigid spine. Mutations in *SEPN1* (AR). CK normal or mildly elevated.
- Congenital myotonic dystrophy. Repeat expansion in the *DMPK* gene (AD). Requests specific DNA testing. Respiratory insufficiency, pronounced facial weakness with tent-shaped mouth, feeding difficulties, joint contractures. Mothers can be only mildly affected and hence undiagnosed.
- Pompe disease. Severe infantile form with presentation at or soon after birth. Mutations in *GAA* lead to acid α-glycosidase (acid maltase) deficiency (AR). Cardiomegaly. Hepatomegaly.

Box 3.21 Cardiac involvement in neuromuscular disorders

Clinically relevant cardiac involvement in neuromuscular disorders can be distinguished in (1) cardiomyopathy and (2) conduction defects with arrhythmias. Cardiomyopathy and arrhythmias may coexist. Cardiac involvement may be a predominant feature or the first manifestation.
Cardiac manifestations may also occur without (prominent) muscle involvement, e.g., due to variant in *DMD* (XR), *LMNA* (AD/AR), *MYH7* (AD).

Prominent feature and sometimes first manifestation

- Dystrophinopathies XR, *DMD* – DMD, BMD, female carriers
- Dilated cardiomyopathy (DCM). In DMD, age of development of abnormal left ventricular ejection fraction is on average 14 years. Correlation between increasing cardiac dysfunction, increasing age, and severity of skeletal muscle disease. DCM virtually present in all DMD patients > 18 years, leading to advanced heart failure and premature death. For BMD, only small proportion of subjects < 16 years of age have symptomatic cardiac involvement. Up to 70% develop symptomatic heart failure by age 40. Nine percent of female carriers may have DCM, may even be the presenting feature. Gadolinium enhancement on MRI shows subclinical DCM in 48%. **Cases 36, 37**
- LGMDR9. **Case 42** AR *FKRP*
- DCM frequent feature, which increases with age, can be present in early childhood.
- Sarcoglycanopathies (LGMDR3–6)
  AR *SCGA*, *SCGB*, *SCGG*, 6–19% of patients have DCM irrespective of severity of muscle weakness.
- Myotonic dystrophy, type 1 **Case 39**
  AD *DMPK*; conduction defects (AV-block, intraventricular) and dysrhythmias; DCM during course of disease. Association between cardiac conduction disturbances and age, duration of neurological disease and male gender. Sudden death in ~30%, also as first manifestation. DM1 > DM2 patients need a pacemaker/implanted cardioverter.
- Myotonic dystrophy, type 2. **Case 40**
  AD *CNBP*; similar to DM1, cardiomyopathy rare. Sudden death may occur.
- X-linked Emery–Dreifuss muscular dystrophy (*EDMD*, *EMD*)
  Conduction abnormalities. Atrial paralysis is pathognomonic. May occur early. Conduction defects in 3rd decade require pacing by age 30; sudden cardiac death may be initial manifestation of disease. Female carriers rarely have conduction defects. **Case 45**

Box 3.21 (cont.)

- AD/AR EDMD (*LMNA*)
  Ventricular dysrhythmias, conduction defects, dilated or hypertrophic cardiomyopathy. Conduction abnormalities in 18% of patients < 10 years. Cardiomyopathy occurs later, reaching 60% in patients > 50 years. Sudden death as result of fatal arrhythmia.
- *FHL1*-related AD EDMD
  Hypertrophic cardiomyopathy, atrial fibrillation or flutter common; risk of cardio-embolic complications. Some patients at high risk for sudden cardiac death.
- Myofibrillar myopathies (*DES* (AR/AD)), **Case 49**, *CRYAB* (AR/AD), *FLNC* (AD), *LBD3* (AD), *BAG3* AD)). Dysrhythmia; dilated, hypertrophic or restrictive cardiomyopathy. Sudden death may occur.
- Pompe disease. **Case 52**
  AR *GAA*; in infantile onset Pompe disease hypertrophic cardiomyopathy.
- Danon disease
  XD *LAMP-2*. Males and females (carriers) may have severe hypertrophic/dilated cardiomyopathy. Sudden death may occur as first manifestation.
- Mitochondrial myopathies
  Hypertrophic, dilated, or restrictive cardiomyopathy, and left ventricular noncompaction; arrhythmia, Wolf–Parkinson–White syndrome. Cardiac structural (29%) and conduction abnormalities (39%), also in children. Sudden death may occur in Kearns–Sayre syndrome and Barth syndrome (XR *TAZ*). **Case 55**
- Neutral lipid storage disease
  AR *PNPLA2*; hypertrophic cardiomyopathy and dysrhythmia
- *MYH7*-related disease
  AD *MYH7*; onset distal leg weakness ('hanging big toe'), with or without hypertrophic cardiomyopathy.
- Channelopathies (Andersen–Tawil syndrome: potassium-sensitive periodic paralysis)
  AD *KCNJ2*; ventricular arrhythmia (syncope, sudden death).
- Congenital myopathies
  AD *ACTA1* (DCM, arrhythmias, sudden death); AR/AD *TTN* (early and late onset); AR *SPEG*, centronuclear myopathy, DCM; AR *MYPN*, nemaline myopathy, **Case 58**; hypertrophic cardiomyopathy; AD/AR *BIN1*, DCM; AR *MYO18B*
- Distal myopathies (*MYH7* variant)
  Dilated, hypertrophic or non-compacted left ventricle cardiomyopathy, and dysrhythmia (50%). Sudden death may occur.
- Amyloidosis
  Major cause of death in patients with hereditary transthyretin (TTR) amyloidosis. (AD *TTR*), **Case 30**; and in amyloid light chain amyloidosis, in which predominantly the heart, kidneys, or both are affected.
- Guillain–Barré syndrome (acute phase). Arrhythmias. **Case 9**

Rare occurrence of cardiac involvement or only subclinical involvement – screening for cardiac involvement is to the discretion of the treating physician

- Anoctamin 5-related myopathies
  AR *ANO5*; dilated cardiomyopathy, ventricular arrhythmia. **Case 49**
- Caveolinopathy
  AD *CAV3*; atrioventricular conduction defects, long QT-syndrome, dilated and hypertrophic cardiomyopathy. **Case 46**
- Facioscapulohumeral dystrophy types 1 and 2
  AD *DUX4*, *SMCHD1*; conduction abnormalities (right bundle branch block, RBBB). Low prevalence: 7% complete RBBB, 5% incomplete RBBB. **Case 38**
- Idiopathic inflammatory myopathies (myositis)
  Subclinical cardiac involvement (heart function, rhythm, and conduction abnormalities in 75% of IIM). If no clinical suspicion (chest pain, shortness of breath, arrhythmias): cardiac troponin (cTnI); if clinical suspicion transthoracic echocardiography and Holter should be performed. If these tests are normal there is no indication for MRI, **Cases 60, 61**. No cardiac involvement in inclusion body myositis (IBM).
- Lyme radiculoneuritis
  1st–3rd degree atrioventricular block, pericarditis and myocarditis can occur. Generally good prognosis with treatment. **Case 25**

Box 3.22 Asymptomatic/paucisymptomatic hyperCKaemia

Values beyond the 97.5th percentile are considered hyperCKaemia: in non-Black women ≥ 217 IU/L; in non-Black men ≥ 336; in Black women: ≥ 414; in Black men: ≥ 801.

First, rule out the most common and treatable non-neuromuscular causes

- Physical exercise, sports
- Trauma, compression
- Iatrogenic (IM injection, EMG, surgery)
- Medication (statins, fibrates, immune checkpoint inhibitors, beta blockers, angiotensin-II receptor blockers, clozapine, hydroxychloroquine, isotretinoin, colchicine)
- Toxins (alcohol, cocaine, heroin)
- Metabolic (hypothyroidism, hyperthyroidism, hyperparathyroidism)
- Seizures
- Cramps
- Myocardial infarction
- McLeod syndrome (ultrarare, X-linked recessive, *XK*; progressive movement disorder features such as chorea and dystonia, epilepsy, peripheral neuropathy, muscle involvement, typically with CK elevation and cardiomyopathy). In almost all patients misshapen red blood cells (acanthocytes)

Neuromuscular causes – CK > 10 × ULN

- Dystrophinopathies XR *DMD* DMD, carrier. **Case 36**
- LGMD AR α-*SG*, *DYSF*, *ANO5*, *CAV3*, *CAPN3*, *FKRP*, *POMT2*. **Cases 41, 42, 47**
- McArdle disease AR *PGYM*. **Case 53**
- Danon disease AD *LAMP-2*. Age at onset infancy–5th decade, mostly childhood, mild proximal muscle weakness, hypertrophic cardiomyopathy, often mental retardation.
- Myositis, in particular paediatric- and adult-onset immune-mediated necrotizing myopathy, associated with anti-SRP and anti-HMGCR autoantibodies. **Cases 60, 61**

Neuromuscular causes – CK > 2 and < 10× ULN

- Dystrophinopathies XR *DMD* BMD, carrier. **Case 37**
- Myotonic dystrophy type 2 AD *CNBP*. **Case 40**
- Pompe disease AR *GAA*. **Case 52**
- Central core disease AD/AR *RYR1* – risk of malignant hyperthermia. **Case 56**
- Myositis. **Cases 59, 60, 61**
- Mitochondrial myopathies, maternal inheritance, AR, AD. **Case 55**
- Myofibrillar myopathies AR/AD, a.o.: *DES*, *CRYAB*, *LDB3*, *TTN*, *FLNA*, *BAG3*. **Case 49**
- Neutral lipid storage disease with myopathy AR *PNPLA2*, associated with Jordan anomaly in leukocytes
- ALS/MND. **Case 1**
- Spinal and bulbar muscular atrophy (carrier included) XR Androgen receptor gene, repeat disorder. **Case 5**
- SMA type 3–4 (AR *SMN*). **Case 7**

Box 3.23 Rhabdomyolysis

Rhabdomyolysis is defined as a clinical syndrome of acute muscle weakness, myalgia, and muscle swelling, combined with a CK cut-off value of > 1000 IU/L or CK > 5 × ULN. Serum CK activity rises 2–12 hours after onset of muscle injury, peaks at 3–5 days after injury, and declines over the subsequent 6–10 days. Myoglobinuria is only present in half of the cases and thus its absence does not rule out the diagnosis.

Rhabdomyolysis can be triggered by physical, chemical, and pharmacological hazards or is a manifestation of a (hereditary) myopathy and as such triggered by exercise, a febrile illness. In case of disorders of fatty acid metabolism fasting is often a trigger.

Recurrent rhabdomyolysis: a positive family history for attacks or persistent hperCKaemia should raise suspicion of a hereditary neuromuscular disease. In most patients with presumed underlying genetic disease, a genetic defect cannot be identified as to date.

Non-neuromuscular causes – the most common are marked with an asterisk (*)

Traumatic causes

- *Vascular/orthopaedic surgery (intraoperative use of tourniquets, tight dressings or casts, prolonged application of air splints or pneumatic anti-shock garments, and clamping of vessels during surgery)

Box 3.23 (cont.)

- *Prolonged immobility (immobilization after trauma, anaesthesia, coma, drug- or alcohol-induced unconsciousness)
- *Muscle ischaemia/anoxia (including vascular occlusion, thrombo-mbolism, shock, aortic dissections, or asphyxia)
- *Traumatic: multiple injury, crush injury (bombings, earthquakes, building collapse, mine accidents, train or motor vehicle accidents)
- Compartment syndrome
- High-voltage electrical injury
- Extensive third-degree burns

Non-traumatic exertional causes
- Extreme physical exertion
- Eccentric exercise
- Hyperkinetic states (e.g., seizures, psychotic agitation, delirium tremens)
- Sickle cell disease (crisis)
- Status asthmaticus
- Exertional heat stroke

Non-traumatic non-exertional causes
- *Infections or sepsis; Viral: influenza A and B, human immunodeficiency virus, enterovirus (Coxsackie, echo), adenovirus, Epstein–Barr virus, cytomegalovirus, herpes simplex virus, varicella-zoster virus, West Nile virus, SARS-C0V-2; Bacterial: *Legionella* species, *Salmonella* species, *Francisella* species, *Streptococcus pneumoniae*, *Staphylococcus aureus*, *Enterococcus*, *Pseudomonas aeruginosa*, *Neisseria meningitidis*, *Haemophilus influenzae*, *Coxiella burnetii*, *Leptospira* species, *Mycoplasma* species, *Escherichia coli*; fungal and malaria infections.
- *Drugs: salicylates, fibric acid derivates (bezafibrate, clofibrate, fenofibrate, gemfibrozil), neuroleptics/antipsychotics (neuroleptic malignant syndrome is associated with haloperidol, fluphenazine, perphenazine, chlorpromazine), quinine, corticosteroids, statins (atorvastatin, fluvastatin, lovastatin, pravastatin, rosuvastatin, simvastatin, cerivastatin), theophylline, cyclic antidepressants, selective serotonin reuptake inhibitors, antibiotics (fluroquinolones, pyrazinamide, trimethoprim/sulphonamide, amphotericin B, itraconazole, levofloxacin), zidovudine, benzodiazepines, antihistamines, aminocaproic acid, phenylpropanolamine.
- *Substance abuse (excessive alcohol intake, amphetamines, heroin, methadone, barbiturates, cocaine, caffeine, amphetamine, lysergic acid diethylamide (LSD), 3,4-methylenedioxymethamphetamine (MDMA, ecstasy), phencyclidine, benzodiazepines, toluene (from glue sniffing), gasoline/paint sniffing).
- Anaesthetics and neuromuscular blocking agents: barbiturates, benzodiazepines, propofol, succinylcholine in patients with Duchenne/Becker muscular dystrophies.
- Toxic agents: carbon monoxide, hemlock herbs from quail, snake bites, spider venom, massive honeybee envenomations, *Tricholoma equestre* (mushroom), buffalo fish.
- Electrolyte disturbance: hyponatraemia, hypernatraemia, hypokalaemia, hypophosphataemia, hypocalciaemia, hyperosmotic conditions.
- Endocrine disorders: hypothyroidism, hyperthyroidism, diabetic ketoacidosis, non-ketotic hyperosmolar diabetic coma, hyperaldosteronism.

Neuromuscular causes

Disorders of glycogen metabolism
- Myophosphorylase deficiency (McArdle disease/GSDV, *PYGM*) AR. **Case 53**
- Phosphofructokinase deficiency (Tarui disease/GSDVII, *PFKM*) AR.
- Phosphoglycerate mutase deficiency (GSDX, *PGAMM*) AR.
- Phosphoglycerate kinase deficiency (*PGK1*) XR; also haemolytic anaemia, CNS dysfunction, myalgia, cramps, slowly progressive muscle weakness.
- Aldolase A deficiency (GSDXII, *ALDOA*) AR; childhood onset; haemolytic anaemia, recurrent rhabdomyolysis, ultrarare).
- Lactate dehydrogenase A deficiency (GSDXI, *LDHA*) AR.
- ß-Enolase deficiency (GSDXIII, *ENO3*) AR.

Disorders of fatty acid metabolism
- Carnitine-palmityl-transferase deficiency (*CPT2*) AR. **Case 54**
- Very long chain acetyl-CoA-dehydrogenase deficiency (*ACADVL*) AR.
- Phosphatidic acid phosphatase deficiency (*LPIN1*) AR.
- Glutaric aciduria type I (*GCDH*) AR; rare, encephalopathic crises, triggered by viral infections, macrocephaly.
- Multiple acyl-coenzyme A dehydrogenase deficiency (MADD) (*ETFB*, *ETFDH*) AR.
- Mitochondrial trifunctional protein (MTP) deficiency/ LCHAD deficiency (*HADHA*, *HADHB*) AR; wide clinical spectrum, ranging from severe neonatal conditions associated with cardiomyopathy, hypoglycaemia, muscle weakness, neuropathy, and liver disease leading to death to a mild phenotype with peripheral neuropathy and pigmentary retinopathy.

Box 3.23 (cont.)

Primary mitochondrial disorders
- Cytochrome b deficiency (Complex III) (*MTCYB*) sporadic; exercise intolerance, proximal weakness.
- Cytochrome-C-oxidase deficiency (*MTCO1, MTCO2, MTCO3*) maternal inheritance; exercise intolerance +/× muscle weakness.
- Thymidine kinase 2 (TK2) deficiency (*TK2*) AR.

Miscellaneous
- *RYR1*-related exertional rhabdomyolysis, see **Case 56,** AR/AD. Relatively frequent cause.
- Limb girdle muscular dystrophies (LGMDs), i.e., dysferlin-related LGMD AR *DYSF*, anoctamin 5-related LGMD (AR *ANO5*), fukutin-related protein-related LGMD AR *FKRP*, sarcoglycanopathies AR *SGCA, SGCC*. **Cases 41, 42, 47**
- Duchenne/Becker muscular dystrophies/carrier XR *DMD*. **Cases 36, 37**
- Brody disease AR *SERCA1*; stiffness, cramps, myalgia.
- TANGO2-syndrome. Childhood-onset. AR *TANGO2*; cardiac arrythmias, rhabdomyolysis, neurodegeneration.
- LPIN1 deficiency. Recurrent rhabdomyolysis, early childhood; may be life-threatening; AR *LPIN1*.
- Marinesco–Sjögren syndrome AR *SIL1*; weakness, cerebellar dysfunction, cataracts, polyneuropathy, hypogonadism.
- Myositis (rare): dermatomyositis, immune-mediated necrotizing myopathy. **Cases 59, 60, 61**

Chapter 4

Electrodiagnostic Studies

Stephan Goedee

Introduction

Electrodiagnostic studies are often at the centre of diagnostic strategies in neuromuscular disorders. The basic electrophysiological techniques commonly used are focused on documenting sufficient proof of dysfunction emanating from different parts of the peripheral nervous system: peripheral motor neuron, nerve root, plexus and peripheral nerve, neuromuscular junction, and skeletal muscle. In short, dedicated nerve conduction studies and needle myography or a combination of these may be needed to help accurately identify the site and nature of the neuromuscular disorder (Fig. 4.1A–C). Appropriate and standardized instrumentation, including control of temperature and uniform sampling, is essential for meaningful interpretation. The electrodiagnostic techniques aligned with the main anatomical correlates underlying different neuromuscular disorders are discussed in this chapter.

Motor Neuron Disorders

Needle myography is often required to establish the pattern of loss of peripheral motor neurons. Characteristic electrophysiological features include, at rest: fibrillation potentials and/or positive sharp waves (compatible with denervation; **Video 1**), and upon volitional contraction: polyphasic motor unit potentials (MUPs) with long duration or giant potentials (compatible with re-innervation; **Video 2**). Fasciculation potentials have been assigned the same weight as signs of denervation in the recent amyotrophic lateral sclerosis (ALS) consensus guidelines, but they have lower specificity since fasciculations can also be present in healthy subjects. A standardized myography protocol, sampling muscles from distinct spinal segments and nerves, is warranted to establish sufficient proof of generalized loss of peripheral motor neurons (Table 4.1). In addition, sensory nerve conduction studies can facilitate distinction between ALS, facial onset sensory and motor neuronopathy (FOSMN), Kennedy disease (bulbospinal muscular atrophy), distal spinal muscular atrophy, and the axonal form of Charcot–Marie–Tooth disease (type 2). The list of possible ALS mimics is extensive, several of which may show similar electrophysiological abnormalities. Examples include spinal canal stenosis and Hirayama disease (abnormalities often limited to one spinal body region (cervical/lumbosacral)), inclusion body myositis (IBM, apparent lack of 'myopathic' MUPs), primary lateral sclerosis (PLS, may have regions with limited long-duration polyphasic MUPs), multifocal motor neuropathy (MMN, conduction blocks on dedicated studies of motor conduction), and post-polio syndrome (PPS, abnormalities often limited to initially affected areas). Consequently, thorough clinical evaluation and complete overview of other relevant ancillary test results are mandatory, and caution is warranted when interpreting the results of needle myography.

Neuropathies

Loss of sensory and motor axons in neuropathies can be evaluated with routine nerve conduction studies (NCS), albeit with varying sensitivity. Characteristic findings are decreased sensory nerve action potentials (SNAPs) and compound motor action potentials (CMAPs). Focal conduction slowing over a known compression site is a typical feature of mononeuropathies, but can also be seen in more generalized neuropathies including hereditary neuropathy with liability to pressure palsies (HNPP), IgM neuropathy (+/−) anti-MAG antibodies, and amyloid neuropathy.

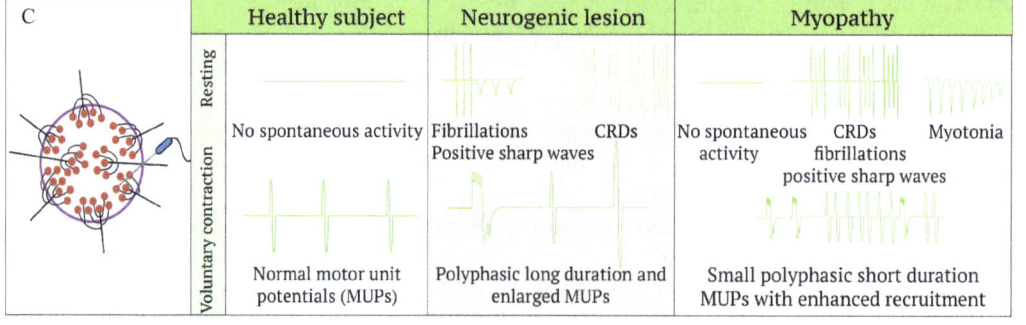

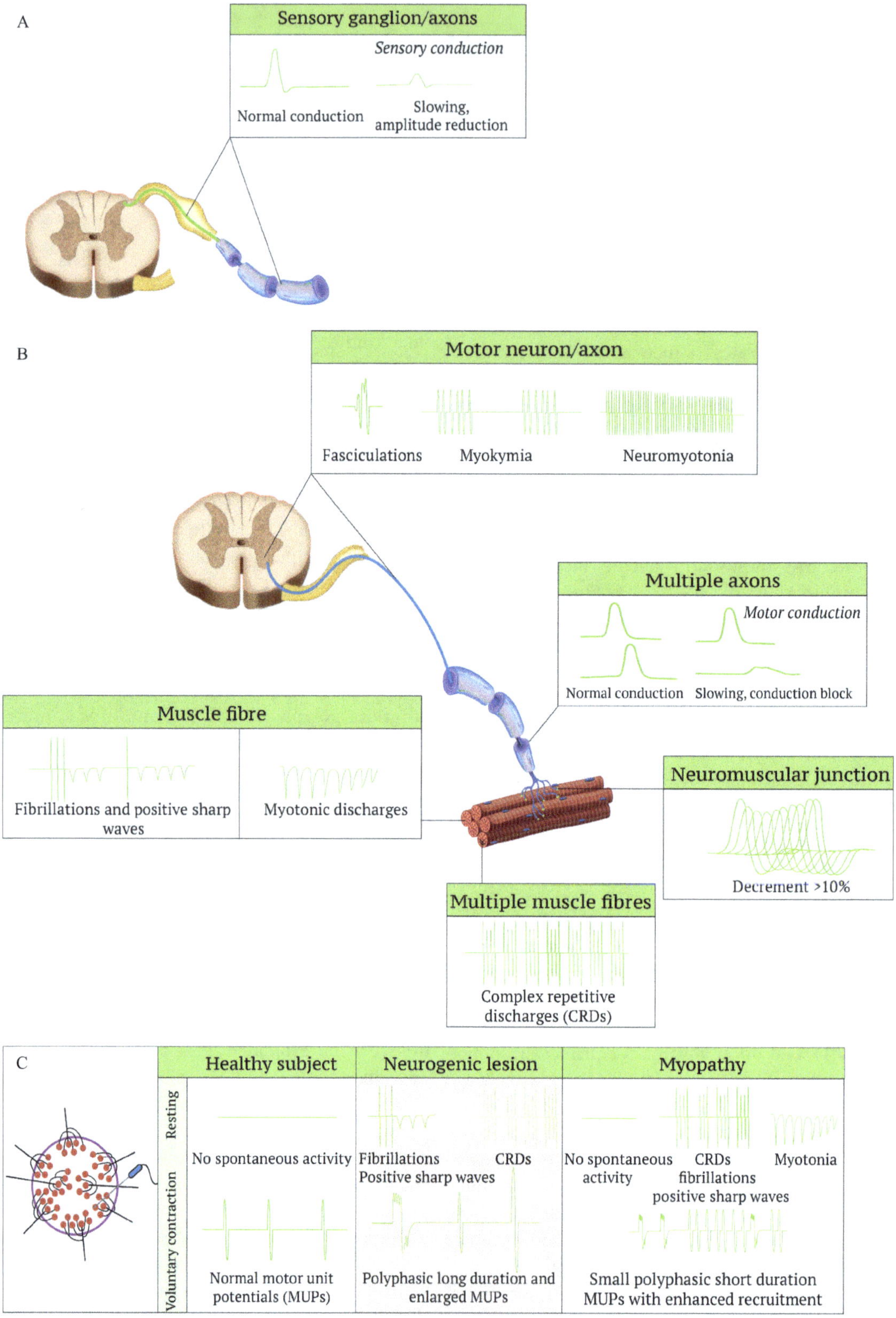

Figure 4.1 A–C Summary electrodiagnostic features in neuromuscular disorders.

Table 4.1 Summary electrodiagnostic criteria for ALS

	Denervation	Re-innervation	Scoring criteria per body region
El Escorial criteria	Fibrillation potentials and/or positive sharp waves	Large polyphasic MUPs with long duration	Lumbosacral/cervical: both de- and re-innervation ≥ 2 muscles innervated by different spinal segments and nerves Bulbar/thoracic: both de- and re-innervation ≥ 1 muscle
Awaji/Gold Coast criteria	Fibrillation potentials, positive sharp waves and/or fasciculations	Large polyphasic MUPs with long duration	Lumbosacral/cervical: both de- and re-innervation ≥ 2 muscles innervated by different spinal segments and nerves Bulbar/thoracic: both de- and re-innervation ≥ 1 muscle

Motor unit potentials (MUPs); note that complex repetitive discharges (CRDs) are not formally included here but can be seen in motor neuron syndromes and therefore could be regarded as a similar sign of denervation. Electrodiagnostic signs of denervation and re-innervation are required to be present in the same muscle to fulfil the consensus criteria. Importantly, the same muscle on the contralateral side should not be considered a different spinal segment. Unfortunately, the Awaji/Gold Coast criteria do not specify the desired balance between presence of fibrillation potentials/positive sharp waves and fasciculations. As a practical rule, fasciculations should only add 1–2 muscles (overall) to fulfil the scoring criterion. In contrast, the relative lack of the fibrillation potentials/positive sharp waves should raise suspicion for potential mimics.

Polyneuropathies

Axonal neuropathies are the most common form of polyneuropathies, typically with symmetrically decreased/absent SNAPs and CMAPs, and no or only mild to moderate conduction slowing. NCS appear to have little added diagnostic value in well-known causes such as diabetes and vitamin deficiencies. In contrast, vasculitic neuropathy classically presents with asymmetric or multifocal abnormal SNAPs and CMAPs, and occasionally a pseudoconduction block (i.e., initial relative drop in proximal CMAP amplitude with temporarily preserved distal CMAP amplitude; the latter also dropping with time as Wallerian degeneration takes place).

Traditionally, the distinction between demyelinating and axonal hereditary neuropathies is based on conduction slowing in the median or ulnar nerve, with homogeneous motor conduction slowing > 60% of lower limit of normal (i.e., ≤ 38 m/s) found exclusively in demyelinating forms. More localized severe motor conduction slowing, distant from compression sites, can be seen in dysimmune and paraproteinaemic neuropathies (Fig. 4.2). Other characteristic electrophysiological features of dysimmune neuropathies such as Guillain–Barré syndrome (GBS) and chronic inflammatory demyelinating polyneuropathy (CIDP) include temporal dispersion and conduction block (CB), and in multifocal motor neuropathy (MMN) CB with normal sensory conduction including in the segment with motor CB (Fig. 4.3). Extensive NCS are often needed, as these abnormalities are focal and patchily distributed. Although the sensory sparing pattern (abnormal median/radial with normal sural) is highly specific for GBS and CIDP, its sensitivity is relatively low. International diagnostic consensus criteria have been published for CIDP, GBS, MMN, and IgM (+/−) anti-MAG antibodies neuropathy, which include specific combinations of conduction abnormalities.

Polyradiculopathy/Plexopathy

The hallmark of polyradiculopathy is decreased/absent CMAPs with preserved SNAPs (as sensory ganglia are unaffected). In contrast, in sensory neuronopathies the SNAPs are decreased/absent but CMAPs are normal. In plexopathy, a diverse mix of abnormal CMAPs and SNAPs can be seen, but sensitivity and specificity of such findings are likely low. Myokymia has been reported in post-radiation plexopathy, but its sensitivity and specificity are unknown.

Peripheral Nerve Hyperexcitability Syndromes

Peripheral nerve hyperexcitability syndromes (e.g., Isaac and Morvan) are characterized by presence of neuromyotonic discharges (i.e., brief clusters of

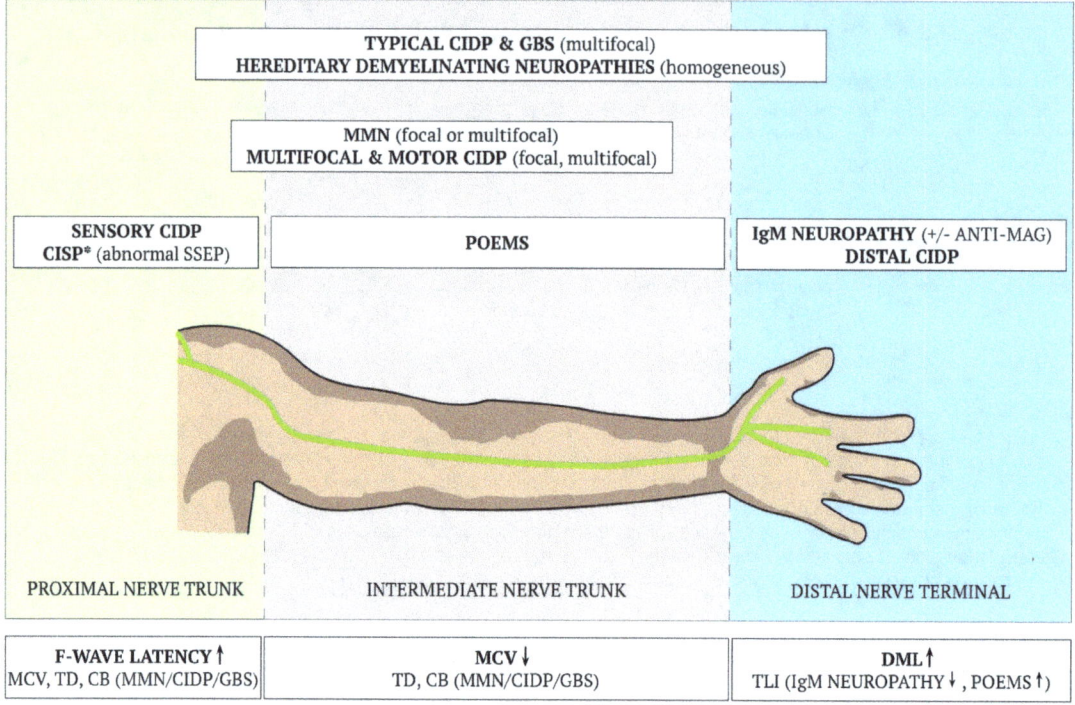

Figure 4.2 Summary distribution demyelinating features in neuropathies. Conduction abnormalities can be focal (limited to 1 nerve segment), multifocal (multiple focal abnormalities), or homogeneous (slowing without significant differences in adjacent nerve segments or nerves and laterality).

Homogeneous conduction slowing is a characteristic feature of hereditary demyelinating neuropathies, without conduction block (CB) or temporal dispersion (TD), but this can be more variable in intermediate forms (e.g., X-linked CMT). Marked conduction slowing and relative lack of CB and TD are also common in POEMS, but distal motor latency (DML) is relatively spared. In contrast, dysimmune neuropathies often have multifocal features compatible with demyelination, including CB and TD. Predominant distal conduction slowing, and loss of longer axons, is typically seen in IgM neuropathy. Sural sparing and terminal latency index (TLI) can help distinguish between CIDP, POEMS (TLI ≥ 0.38) and IgM neuropathy (TLI ≤ 0.25). In the second revision of the international CIDP guidelines, an arbitrary subclassification between sensory (CISP) and sensory-predominant CIDP was established.

CIDP = Chronic inflammatory demyelinating polyneuropathy; CISP = chronic immune sensory polyneuropathy; GBS = Guillain–Barré syndrome; MCV = motor conduction velocity; MMN = multifocal motor neuropathy; POEMS = polyneuropathy, organomegaly, endocrinopathy, M protein and skin changes syndrome.

spontaneous motor units firing rhythmically at high frequencies; often 100–300 Hz), fasciculations that are often in doublet or triplet, and myokymia.

Neuromuscular Junction Disorders

Instability of the function of the neuromuscular junction can be evaluated by repetitive nerve stimulation (RNS), with decrement (Fig. 4.4) representing the classic hallmark of a neuromuscular junction disorder. This can be seen not only in myasthenia gravis (MG) and Lambert–Eaton myasthenic syndrome (LEMS), but also in botulism and congenital myasthenic syndromes. In suspected MG, testing multiple muscles (particularly those clinically affected, such as the nasalis in bulbar presentations) may be needed to capture this decrement. Unfortunately, several other neuromuscular disorders affecting the terminal axon may also show a comparable decrement (e.g., motor neuron disorders). Consequently, decrement with RNS warrants cautious interpretation in the clinical context. RNS has relatively low sensitivity in patients with exclusively ocular symptoms. In such patients, increased jitter and blocking on single-fibre electromyography (SfEMG) may help facilitate the diagnosis. While SfEMG has higher sensitivity compared with RNS, it has lower specificity with positive results also identified in myopathies and disorders with loss of motor neurons. Post-facilitation increment is a highly specific finding for LEMS. As such, a low distal CMAP with normal sensory conduction

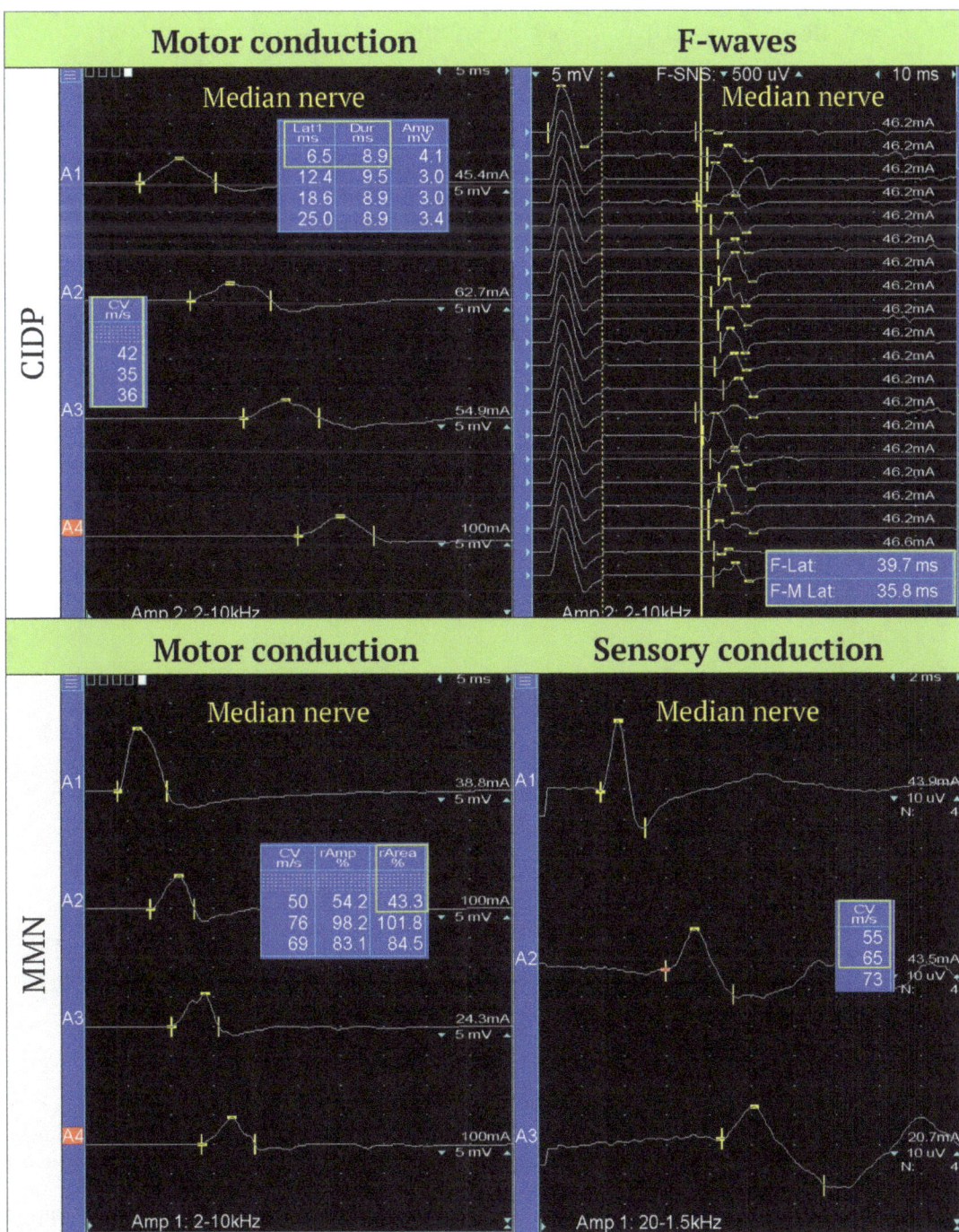

Figure 4.3 Characteristic EMG findings in patients with CIDP (upper panels) and MMN (lower panels). The EMG in the patient with CIDP shows multifocal motor conduction slowing, that is, prolonged DML, increased duration of distal compound muscle action potential (CMAP), segmental conduction slowing, and increased F-wave latencies, all compatible with patchy demyelination. In contrast, the MMN patient has a focal motor conduction block with normal sensory conduction across the same segment. For abbreviations, see Fig. 4.2 caption.

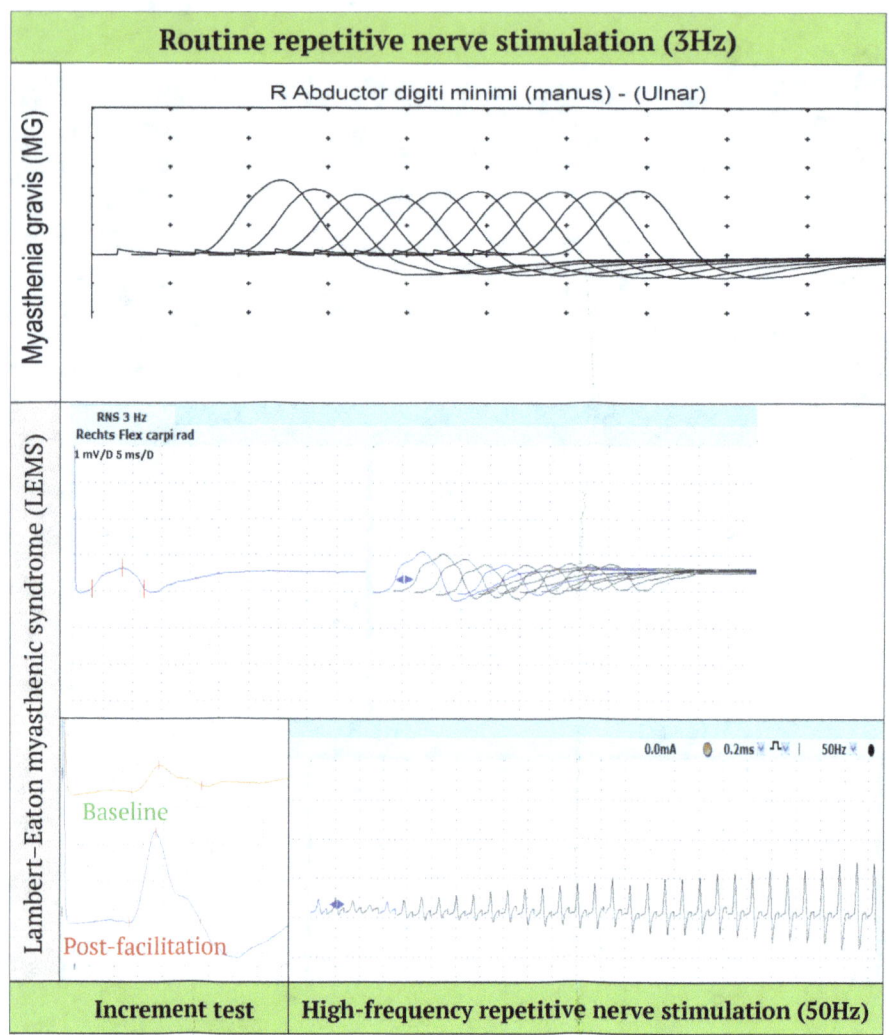

Figure 1.4 EMG examples of myasthenic syndromes. The patients with myasthenia gravis (MG) and Lambert–Eaton myasthenic syndrome (LEMS) both show significant decrement (> 10% amplitude drop between first and fourth CMAP of a series of 10 repetitive stimuli of standard repetitive nerve stimulation). In addition, the LEMS patient also shows significant increment (> 100% amplitude increase) post-facilitation and with high-frequency nerve stimulation.

should prompt consideration of LEMS and subsequent testing for presence of increment. Finally, a double CMAP has been reported in several congenital myasthenic syndromes.

Myopathies

Needle myography can be helpful in diagnosing a myopathy, with small, brief-duration polyphasic MUPs and enhanced recruitment as classic findings. Unfortunately, such small, brief-duration polyphasic MUPs (**Video 3**) are often difficult to capture, even when sampling multiple muscles. In general, electromyography has usually no added value in diagnosing a myopathy when serum creatine kinase (CK) activity is > 10 × the upper limit of normal. The yield of needle myography is also low in metabolic myopathies. Furthermore, these abnormal MUPs may also be seen in some primary neurogenic disorders (e.g., in the early re-innervation phase). Moreover, fibrillation potentials and positive sharp waves can be seen in myopathies with more prominent muscle fibre degradation and separation of these fibres from the terminal axon (e.g., muscular dystrophies, myositis, Pompe disease). In chronic myopathies, even long-duration polyphasic or giant MUPs with poor recruitment can be expected, further challenging their distinction with neurogenic disorders. Complex repetitive discharge (CRD; **Video 4**) can be seen in a diverse set of myopathies, but may also occur in neurogenic disorders, including motor neuron disorders. Myotonic discharges (**Video 5**) are specific for a subset of myopathies, including myotonic dystrophy and congenital myotonia. As such, electromyography should only be considered in a selected set of suspected myopathies, dictated by the appropriate clinical context.

Suggested Reading

Bromberg MB. Review of the evolution of electrodiagnostic criteria for chronic inflammatory demyelinating polyradicoloneuropathy. *Muscle Nerve* 2011;43(6):780–794. doi: 10.1002/mus.22038. PMID: 21607962.

de Carvalho M. Electrodiagnosis of amyotrophic lateral sclerosis: a review of existing guidelines. *J Clin Neurophysiol* 2020 Jul;37(4):294–298. doi: 10.1097/WNP.0000000000000682. PMID: 33151660.

Fournier E, Tabti N. Clinical electrophysiology of muscle diseases and episodic muscle disorders. *Handb Clin Neurol* 2019;161:269–280. doi: 10.1016/B978-0-444-64142-7.00053-9. PMID: 31307605.

Franssen H, Notermans NC. Length dependence in polyneuropathy associated with IgM gammopathy. *Ann Neurol* 2006;59(2):365–371. doi: 10.1002/ana.20785. PMID: 16437567.

Joint Task Force of the EFNS and the PNS. European Federation of Neurological Societies/Peripheral Nerve Society Guideline on management of paraproteinemic demyelinating neuropathies. Report of a Joint Task Force of the European Federation of Neurological Societies and the Peripheral Nerve Society–first revision. *J Peripher Nerv Syst* 2010;15(3):185–195. doi: 10.1111/j.1529-8027.2010.00278.x. PMID: 21040140.

Katzberg HD, Abraham A. Electrodiagnostic assessment of neuromuscular junction disorders. *Neurol Clin* 2021;39(4):1051–1070. doi: 10.1016/j.ncl.2021.06.013. Epub 2021 Sep 3. PMID: 34602214.

Nasu S, Misawa S, Sekiguchi Y, et al. Different neurological and physiological profiles in POEMS syndrome and chronic inflammatory demyelinating polyneuropathy. *J Neurol Neurosurg Psychiatry* 2012;83(5):476–479. doi: 10.1136/jnnp-2011-301706. Epub 2012 Feb 15. PMID: 22338030.

Preston DC, Shapiro BE. *Electromyography and Neuromuscular Disorders: Clinical-Electrodiagnostic-Ultrasound Correlations*. 4th edn. Elsevier; 2020.

Van Asseldonk JT, Van den Berg LH, Kalmijn S, Wokke JH, Franssen H. Criteria for demyelination based on the maximum slowing due to axonal degeneration, determined after warming in water at 37 degrees C: diagnostic yield in chronic inflammatory demyelinating polyneuropathy. *Brain* 2005;128:880–891. doi: 10.1093/brain/awh375. Epub 2005 Feb 2. PMID: 15689367.

Van den Bergh PYK, van Doorn PA, Hadden RDM, et al. European Academy of Neurology/Peripheral Nerve Society guideline on diagnosis and treatment of chronic inflammatory demyelinating polyradiculoneuropathy: Report of a joint Task Force-Second revision. *Eur J Neurol* 2021 Nov;28(11):3556–3583. doi: 10.1111/ene.14959. Epub 2021 Jul 30. Erratum in: Eur J Neurol 2022;29(4):1288. PMID: 34327760.

Vlam L, van der Pol WL, Cats EA, et al. Multifocal motor neuropathy: diagnosis, pathogenesis and treatment strategies. *Nat Rev Neurol* 2011 22;8(1):48–58. doi: 10.1038/nrneurol.2011.175. PMID: 22105211.

Chapter 5

Imaging

Stephan Goedee

Introduction

Magnetic resonance imaging (MRI) and ultrasound (US) of nerves and muscles are increasingly used as complementary tools in the diagnosis of neuromuscular disorders. Ultrasound has superior image resolution over MRI, a flexible field of view, and relatively low cost. US is also the preferred imaging modality when evaluating superficial structures. In contrast, MRI has the advantage of dedicated sequences with unique tissue-discriminating properties, and coverage of more deeply located structures. However, MRI requires dedicated protocols and visual assessment is limited by a high interobserver variability. US is device- and operator-dependent, and less suitable for evaluating much deeper structures. Visual assessment is, like MRI, subject to interobserver variability. Qualitative US has the ability to obtain more objective and repeatable measures.

Motor Neuron Disorders

Magnetic resonance imaging of the cranio-cervical region and spinal cord can help exclude important mimics of motor neuron disorders (MND). Muscle MRI may reveal patchy atrophy (T1-weighted imaging) and hyperintense signal (T2-weighted imaging).

Muscle ultrasound (MUS) can also be used to assess the presence and distribution of muscle atrophy and compatible patchy denervation (often referred to as a 'moth-eaten' appearance), and help improve detection of fasciculations (**Video 6**). However, at present consensus is lacking with regard to which muscle groups should be sampled, criteria to rate fasciculations as abnormal (e.g., distribution across and within muscles), and how to combine these MUS findings with needle myography. Importantly, the presence of fasciculations is certainly not exclusive for MND, as these can also be seen on MUS in both a healthy population as well as a diverse range of other neuromuscular disorders. Hence, there is also a temporal evolution of presence of fasciculations, likely varying between patients and muscles, all further complicating the interpretation of MUS.

Finally, the utility of nerve imaging has also been explored in smaller amyotrophic lateral sclerosis (ALS) cohorts, but this has resulted in mixed findings. At present, the appropriate reference values for the lower limit of normal nerve size are lacking. As such, muscle and nerve imaging is not recommended routinely in the diagnosis of ALS.

Neuropathies

Nerve ultrasound (NUS) is increasingly used as a practical complement to nerve conduction studies (NCS) in an expanding spectrum of neuropathies. Focal nerve enlargement at common entrapment sites is a typical finding in mononeuropathies, but is also observed in more generalized neuropathies and even in ALS. Enlargement of leg nerves is common in many polyneuropathies, whereas nerve enlargement in more proximal segments of the arm may point to more specific causes (Figs. 5.1 and 5.2). In chronic inflammatory demyelinating polyneuropathy (CIDP) and multifocal motor neuropathy (MMN), prominent enlargement of the median nerve in upper arm and forearm segments (regional or diffuse, occasionally only focal) as well as of the brachial plexus (**Video 7**) is a common finding, even in cases with equivocal electrodiagnostic findings. However, paraproteinaemic neuropathies (IgM neuropathy (+/−) anti-MAG antibodies, amyloid neuropathy, and polyneuropathy, organomegaly, endocrinopathy, M-protein, and skin changes (POEMS)) may have a comparable pattern of nerve enlargement, representing important imaging mimics of CIDP and MMN. Hereditary demyelinating neuropathies often display more homogeneous and striking nerve enlargement, but this can also be limited to a more regional distribution. Importantly, the

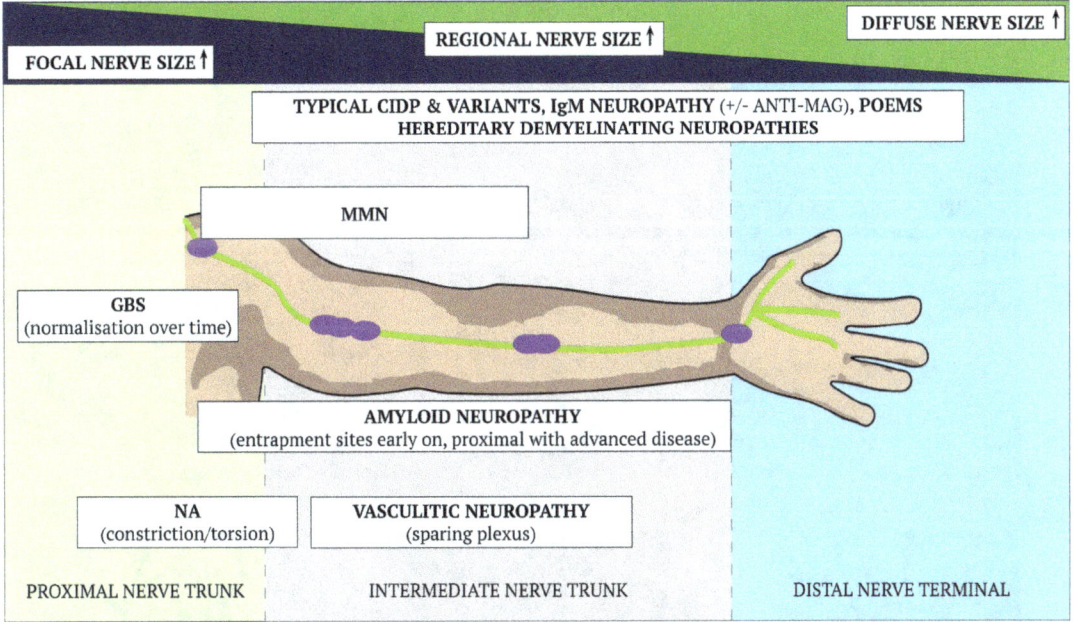

Figure 5.1 Summary distribution nerve enlargement on imaging in neuropathies. Nerve enlargement in polyneuropathies can be focal (one area only), multifocal (multiple focal areas in > 1 nerve), regional (extended along nerve segment), or diffuse (multiple adjacent nerve segments and different nerves) affecting the arm nerves and brachial plexus.
Of note, neurolymphomatosis and radiculoplexus neuropathy may show variable nerve enlargement that can be similar to the pattern seen in dysimmune neuropathies. The majority of the reported nerve enlargement in hereditary neuropathies is based on findings in adult patients with Charcot–Marie–Tooth (CMT) type 1A. Comparable findings have been noted in other demyelinating CMT types, whereas variable enlargement has been found in, e.g., X-linked CMT, adrenomyeloneuropathy, and Noonan syndrome. In neurofibromatosis, there appears to be a mixed pattern of focal nerve enlargement, neurofibromas, plexiform neurofibromas, and schwannomas, often affecting multiple nerves and/or nerve segments. Consequently, in order to accurately interpret abnormal nerve size, the clinical context and, where appropriate, other aspects of nerve architecture should all be carefully considered. NA = neuralgic amyotrophy. See Fig. 4.2 in Chapter 4 for other abbreviations.

currently available reference values for nerve size in children are limited. As such, the exact evolution of pathological nerve enlargement in the paediatric setting is still largely unknown, as nerve size increases with increasing age and reliable cut-offs for disease are lacking (hereditary and even rarer dysimmune neuropathies). Interestingly, in vasculitic neuropathy arm nerves may also harbour regional enlargement, but the brachial plexus is usually spared. In contrast, in Guillain–Barré syndrome (GBS) the spinal nerve roots appear to be primarily affected and enlarged on imaging, whereas arm nerves appear to be relatively spared. The latter sonographic finding potentially may help to distinguish patients with acute-onset CIDP from GBS. Other peripheral nerve disorders with a diverse range of nerve enlargement are polyradiculoneuropathy, neurolymphomatosis, and neuralgic amyotrophy (NA). Additionally, focal constriction is reportedly a unique finding in NA, but its prevalence is likely lower than the more commonly seen segmental enlargement of brachial plexus and arm nerves. A significant reduction of nerve size in the arms has been shown in several neuronopathies, but the lack of adequate reference values here also limits the utility of this finding.

Magnetic resonance imaging of the plexus (brachial/lumbosacral) can be considered in patients with suspected dysimmune neuropathies. Nerve enlargement and hyperintense signal on MRI (Fig. 5.2) are considered supportive in diagnostic consensus criteria for CIDP and MMN. However, the reliability of such MRI findings using the common qualitative rating appears to be low, even among experienced neuroradiologists. In line with NUS, this pattern of plexus enlargement (regional or diffuse) can also be seen using MRI. Contrast enhancement is a nonspecific finding, with no uniform protocol and low yield in CIDP/MMN, and therefore only useful if the differential diagnosis includes specific alternative causes such as a tumour.

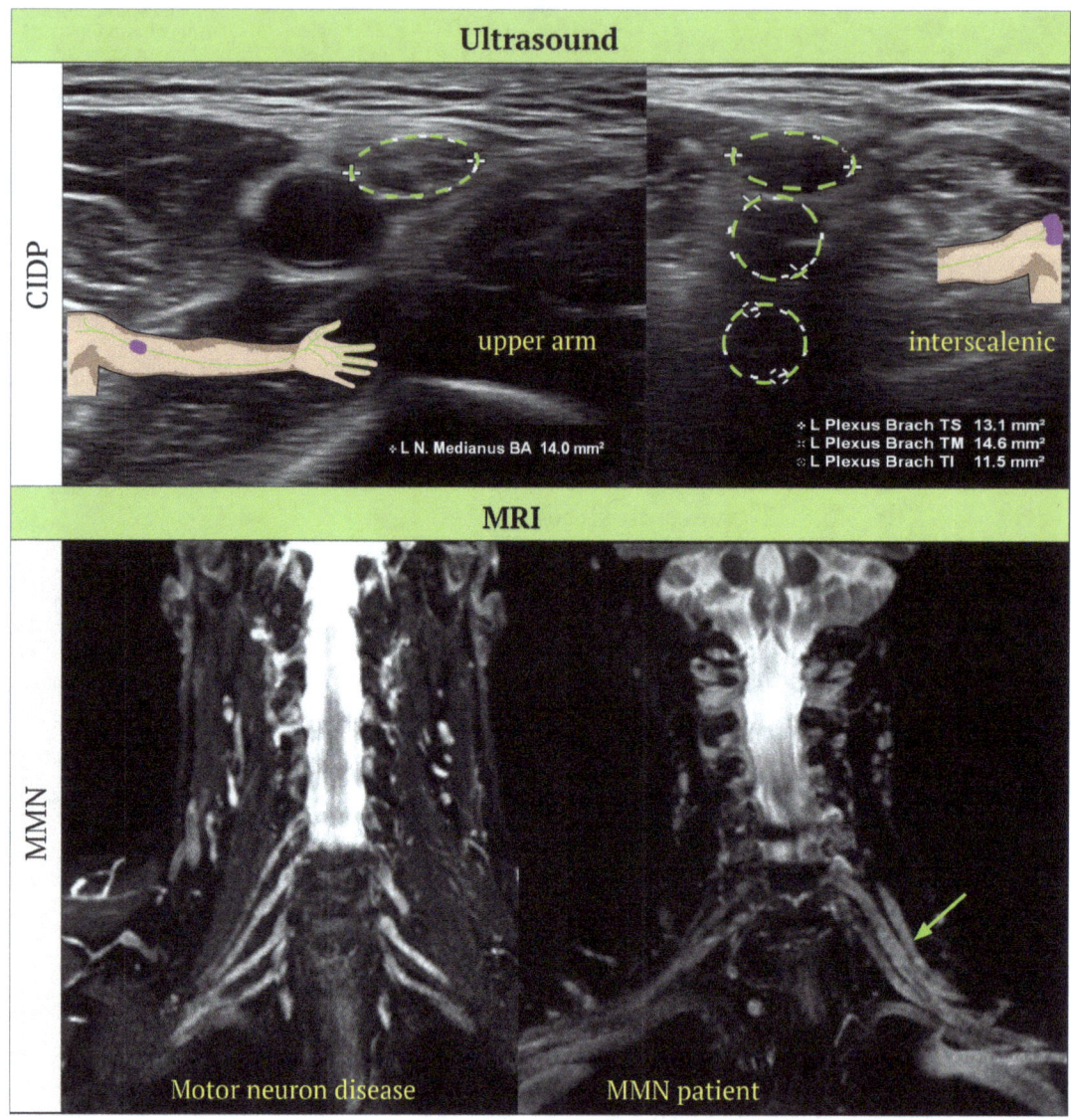

Figure 5.2 Examples of nerve enlargement on imaging in neuropathies. Note the enlarged median nerve in upper arm and brachial plexus on nerve ultrasound in a patient with chronic inflammatory demyelinating polyneuropathy (CIDP) and asymmetrically enlarged brachial plexus on MRI (maximal intensity projection; MIP sequences) (green arrow) in a patient with multifocal motor neuropathy (MMN), in contrast to the normal size of the brachial plexus in motor neuron disease.

Myopathies

Muscle imaging has advanced to a more prominent role in the evaluation of patients with suspected myopathies, complementing the clinical characterization of involved versus spared muscles. As such, MRI and MUS can help to detect the pattern of muscles with atrophy or replacement of muscle fibres by fat, and on MRI also the presence of oedema (i.e., increased T2 signal, similar to 'denervation' in neurogenic conditions). Of note, an increased T2 signal is not only found in inflammatory disease such as myositis, but can also be seen in hereditary disorders. The patterns of muscle involvement in hereditary myopathies are best appreciated as fatty replacement of muscle tissue in T1 sequences of a whole-body MRI and include involvement of shoulder and pelvic girdle muscles, anterior and posterior compartments of the legs and paraspinal muscles, asymmetry, and in certain muscle disorders, the sparing of specific muscles (Table 5.1). On MUS, muscle echogenicity can be determined

Table 5.1 Reported imaging patterns in selected myopathies with limb girdle/proximal weakness

	Upper leg		Lower leg			
	Ant.	Post.	Ant.	Post.	Selective involvement	Other features[a] Sparing

	Ant.	Post.	Ant.	Post.	Selective involvement (genes)	Sparing (genes)
Hereditary myopathies						
Limb girdle muscular dystrophies (LGMDs)	+/−	++	+/−	++	Medial gastrocnemius (all, except DYSF, SGCs) Adductor magnus (CAPN3, DYSF, SGCs) Quadriceps, patchy (DYSF, ANO5, SGCs) Post. Thigh (SGCs) Peroneal + tibial ant. (DYSF, FKRP)	Gracilis Sartorius (DYSF, ANO5, FKRP) Calf hypertrophy (FKRP) Calf muscles (SGCs)
Duchenne and Becker muscular dystrophies	+/−	++	+/−	++	Posteromed. thigh + gastrocnemius. Hypertrophy of sartorius, gracilis, semitendinosus, gastrocn., rectus fem.	Gracilis, Sartorius
Facioscapulohumeral dystrophy (FSHD)	+/−	+	++	+/−	Trapezius + serratus anterior, latissimus dorsi + pectoralis major	Spinati; subscapular
Myotonic dystrophy type 2	+	+/−	+/−	++	Erector spinae + gluteus max.	
Emerinopathies/Laminopathies	+/−	++	+/−	++	Medial gastrocnemius (LMNA, EMD)	
Collagen VI disorders (Ullrich, Bethlem)	+/−	++	+/−	++	Central part rectus femoris (target sign), peripheral parts with central sparing in other muscles (sandwich sign) (Case 43, Fig. 43.2). Rim between soleus & gastrocn.	Forearm
Congenital myopathies	+	+/−	+/−	+	Vasti, add. magnus + sartorius (RYR1) Sartorius > gracilis + diffuse post. lower leg (SELENON/SEPN1) Sternocleidomastoid (SELENON/SEPN1) Neck extensors, paraspinal + deep forearm muscles (DNM2)	Rectus fem, add. longus & gracilis, tibialis ant. (RYR1) Gastrocn., gracilis + sartorius (DNM2)
Pompe disease	+	+/−	−	−	Paraspinal + quadriceps, gluteal + add. magnus. Tongue & subscapular	Rectus femoris Lower leg
Acquired myopathies						
Dermatomyositis (DM), immune-mediated necrotizing myopathy (IMNM), anti-synthetase syndrome (ASS)	+	+/−	+/−	+/−	Oedema[b] (ASS: ant. thigh; IMNM: ant.-medial thigh + paraspinals; DM: focal and patchy, anterior thigh) Fatty replacement in post. thigh (ASS, IMNM), paraspinals (IMNM) Fascial oedema (ASS, DM) Subcutaneous oedema (DM)	
Inclusion body myositis (IBM)	+	+/−	+/−	+	Asymm. deep finger flexors, distal quadriceps, ant. thigh > post.; sartorius; gastrocnemius medialis most involved muscle in lower leg.	Rectus femoris
Motor neuron syndromes						
Spinal muscular atrophy	++	+/−	+	+/−	Triceps, iliopsoas + quadriceps	Biceps, deltoid, gluteal + add. longus

The reported ranges of muscle abnormalities on imaging in myopathies are often based on selected cohorts with small sample sizes. Studies evaluating the yield in consecutive patients with suspected myopathy are lacking; thus, sensitivity and specificity are unknown, limiting the generalizability of imaging findings to routine clinical practice. Moreover, the optimal window to detect abnormalities remains unknown, but ultimately in advanced stages these patterns all converge. Muscle abnormalities can also be seen in ALS and polyneuropathies. Of note, selective involvement of deep finger flexors in IBM (MRI/US) has been suggested to be supportive for the diagnosis.

[a] See also, e.g., https://neuromuscular.wustl.edu/pathol/diagrams/musclemri.htm
[b] Oedema is not restricted to myositis. It can also be found in genetic myopathies and in neurogenic disorders.

visually or quantitatively. Visual assessment has lower sensitivity and reproducibility, whereas datasets on quantitative imaging are not easily transferable across different devices. Similar limitations apply to assessment of muscle vascularization. While MUS and MRI can be used to screen children with suspected myopathy, the diagnostic yield of imaging is low in young children and metabolic myopathies. When available, MRI is the preferred imaging modality to evaluate suspected myopathies, given the larger coverage of muscle groups and utility of different sequences adding further information.

Establishing the pattern of affected muscles can guide the further diagnostic process, but muscle MRI is increasingly also used for reverse phenotyping to help determine pathogenicity of genetic variants with uncertain significance (VUS). However, caution is highly warranted for such practice, as the accuracy of such inverse fitting is as yet unknown.

Muscle MRI and MUS can also be used to help optimize selection of the muscle biopsy site, highlighting areas of abnormal muscle but also avoiding sampling areas with end-stage muscle disease.

Quantitative neuromuscular imaging can potentially also be used to monitor the disease activity and assessment of treatment efficacy, but similar to more detailed muscle structure imaging with advanced MRI techniques such as diffusion tensor imaging (DTI), these are all still reserved for research settings only.

Suggested Reading

Aivazoglou LU, Guimarães JB, Link TM, et al. MR imaging of inherited myopathies: a review and proposal of imaging algorithms. *Eur Radiol* 2021;31(11):8498–8512. doi: 10.1007/s00330-021-07931-9. Epub 2021 Apr 21. PMID: 33881569.

Goedee HS, van der Pol WL, Hendrikse J, van den Berg LH. Nerve ultrasound and magnetic resonance imaging in the diagnosis of neuropathy. *Curr Opin Neurol* 2018;31(5):526–533. doi: 10.1097/WCO.0000000000000607. PMID: 30153189.

Goedee HS, van der Pol WL, van Asseldonk JH, et al. Diagnostic value of sonography in treatment-naive chronic inflammatory neuropathies. *Neurology* 2017;88(2):143–151. doi: 10.1212/WNL.0000000000003483. Epub 2016 Dec 7. PMID: 27927940.

Gómez-Andrés D, Oulhissane A, Quijano-Roy S. Two decades of advances in muscle imaging in children:
from pattern recognition of muscle diseases to quantification and machine learning approaches. *Neuromuscul Disord* 2021;31(10):1038–1050. doi: 10.1016/j.nmd.2021.08.006. Epub 2021 Oct 9. PMID: 34736625.

Herraets IJT, Goedee HS, Telleman JA, et al. Nerve ultrasound for diagnosing chronic inflammatory neuropathy: a multicenter validation study. *Neurology* 2020 ;95(12):e1745–e1753. doi: 10.1212/WNL.0000000000010369. Epub 2020 Jul 16. PMID: 32675082.

Hobson-Webb LD, Simmons Z. Ultrasound in the diagnosis and monitoring of amyotrophic lateral sclerosis: a review. *Muscle Nerve* 2019;60(2):114–123. doi: 10.1002/mus.26487. Epub 2019 Apr 25. PMID: 30989697.

Telleman JA, Herraets IJ, Goedee HS, van Asseldonk JT, Visser LH. Ultrasound scanning in the diagnosis of peripheral neuropathies. *Pract Neurol* 2021;21(3):186–195. doi: 10.1136/practneurol-2020-002645. Epub 2021 Feb 4. PMID: 33541914.

Ten Dam L, van der Kooi AJ, Verhamme C, Wattjes MP, de Visser M. Muscle imaging in inherited and acquired muscle diseases. *Eur J Neurol* 2016;23(4):688–703. doi: 10.1111/ene.12984. PMID: 27000978.

van Rosmalen MHJ, Goedee HS, van der Gijp A, et al. Low interrater reliability of brachial plexus MRI in chronic inflammatory neuropathies. *Muscle Nerve* 2020;61(6):779–783. doi: 10.1002/mus.26821. Epub 2020 Feb 21. PMID: 32012299; PMCID: PMC7317832.

de Visser M, Carlier P, Vencovský J, Kubínová K, Preusse C; ENMC Muscle Imaging in Idiopathic Inflammatory Myopathies workshop study group. 255th ENMC workshop: Muscle imaging in idiopathic inflammatory myopathies. 15th January, 16th January and 22nd January 2021 - virtual meeting and hybrid meeting on 9th and 19th September 2022 in Hoofddorp, The Netherlands. Neuromuscul Disord. 2023 Oct;33(10):800-816. doi: 10.1016/j.nmd.2023.08.014. Epub 2023 Sep 3. PMID: 37770338.

Wattjes MP, Fischer D. *Neuromuscular Imaging*: Springer; 2016.

Weber MA, Wolf M, Wattjes MP. Imaging patterns of muscle atrophy. *Semin Musculoskelet Radiol* 2018;22(3):299–306. doi: 10.1055/s-0038-1641574. Epub 2018 May 23. PMID: 29791958.

Wijntjes J, van Alfen N. Muscle ultrasound: present state and future opportunities. *Muscle Nerve* 2021;63(4):455–466. doi: 10.1002/mus.27081. Epub 2020 Oct 13. PMID: 33051891; PMCID: PMC8048972.

Chapter 6
Muscle and Nerve Pathology

Muscle Biopsy

For decades, muscle biopsy has been considered an essential part of the work-up of patients suspected of a neuromuscular disease, alongside the physical examination, laboratory testing, electromyography, muscle imaging, and molecular investigations.

However, muscle biopsy is usually not the first diagnostic test requested when the clinical phenotype of a myopathic patient is clear ('Gestalt') and the molecular diagnosis is straightforward. For example, for patients with a phenotype of facioscapulohumeral dystrophy, Duchenne muscular dystrophy, or myotonic dystrophy, genetic investigations are the primary requested diagnostic tests. Since next-generation sequencing (NGS) has entered the diagnostic arena, a muscle biopsy is no longer a first-tier examination if a hereditary neuromuscular disorder – be it a myopathy, neurogenic disorder, or congenital myasthenic syndrome – is considered. Likewise, in patients with subacute weakness, especially if accompanied by skin abnormalities, the introduction of new serological markers has made the position of the applicability of muscle biopsy questionable according to some clinicians.

A muscle biopsy should be considered when genetic testing did not yield a cause or in suspected acquired myopathies like seronegative immune-mediated or drug-induced myopathies. Other considerations include suspected peripheral nerve vasculitis (combined nerve and muscle biopsy, see further), possible neurosarcoidosis, or intravascular lymphoma (muscle or skin).

If the decision has been taken to perform a muscle biopsy, there should be a strict protocol for how to obtain a muscle specimen and standards for muscle pathology procedure and analysis (see Fig. 6.1). All the three stages of the protocol require extensive skills and experience. Not only should the muscle biopsy be read by an experienced neuromuscular pathologist, preferably it should be done

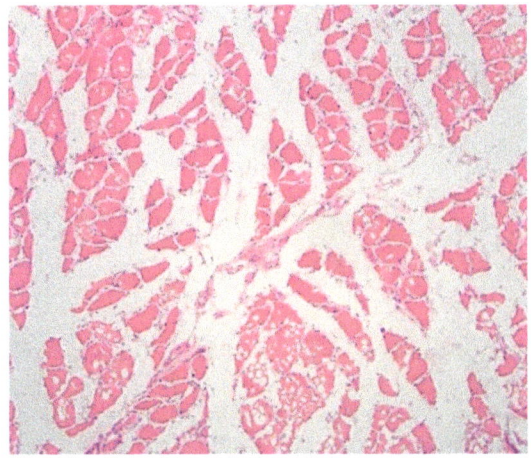

Figure 6.1 Haematoxylin & eosin (H&E) stain. The optically clear spaces within the muscle fibres represent freezing artefacts, which hampers the morphologic evaluation of muscle biopsies Courtesy Professor Eleonora Aronica.
Typically, muscle biopsies are 'snap frozen' by plunging the tissue into isobutene (2-methylbutane) cooled to ~ − 155°C by liquid nitrogen. A number of small missteps in the freezing process may cause slow freezing and lead to freezing artefacts.
Freezing artefact can be partially corrected by briefly (but completely) thawing the biopsy tissue followed by re-freezing in liquid nitrogen-cooled isobutane.

together with the clinician who examined the patient. Don't forget to ask the patient whether they are being treated with anticoagulants or antiplatelet drugs, which have to be stopped for one or more days, depending on the surgeon's instructions. Muscle biopsies should be taken from symptomatic – mildly to moderately weak – muscles, preferably the quadriceps femoris, the deltoid, or an upper arm muscle. In case of predominantly distal muscle weakness, muscle imaging may reveal subclinical proximal involvement, or a muscle biopsy from the anterior tibial or gastrocnemius muscle may be considered. The muscle should not be too weak or show fatty changes on imaging, because in that case one might end up with an 'end-stage' biopsy (Fig. 6.2). It is important to avoid muscle that has undergone recent electromyographic (EMG) assessment.

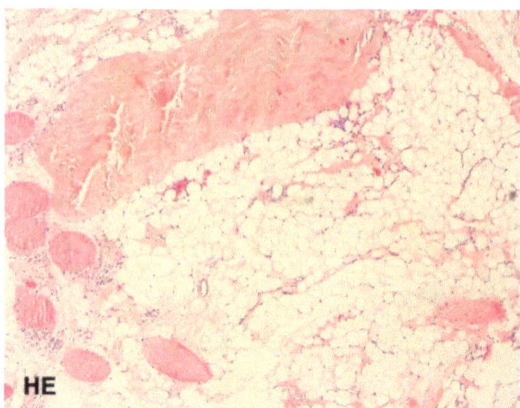

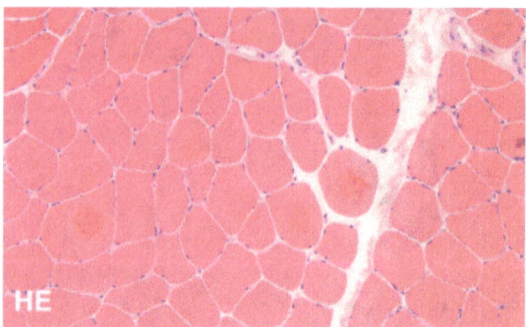

Figure 6.2 Muscle biopsy taken from a vastus lateralis muscle of a patient with inclusion body myositis without performing muscle imaging prior to the biopsy, and therefore nearly almost all muscle tissue has been replaced by fat. Courtesy Professor Eleonora Aronica.

Figure 6.3 Normal adult skeletal muscle: subsarcolemmal located nuclei, average fibre size about 35–85 μm, surrounded by sparse endomysial connective tissue and a visible perimysial septum (H&E). Courtesy Professor Eleonora Aronica.

Muscle imaging may help select the most suitable biopsy site.

The European Reference Network on Neuromuscular Diseases (ERN EURO-NMD) published recommendations on Standard Methods for muscle biopsies in 2018, for example How to secure best tissue quality, Specimen preparation, Routine stains for all new biopsies, Recommended extended methods – context-dependent.

Biopsy Technique, Tissue Preparation, Stains

In order to increase diagnostic yields, muscle specimens can be obtained by an open surgical technique, which allows for acquisition of a potentially larger sample, though some clinicians prefer to use percutaneous techniques, such as a Bergström needle or conchotome forceps. All procedures are conducted under local anaesthesia in adults. In children and rarely in adults, use of general anaesthesia is required.

There is a small risk of haemorrhage or infection, but such complications are rare. Following an open procedure, it is not uncommon to have a small area of numbness or hyperaesthesia around the scar, which may last for a few weeks to months. Muscle specimen dimensions are usually approximately 1 × 0.5 × 0.5 cm.

Histological and (immune)histochemical studies are performed on frozen material.

Six to ten μm sections are cut and stained with a panel of (immune)histochemical stains (see Table 6.1).

Electron microscopy (EM) can be used in samples without diagnostic findings by other methods to clarify abnormalities observed or not visible on light microscopy, especially in unclear sarcoplasmic abnormalities, toxic, and myofibrillar myopathies, and in neonatal muscle biopsies.

Nerve Biopsy

In 12–28% of patients with peripheral neuropathy no cause is found ('idiopathic'), and therefore, clinicians may be inclined to perform a nerve biopsy, especially if the condition is clearly progressive. However, a nerve biopsy is an invasive procedure that may be complicated by persistent numbness, dysaesthesia, paraesthesia, or pain in the territory of the biopsied nerve in ~10%. These complaints may be present after full thickness and after fascicular biopsies. Major complications, such as neuroma formation or wound infections, occur in 1% of patients, and in patients affected by vasculitis receiving corticosteroid therapy, this may result in delayed healing.

Diagnostic developments and in particular NGS, nerve imaging (MRI and ultrasound (US)), neurophysiological investigations, and skin biopsy have dramatically decreased the number of nerve biopsies, similar to the advents in genetic testing in myopathies leading to narrowing of the indication for a muscle biopsy.

The yield of a nerve biopsy in peripheral neuropathy of unknown aetiology is 27–35%. In

Chapter 6 Muscle and Nerve Pathology

Table 6.1 (Immuno)histochemical stains – modified according to ERN-EURO-NMD recommendations

Conventional histology

- Haematoxylin & eosin (HE) (Fig. 6.3)
- Modified trichrome Gomori – mitochondrial myopathy (ragged red fibres), tubular aggregates, rods
- Oil-red-O or Sudan Black (lipid)
- Periodic acid-Schiff (PAS) (glycogen)
- Congo red – amyloid myopathy

Enzyme histochemistry (EHC)

ATPases   Type 1 and types 2A, 2B, and 2 C fibres (pH 9.4, 4.6, and 4.3)
Alternatively, for fibre typing: Myosin heavy chain immunohistochemistry (IHC) with antibodies to slow beta and fast IIA with haematoxylin counterstain for fibre types I (MyHC isoform, *MyHC7*), IIA (MyHC isoform IIA, *MyHC2*), IIX (MyHC isoform IIA, *MyHC1*), and hybrids I+IIA (corresponding to 1–2A–2B–2 C, respectively, with ATPase)

Oxidative enzymes

- Nicotinamide adenine dinucleotide dehydrogenase (NADH-TR) – congenital myopathy (rods, (mini)cores), neurogenic pathology (target fibres))
- Succinate dehydrogenase (SDH) – mitochondrial myopathy, tubular aggregates
- Cytochrome oxidase (COX)-SDH – mitochondrial myopathy
- Acid phosphatase
- Nonspecific esterase

Immunohistochemistry (IHC) – routine

- Myosin heavy chain neonatal/fetal
- Myosin heavy chain developmental/embryonic
- Myosin heavy chain MyHC fast
- Myosin heavy chain MyHC slow/beta cardiac
- MHC class 1
- P62 – immune-mediated myopathy, vacuolar and protein aggregate myopathy

Context-dependent

In case of suspected immune-mediated myopathy

- IHC: P62, CD68 (macrophages), CD8 (cytotoxic T-cells), CD20 (B-cells), C5b–9 (membrane attack complex), CD31 (endothelial cells), major histocompatibility antigen 1 (MHC1)
- EHC: alkaline phosphatase

In case of suspected muscular dystrophy, congenital and progressive myopathies

- For sarcolemmal protein defects (use beta spectrin as positive control): dystrophin, N, rod, and C domains, utrophin, sarcoglycans α, β, γ, δ, αDG (dystroglycan) glycosylated (always together with β-dystroglycan), α2-laminin 80 & 300 kDa, caveolin-3, emerin, telethonin, COL VI (use together with perlecan or COL IV as control). Paediatric biopsies: laminin β1, laminin γ1, laminin α5

In case of suspected vacuolar and protein aggregate myopathy (myofibrillar myopathy)

- IHC: P62, desmin, TDP-43, LAMP-2, Dys1, MHC class1, C5b-9, myotilin, ubiquitin

In case of suspected glycogenosis

- EHC: phosphorylase, phosphofructokinase, lactate dehydrogenase
- EHC: PAS-diastase (PAS-D)

---

a prospective study on patients with a clinically significant neuropathy of unclear pathogenesis, the sural nerve biopsy was contributory and changed management in 7 out of 50 patients (14%, 3 patients were found to have vasculitis, 1 had chronic inflammatory demyelinating polyneuropathy (CIDP), 1 Guillain–Barré syndrom (GBS), 1 lymphomatous neuropathy, and 1 IgM paraproteinaemic demyelinating neuropathy associated with antibodies to myelin-associated glycoprotein).

A review systematically investigated indications for a nerve biopsy in adults and found that this procedure is of high importance in:

- nonsystemic vasculitic neuropathy (sensitivity ~50%, muscle biopsy may increase the yield with ~5% and nerve US may improve

diagnostic yield by guiding the most appropriate nerve to biopsy),
- neurolymphomatosis,
- primary nerve/sheath tumour (MRI and US may be helpful in assessment of tumours),
- AL amyloidosis (if other tissues, e.g., abdominal fat pad, are not amenable to biopsy; concomitant muscle biopsy may increase yield),
- neurosarcoidosis without extraneural involvement (muscle biopsy may improve yield),
- pure neuritic leprosy, and
- IgG4-related perineural disease/neuropathy (in case of an atypical phenotype, no tissue evidence of extraneural IgG4-related disorder and poor response to steroids).

The authors also listed disorders in which the nerve biopsy is not helpful: paraproteinaemic neuropathy, CIDP, hereditary neuropathies, acute motor neuropathies, and adult polyglucosan body disease.

The site of the biopsy is dependent on the indication. A diagnosis by nerve biopsy is more likely if performed within 6 months after onset of symptoms. The yield is also higher in patients with an asymmetric or multifocal manifestation.

The biopsy specimen should preferably be obtained from a nerve identified as clinically or electrophysiologically affected. Imaging (MRI or US) may be helpful in localizing nerve damage.

For a combined nerve–muscle biopsy when a vasculitis or neurosarcoidosis is suspected, the superficial peroneal nerve (a sensory branch of the lateral popliteal nerve)/peroneus brevis biopsy via a single skin incision on the antero-lateral surface of the leg is recommended. The superficial radial nerve or the dorsal cutaneous branch of the ulnar nerve may also be biopsied. Otherwise, the easily accessible sural nerve (another sensory branch of the lateral popliteal nerve) is the preferred site. It is recommended that 4–5 cm of nerve be removed for sufficient diagnostic value, noting that the post-biopsy neurological deficit is independent of specimen length. As with the muscle biopsy, the skills and expertise of the clinician performing the nerve biopsy are paramount. In ~4%, a blood vessel instead of a nerve is removed.

In selected cases, a high diagnostic yield and acceptable adverse events have been described for targeted fascicular biopsies of the plexus brachialis and the sciatic nerve. This should only be performed in highly specialized laboratories.

Teased fibre preparations (osmium tetrachloride) are used to show axonal degeneration and demyelination; paraffin sections stained with H&E for inflammation, neovascularization, and haemosiderin; Masson's trichrome for fibre density, axonal degeneration, and fibrinoid necrosis; and Luxol fast blue (LFB) stain for density, perineural thickening, and polyglucosan bodies. Immunohistochemistry is performed for inflammation and neoplasm.

Epoxy preparations (semithin sections) with methylene blue stain are used for density, fibre size and distribution, axonal degeneration, regenerating clusters, demyelination, onion bulbs, naked axons, perineural thickening, and injury neuroma.

In conclusion, although the utility of nerve biopsy in the clinical setting may have decreased, it continues to play a role in the diagnostic work-up of highly selected patients.

Skin Biopsy

Skin biopsy to quantify skin innervation by measurement of the density of intra-epidermal nerve fibres (IENFD) has gained much interest over the past decades. Indeed, in suspected small nerve fibre neuropathy (SFN) it is an important tool and considered the gold standard for diagnosis, since clinical examination and EMG are usually normal and other evaluations such as measurement of thermal thresholds and autonomic function assessment have limitations.

However, as also mentioned in Part II, Case 15, there is a practical disadvantage of using skin biopsies as a routine diagnostic tool, because determination of IENFD is a time-consuming and technically challenging procedure that is only available in a limited number of, usually academic, laboratories.

Skin punch biopsies can be taken from different sites, for example the lower abdomen, mid-lateral thigh, distal lateral leg, and dorsal foot. Two sites may be biopsied (one distal and one proximal site) in order to distinguish between a length-dependent SFN or small-fibre ganglionopathy (e.g., the following causes: paraneoplastic, Sjögren syndrome, some viral infections, and chemotherapies). However, normative reference values are publicly available for the distal leg, but not for the other sites, and therefore routinely only a biopsy at the ankle is taken. Expert centres usually have their own normative values.

Skin biopsies may also be used to identify the underlying cause of SFN, for example amyloidosis.

However, a word of caution regarding the use of a skin biopsy in search of a cause. Loss of IENFD has been claimed to be associated with fibromyalgia, postural orthostatic tachycardia syndrome, and many other diseases. The use of commercial labs has led to a steep increase in the diagnosis of SFN. Reduced IENFD is not synonymous with SFN and should be interpreted within the clinical context.

Suggested Reading
Muscle Biopsy

Nix JS, Moore SA. What every neuropathologist needs to know: the muscle biopsy. *J Neuropathol Exp Neurol* 2020;79(7):719–733. doi: 10.1093/jnen/nlaa046. Erratum in: J Neuropathol Exp Neurol. 2021 Mar 22;80(4):387. PMID: 32529201; PMCID: PMC7304986.

Udd B, Stenzel W, Oldfors A, et al. 1st ENMC European meeting: the EURO-NMD pathology working group Recommended Standards for Muscle Pathology Amsterdam, The Netherlands, 7 December 2018. *Neuromuscul Disord* 2019;29(6):483–485. doi: 10.1016/j.nmd.2019.03.002. Epub 2019 Mar 15. PMID: 31101462.

Walters J, Baborie A. Muscle biopsy: what and why and when? *Pract Neurol* 2020;20(5):385–395. doi: 10.1136/practneurol-2019-002465. Epub 2020 Jun 5. PMID: 32503899.

Nerve Biopsy

Dyck PJ, Dyck PJB, Engelstad J. (2005) Pathologic alterations of peripheral nerves. In: *Peripheral Neuropathy: 2-Volume Set with Expert Consult Basic* (pp. 733–829). Elsevier.

Gabriel CM, Howard R, Kinsella N, et al. Prospective study of the usefulness of sural nerve biopsy. *J Neurol Neurosurg Psychiatry* 2000;69(4):442–446. doi: 10.1136/jnnp.69.4.442. PMID: 10990501; PMCID: PMC1737127.

Lehmann HC, Wunderlich G, Fink GR, Sommer C. Diagnosis of peripheral neuropathy. *Neurol Res Pract* 2020;2:20. doi: 10.1186/s42466-020-00064-2. PMID: 33324924; PMCID: PMC7650053.

Nathani D, Spies J, Barnett MH, et al. Nerve biopsy: current indications and decision tools. *Muscle Nerve* 2021;64(2):125–139. doi: 10.1002/mus.27201. Epub 2021 Feb 25. PMID: 33629393; PMCID: PMC8359441.

Tracy JA, Engelstad JK, Dyck PJB. Microvasculitis in diabetic lumbosacral radiculoplexus neuropathy. *J Clin Neuromusc Dis* 2009, 11:44–48.

Skin Biopsy

Lauria G, Faber CG, Cornblath DR. Skin biopsy and small fibre neuropathies: facts and thoughts 30 years later. *J Neurol Neurosurg Psychiatry* 2022;93(9):915–918. doi: 10.1136/jnnp-2021-327742. Epub 2022 Mar 4. PMID: 35246491; PMCID: PMC9380509.

Sommer C. Nerve and skin biopsy in neuropathies. *Curr Opin Neurol* 2018;31(5):534–540. doi: 10.1097/WCO.0000000000000601. PMID: 30080717.

Chapter 7

Genetic Testing

Wouter van Rheenen

Driven by technological advances, an ever-increasing number of genes and mutations are implicated in neuromuscular diseases. This has led to revised classifications of neuromuscular diseases and expanding phenotypic spectra related to single genes. As a result, gene-targeted therapies are emerging. Combined with the reduction in costs of genome sequencing, genetic testing plays an increasingly important role in the diagnostic process of neuromuscular diseases. Nevertheless, caution is warranted since results of genome sequencing can be challenging regarding the interpretation of the results. Here we discuss general principles that aid the efficient use of genetic testing that may improve the interpretation of results (see Table 7.1).

Table 7.1 Approach to suspected genetic neuromuscular disease

1. Take detailed family history
    - Neuromuscular diseases in relatives (up to third degree)
    - Mode of inheritance (autosomal dominant, autosomal recessive, X-linked recessive/dominant, maternal inheritance)
    - Determine family size
    - Presence of related phenotypes

2. Discuss consequences of genetic diagnosis
    - Confirm suspected diagnosis
    - Genetic counselling
    - Burden of knowledge
    - More accurate prognosis?
    - Future gene-targeted therapies?

3. Choose appropriate genetic test

Primary genetic analyses:
   - *NGS panel:* tests multiple genes, but exonic SNVs and indels only. Indels causing CMT1A and HNPP (*PMP22*), and CMTX1 (*GJB1*) are captured with NGS panel analysis.
   - *Repeat analysis:* DM1 (*DMPK*), DM2 (*CNBP*), OPMD (*PABPN1*), C9-ALS/FTD (*C9orf72*), SBMA (*androgen receptor*), FSHD1 (contraction D4Z4 repeat chr 4q35), FRDA (*FXN*)
   - *CNV analysis:* SMA (*SMN1*), DMD and BMD (*DMD*)
   - *Mitochondrial DNA:* e.g., CPEO, KSS, MERRF, NARP

Secondary genetic analyses:
   - *Trio analysis (patient and parents):* suspected *de novo* mutation; suspected compound heterozygous mutation
   - *Runs of homozygosity:* suspected recessive inheritance
   - *WGS + RNAseq:* intronic or splice site mutations (esp. collagen VI-related muscular dystrophies).

4. Interpretation of results
    - Exact mutation described in similar phenotype?
    - Phenotype compatible with published genotype–phenotype association?
    - Occurrence in population databases?
    - Functional consequence?
    - Co-segregation of mutation and phenotype within family?

BMD = Becker muscular dystrophy; CMT1A, CMTX1 = Charcot–Marie–Tooth disease variants; CPEO = chronic progressive external ophthalmoplegia; DM = diabetes mellitus; DMD = Duchenne muscular dystrophy; HNPP = hereditary neuropathy with pressure palsies; KSS = Kearns–Sayer syndrome; MERRF = myoclonic epilepsy and ragged red fibres syndrome; NARP = neuropathy, ataxia, retinitis pigmentosa syndrome; OPMD = oculopharyngeal muscular dystrophy; SBMA = spinal-bulbar muscular atrophy; SMA = spinal muscular atrophy. Other abbreviations are defined in the text.

Consequences of a Genetic Diagnosis

The first question that needs to be answered before any diagnostic test, and genetic testing in particular, is ordered is what the consequences are of its result. To many clinicians the answer may seem obvious: to diagnose a genetic neuromuscular disease. A precise diagnosis may help to provide a more accurate prognosis and risk assessments of comorbidities such as cardiomyopathy in Duchenne carriers may lead to a targeted therapy. To patients and their families, however, establishing a genetic neuromuscular disease may have additional consequences. Whereas it might help in advance family planning, prenatal diagnostic testing, or recognition of early symptoms in some, others can find this knowledge to be a burden that has a negative effect on quality of life. Furthermore, depending on the chosen technology, genetic testing can result in unsolicited findings, or findings with uncertain significance, as outlined below. It is good practice to discuss this with patients and relatives prior to ordering any of these tests.

Family History

A second step prior to ordering genetic tests is to take a detailed family history. A positive family history greatly increases the chances of finding a genetic diagnosis. Sometimes the genetic disease has already been diagnosed in family members and genetic testing can be limited to a single mutation, minimizing the chance of unsolicited findings. Furthermore, a family history can help to order nonstandard genetic tests such as analysing regions of increased homozygosity (in suspected recessive traits), mitochondrial DNA (maternal inheritance), screening de novo mutations in trios (in case of a negative family history in apparently sporadic disease), or genome-wide screens using linkage analyses (in large pedigrees). Even in standard diagnostic testing a family history can be crucial, as co-segregation of a putative causal mutation with the neuromuscular disease of interest may enable definitive genetic diagnosis. Key elements of a family history include the presence of the neuromuscular disease in family members, ideally up to second or third degree (first cousins), determining the family size (smaller family size reduces the chance of a positive family history), estimating the risk of unknown consanguinity (isolated populations), and acknowledging the unknowns (due to lost contact with relatives or early deaths). Furthermore, the family history should not only include neuromuscular diseases. Pleiotropy, where a single mutation causes multiple phenotypes, is common. Asking for related phenotypes should depend on the differential diagnosis, for example cataract in myotonic dystrophy, dementia in amyotrophic lateral sclerosis (ALS), or heart failure in transthyretin amyloidosis (ATTR).

Genetic Tests

The first line in genetic tests can routinely be ordered by any clinician and these include next-generation sequencing (NGS) panels, analyses for structural variation such as large copy number variants (deletions/duplications), repeat expansions, and mitochondrial DNA. Following the general principles as discussed below, the trained clinician should be able to interpret the outcome of these tests and communicate them to the patient, including referral to a clinical geneticist if the patient wishes. Although an increasing number of patients with suspected genetic neuromuscular disease can be diagnosed in this way, a fair proportion remains unsolved so far. When first-line genetic tests do not yield a definite diagnosis, second-line genetic tests can be performed. These tests include trio analyses (proband plus parents), homozygosity mapping, genome sequencing, or RNA sequencing and are usually reserved for clinical geneticists. Although we provide some indications for these tests, their interpretation falls beyond the scope of this chapter.

First-Line Genetic Tests

NGS panels. Over the past years, genetic testing has evolved from Sanger sequencing one gene at a time to next-generation sequencing (NGS), interrogating multiple genes or the entire exome (~22 K genes) at once. Exome sequencing is usually more cost-effective than Sanger sequencing multiple genes and therefore the method of choice in most instances. In the neuromuscular clinic, genes causing neuromuscular diseases can be grouped in so-called NGS panels such that they can be ordered at once. When these panels are ordered, laboratories usually perform whole exome sequencing (WES) but the genes not included in these panels are masked from the analyses and thus variants in these genes are not reported to the clinician or patient. This reduces the chance of unsolicited findings. A benefit of this approach to first generate exome sequencing is that the results can be re-analysed when panels are updated and newly discovered genes are included. Because of technical aspects of NGS, these panels can detect single base-pair alterations (single nucleotide variants or polymorphisms, SNV, SNP) and small insertions and deletions (indels). NGS is, however, not always suited for structural variation such as repeat expansions and (larger) deletions/duplications, although bioinformatic solutions for this are being introduced in the clinic. Finally, not all regions in the genome are well suited for NGS due to repetitive sequences (e.g., *SELENON1* gene), complex rearrangements of DNA (e.g., *SMN* locus), or regions for which no high-quality reference sequence exists (telomeric and centromeric regions).

Structural variation. NGS panels do not routinely identify structural variations. First, repeat expansions are generally not found through NGS panels. This is relevant for some more common neuromuscular diseases such as myotonic dystrophy type 1, myotonic dystrophy type 2, oculopharyngeal muscular dystrophy, ALS, spinobulbar muscular atrophy, facioscapulohumeral dystrophy (FSHD) type 1, and Friedreich ataxia (FRDA). Depending on the type of repeat a targeted (repeat-primed) polymerase chain reaction (PCR) or Southern blotting (FSHD type 1) should be performed. Second, copy number variants (CNVs, i.e., larger insertions and deletions of DNA) can be easily missed in NGS panels. Common neuromuscular diseases that warrant specific CNV analyses include spinal muscular atrophy (SMA) and dystrophinopathies. For many of these genes, multiplex ligation-dependent probe amplification (MLPA) is still the gold standard. While methods for detecting structural variants from NGS are being developed, they have not yet made their way to routine testing in the clinic.

Mitochondrial DNA. Mitochondrial DNA (mtDNA) is maternally inherited. Whereas most of the mitochondrial proteins (> 1000) are encoded by nuclear DNA, mitochondria themselves contain a small amount (16.6 kilobases) of circular DNA encoding 37 genes that are involved in oxidative phosphorylation and ancillary processes. Cells contain multiple mitochondria, and each mitochondrion contains multiple copies of the mtDNA. Due to de novo mutations and purifying selection in dividing cells, heteroplasmy (coexistence of mutated and wild-type mtDNA genotype within the same mitochondrion, cell, or tissue) can occur. Heteroplasmy is more pronounced in mitochondrial disease (increased heteroplasmy). Standard NGS panels do not include the analysis of mtDNA. When suspecting neuromuscular diseases caused by mtDNA mutations (e.g., sporadic chronic progressive external ophthalmoplegia, CPEO), specific analyses of mtDNA should be ordered. Due to the heteroplasmic nature of most mtDNA mutations, testing is most sensitive in affected tissue. Urine sediment cells seem to be fairly representative, and thus urine testing may be a patient-friendly alternative to a muscle biopsy. Currently, mtDNA mutation can also be increasingly detected in leucocytes as well, despite low levels of heteroplasmy in clinically unaffected tissue. Whole genome sequencing (WGS), which includes the mtDNA, may become more widely applicable with improved data storage methods and reducing costs.

Second-Line Genetic Tests

When first-line genetic testing has not yielded a genetic diagnosis, second-line genetic tests can be ordered, usually in consultation with a clinical geneticist. The appropriate test depends on presumed mode of inheritance derived from an adequate family history. In suspected recessive disease or possible (distant) consanguinity, searching for genomic regions with excessive homozygous variants (homozygosity mapping) can narrow the search for homozygous mutations. When there is no clear family history, trio sequencing (of the entire exome) can be performed to search for de novo coding mutations. Finally, standard genetic analyses only include the coding regions of our genome (exome), which comprises only 3% of the genome. Although the functional consequences of non-coding variants are hard to interpret, combination with RNA sequencing can help. For example, intronic variants in *COL6A1* that lead to alternative splicing and inclusion of cryptic exons are a relatively frequent cause of collagen VI-related muscular dystrophy (Bethlem myopathy). These splicing events that alter the protein structure after removal of introns from the pre-mRNA are of interest in other neuromuscular diseases as well.

Interpretation of Results

Genetic variants are abundant in any genome, and the resulting genetic diversity shapes a virtually infinite number of phenotypic traits in the human population. Solely by chance, DNA tests can identify genetic variants in genes that are implicated in neuromuscular diseases. Thus, finding a variant is not proof that it causes the disease. This relates to terminology where a variant can be a benign variant (proven nonpathogenic), likely benign, a variant of uncertain significance (VUS) (unknown pathogenicity), likely pathogenic, or pathogenic (proven pathogenic variant). A general strategy to provide evidence for pathogenicity is to answer the following questions:

1. Has this variant been described before?
A literature search can help identify other patients in which this variant has been found. Besides PubMed, ClinVar and in-house genetic databases can be queried. Assessing the evidence of pathogenicity in these reports is crucial, especially since genotype–phenotype associations from the early genetic era do not meet current standards of evidence. Co-segregation of the variant with the disease (see number 4, below) provides strong evidence. Data that show the variant has functional consequences, such as mislocalization of the mutated protein, can help but are insufficient.

2. Is the phenotype in the tested patient compatible with the reported genotype–phenotype association?
Since multiple genes are tested through NGS, not all genes will match the patient's phenotype equally. If this is clearly not the case, a variant can be dismissed as a pathogenic candidate. Sometimes, additional investigations such as a repeat neurological exam, additional laboratory investigations, or a muscle biopsy can help. One should be careful, however, that this process of 'reverse phenotyping' is inherently biased, as clinicians may be inclined to reason towards pathogenicity of the found genetic variant. On the other hand, now that genetic testing is common practice, certain genes are associated with expanding phenotypic spectra where not all patients with the variant exhibit the classic neuromuscular phenotype.

3. How often is the variant observed in the general population?
The completion of the genome aggregation database (gnomAD) has provided a unique opportunity to assess the frequency of rare genetic variants in a large and diverse population sample. It includes whole-genome sequencing data of 195,000 individuals and provides frequencies for single nucleotide variants, indels, and even structural variations including repeats. As most neuromuscular diseases are rare, the genetic variants causing them are expected to be rare as well. There is no uniform cut-off, but generally speaking, variants that are present in >1:1000 individuals in any population are unlikely to cause a neuromuscular disease. An important exception is for recessive diseases, where carrier frequencies can be up to 1:50 (*SMN1* deletions for SMA carriers). Following the gnomAD database release, numerous genetic variants that were described as pathogenic are now considered benign polymorphisms.

4. What is the (expected) functional consequence of the variant?
Pathogenic variants are expected to alter the function of a gene. Nevertheless, a demonstrated alteration of a gene's function caused by a variant can support but not prove pathogenicity since not all altered gene functions lead to disease. Exceptions exist where a functional assay is very specific for a disease (chloride channel function in cystic fibrosis, in vitro contraction test for muscle biopsies with *RYR1* pathogenic variants for malignant hyperthermia). Data-driven algorithms to predict a variant's pathogenicity may seem accurate at group level but are generally not very well applicable to an individualized approach.

5. Does the variant co-segregate with the disease within the family?
When all affected family members in a pedigree share the same genetic variant, and unaffected family members do not, co-segregation is established. This can be challenging for pathogenic variants with reduced penetrance especially in late-onset diseases and pleiotropy (e.g., *C9orf72*-linked ALS with frontotemporal degeneration). Therefore, the detailed family history is crucial in the genetic diagnostic process. If a family is sufficiently large, this can provide definite proof for a pathogenicity of the variant. However, even in smaller pedigrees, segregation analyses can be used to rule out variants as pathogenic when unaffected family members are shown to carry the variant of interest. Other instances that support pathogenicity of variants are demonstration of a de novo

variant in apparently sporadic disease or proof that two variants in the same gene are compound heterozygous (one variant is inherited from one parent and the other variant from the other parent) in recessive disease.

In conclusion, genetic testing is an increasingly powerful tool in the diagnostic process of neuromuscular diseases. To benefit from its full potential, a precise clinical diagnosis, taking a detailed family history, and choosing the appropriate techniques are crucial. Ultimately, the evidence for pathogenicity of a variant should be appraised critically, so the patient and family can be counselled. This approach is well suited for a multidisciplinary approach that at least includes neuromuscular neurologists and geneticists.

Useful Databases

Genome Aggregation Database, http://gnomad.broadinstitute.org

OMIM: An Online Catalog of Human Genes and Genetic Disorders, omim.org

Chapter 8

Management

Major advances over the past decades have transformed the management landscape of neuromuscular disorders. Increased availability of genetic testing, innovative therapies that target specific disease pathways and mechanisms, and a multidisciplinary approach to care including both transitional and palliative care contribute to timely and more appropriate management of conditions that are associated with a severe disease burden and often also a reduction of life expectancy.

There is an increasing number of consensus recommendations/guidelines that are a useful adjunct for establishing a timely and accurate diagnosis, and enable prognostication of disease-related complications, are a guide for multidisciplinary care and treatment, and expedite initiation of disease-modifying interventions. A number of these guidelines have been referred to in various cases, such as myasthenia gravis (MG), myotonic dystrophy type 1 and 2, chronic inflammatory demyelinating neuropathies (CIDP), and Duchenne muscular dystrophy (DMD), to name a few.

Causative Treatment for Genetic Diseases

Genetic medicines using antisense oligonucleotides (ASOs) or small interfering ribonucleic acids (siRNAs) that target RNA transcripts are precision genetic therapeutics and emerging as a new pharmacological modality for rare neuromuscular diseases. ASO-mediated exon skipping is approved for DMD, spinal muscular atrophy (SMA), and most recently for amyotrophic lateral sclerosis (ALS), and siRNAs for transthyretin amyloidosis (ATTR) and acute hepatic porphyria. The preliminary results of single-dose treatment of ATTR using CRISPR-Cas9–based in vivo gene editing in patients with hereditary TTR with polyneuropathy and with cardiomyopathy, respectively, seem impressive. Current therapeutic strategies for ATTR rely on reducing ongoing amyloid formation through stabilization of the tetrameric form of TTR, *TTR* silencing, or TTR extraction or resorption. Such treatments produce symptom relief and functional improvement and prolong survival but are limited by the requirement for long-term administration, the association with serious side effects (e.g., heart failure, kidney dysfunction, hepatotoxicity), or persistent disease progression.

An impressive therapeutic advance is the treatment of children suffering from SMA type 1 with single-dose intravenous gene-replacement therapy delivering an *SMN1* transgene using a modified AAV9 vector (onasemnogene abeparvovec). Neonates treated pre-symptomatically achieve greater and earlier developmental milestones than untreated patients and symptomatic patients, showing that treatment needs to be started as early as possible. This can only be achieved if a test for SMA is included in the newborn screening (NBS) programme. The aim of the NBS is the early detection of certain serious disorders in newborns to allow for early interventions that can prevent or limit irreparable health damage.

Immunotherapies

In most immune-mediated neuromuscular disorders, corticosteroids, often in combination with a second-line immune-suppressive drug, are standard treatment. In MG, treatment with pyridostigmine only may be sufficient, but many patients require immunotherapy as well. Corticosteroids are surprisingly ineffective in Guillain–Barré syndrome (GBS) and multifocal motor neuropathy (MMN). In a myasthenic crisis and in GBS, IVIg and plasma exchange (PE) are standard treatments. In CIDP, corticosteroids and IVIg are first-line treatment, and PE can be tried, especially if these treatments are ineffective. In MMN and in some MG patients, IVIg is used as chronic treatment. For myositis, clear evidence for effectiveness of IVIg as first-line treatment is not available. Yet, in clinical practice IVIg is increasingly used as first-line chronic treatment. In some countries, IVIg is administered at home.

New treatments are being developed for patients with MG, GBS, CIDP, MMN, and myositis. Examples are rituximab, an anti-CD20 monoclonal antibody for treatment of MG, in particular in association with muscle-specific kinase (MuSK) antibodies. Monoclonal antibodies against the fragment crystallizable neonatal receptor (FcRn), such as efgartigimod, can be of benefit in refractory MG, and the same holds for drugs that inhibit distinct components of the complement system activated by the pathogenic MG antibodies (e.g., eculizumab). Of note, these new drugs, if successful and approved by the regulatory authorities, are very costly and therefore evidence-based algorithms should be developed to guide the clinician.

Rehabilitation and Palliative Care

In most neuromuscular disorders, a causative treatment is not yet available. In those cases, it is of utmost importance to convey the message to the patients, their carers, and/or parents that there are many options for targeting impairments, enabling activities of daily living, and improving quality of life. Referral to a rehabilitation physician is strongly recommended. Modalities such as range-of-motion and mild-to-moderate intensity of exercise (e.g., progressive resistance strength training) may improve endurance and cardiovascular fitness in children with Charcot–Marie–Tooth (CMT) disease delayed worsening of foot extensors has been found. Adaptive devices and surgical intervention, when appropriate, may improve walking 'economy'.

Increased awareness of the neuropsychiatric phenotype of several neuromuscular conditions such as DMD, myotonic dystrophy, and mitochondrial myopathies enables early detection and intervention of specific learning and behavioural difficulties.

Fatigue and pain (see further) are highly prevalent and important problems in both adults and children with neuromuscular disease. Chronic fatigue may lead to reduced social participation. Aerobic exercise training has been found to alleviate chronic fatigue in facioscapulohumeral dystrophy (FSHD) and mitochondrial myopathies. Cognitive behavioural therapy has also proven to diminish chronic fatigue in FSHD and to improve participation in myotonic dystrophy type 1. Energy conservation management, which aims to support fatigue self-management in daily life to enable participation in daily occupations, was found to result in significant improvement of social participation in a heterogeneous group of fatigued patients with neuromuscular disorders as compared with usual care.

There is increasing awareness that palliative care could be provided alongside other treatments, in particular to patients and their carers who are faced with a life-threatening illness characterized by progressive muscle weakness, leading to incapacitating physical disabilities. In ALS, palliative care including Advance Care Planning (ACP) is integrated in multidisciplinary treatment starting right after the patient has been informed about the diagnosis. This addresses not just the physical but also the psychological, practical, and spiritual domains in the course of care. ACP in ALS leads to improvement in symptom burden, emotional issues, and quality of life (QoL) of the patients. Rapid decline in the patients' physical function and emotional distress have a negative impact on QoL among carers. To be able to support and help them, healthcare professionals need to focus as well on the carer's QoL and the factors contributing to their QoL throughout the disease trajectory.

Literature and research on palliative care in neuromuscular disorders other than ALS are sparse. In most neuromuscular disorders, palliative care is still underutilized. There are several reasons for this. First, the knowledge about the appropriateness of palliative care in neuromuscular disorders is just emerging. Healthcare professionals and patients/parents alike need to be educated that palliative care is not synonymous with hospice care or end-of-life care. Second, illness trajectories vary from rapidly progressive to chronic progressive and are therefore associated with different symptom profiles, needs, preferences, and psychosocial issues. Currently, standards of care in which palliative care is integrated are being developed, for example, in DMD and SMA.

Multidisciplinary Care

Chronic neuromuscular disorders may be associated with sometimes life-threatening issues due to involvement of the heart and respiratory weakness. In addition, there may be nutritional or gastrointestinal complications, endocrinological, orthopaedic, and cognitive, behavioural, or psychosocial issues, including sexual health needs.

This calls for guidelines, clear recommendations, and care pathways, which have been published in recent years for a number of diseases, such as DMD, SMA, myotonic dystrophies, ATRR, and *VCP*-related proteinopathy.

Cardiac Involvement

It is common knowledge that dilative cardiomyopathy frequently occurs in DMD and Becker muscular dystrophy (BMD), and conduction abnormalities are a well-known feature of the myotonic dystrophies. However, there are many other myopathies that may develop heart involvement, including limb girdle muscular dystrophies (LGMDs; e.g., sarcoglycanopathies and LGMD9 related to *FKRP*), Emery–Dreifuss muscular dystrophy, mitochondrial myopathies, myofibrillar myopathies, and others.

After diagnosis these individuals should undergo cardiac screening on a regular basis, which is currently not systematically done, except for those diseases for which guidelines have been established. It is a particular concern that sudden death due to dysrhythmias or conduction abnormalities may occur in myotonic dystrophy, type 1 and type 2, Emery–Dreifuss muscular dystrophy, myofibrillar myopathies, BMD, Danon disease, and mitochondrial disease (Kearns–Sayre syndrome and Barth syndrome).

Respiratory Complications

Respiratory weakness is known to occur in advanced stages of numerous neuromuscular diseases, e.g., ALS, SMA, DMD and BMD, DM1, inclusion body myositis (rare), congenital myopathies (X-linked myotubular myopathy, centronuclear myopathies, *RYR1*-related, and selenoprotein (*SEPN1* or *SELENON*)-related myopathies), or in rapidly evolving diseases such as MG and GBS. There are also neuromuscular disorders in which diaphragm weakness does not keep up with limb muscle weakness, like Pompe disease or hereditary myopathy with early respiratory failure (HMERF), a rare, adult-onset autosomal dominant myopathy caused by variants in the titin gene. The presentation of respiratory weakness in chronic diseases is rarely acute, with the exception of acute-on-chronic decompensation.

Acute neuromuscular respiratory failure is a clinical diagnosis and requires a practised skill to recognize. Failure of respiratory mechanics leads to restlessness, tachycardia, tachypnoea, use of sternocleidomastoid or scalene muscles, and failure to string more than a few words together in a sentence. In chronic neuromuscular disorders, the clinical signs of respiratory failure may be very subtle. When there is emerging hypercapnia, the patient may easily fall asleep. History taking should focus on (night-time) hypoventilation, discomfort or inability to lie flat, morning fatigue or headache, vivid dreams, dyspnoea on exertion, as well as on unwanted loss of weight.

Chronic noninvasive ventilation (NIV) should be initiated if:
- There are symptoms of (night-time) hypoventilation AND hypercapnia (pCO_2 > 45 mmHg (6,0 kPa)) OR
- There is orthopnoea with an impaired sleeping pattern consistent with diaphragmatic weakness, even without hypercapnia.

Initiation of chronic ventilation may be *considered* it there is hypercapnia without symptoms of hypoventilation.

Chronic ventilation of patients with neuromuscular disorders can be applied at home (home mechanical ventilation, HMV) by specialized nurses. In the past, initiation of ventilation usually took place in an in-hospital setting. However, recent evidence showed that mechanical ventilation initiation at home combined with the use of telemonitoring of ventilator data, transcutaneous measured gas exchange parameters, and daily nurse-led adjustments of ventilator settings is safe and effective.

Gastrointestinal Involvement

Swallowing difficulty (dysphagia) is frequently found in neuromuscular diseases and often goes unnoticed. It may be the presenting symptom in ALS, Kennedy syndrome, MG, myotonic dystrophy type 1, oculopharyngeal muscular dystrophy, and inclusion body myositis. Dysphagia may lead to undernutrition, aspiration pneumonia, and consequently reduced quality of life.

There are various assessment tools, for example patient-related outcome measures, bedside tests (fluids and/or solids), and instrumental tools (e.g., fibreoptic endoscopic evaluation of swallowing, videofluoroscopic swallowing study), which are still being investigated for reliability and validity.

Numerous management options are available: oral health, changing of diet and eating habits, attention to posture (chin-up), dilation of the upper part of the oesophagus, cricopharyngeal myotomy, percutaneous endoscopic gastrostomy/percutaneous radiographic gastrostomy (PEG/PRG), and Botox administered to the cricopharyngeus muscle. However, there is a lack of evidence on the effect of these treatments, since no proper randomized controlled trials (RCTs) have been conducted.

Pain Management

Pain may be characterized as acute (lasting for a short period of time) or chronic (persistent). Determining the duration of pain has implications with respect to both diagnostic and therapeutic management. Characterizing pain intensity can be achieved through, for example, a visual analog scale, which asks patients to rate their pain on a scale from 0 to 10, with 0 being 'no pain' and 10 being the 'worst pain imaginable'.

A detailed pain history includes the onset, location, duration, quality (i.e., burning, tingling, shooting), and intensity of pain and what provokes the pain.

A physical examination should look for clues causing pain, for example contractures, impaired range of motion, fractures, spinal deformities, and symptoms and signs consistent with neuropathy or spasticity.

In virtually all neuromuscular disorders pain may occur. Neuropathic pain in diseases caused by involvement of the nerve roots (e.g., GBS), plexus (e.g., neuralgic amyotrophy), acute inflammation of the peripheral nerve (e.g., vasculitis), or small-fibre neuropathy (e.g., as a complication of diabetes mellitus (DM)) is most common and usually has a severe intensity. Pain is often not recognized in other neuromuscular disorders, for example ALS was for a long time considered to be a painless disease. There is now robust evidence that pain – mostly of moderate intensity – is an important issue in patients with ALS with a significant impact on quality of life. Causes are manifold, that is, cramps, spasticity, and musculoskeletal. Myalgia is a frequent symptom in subacute-onset myositis, in particular in immune-mediated necrotizing myopathy (IMNM), but there is increasing awareness that also a significant proportion of patients with chronic myopathies, for example DM type 2, FSHD, and Pompe disease may complain about pain.

Unfortunately, neuropathic pain is difficult to treat effectively. A multidisciplinary approach is now advocated, combining pharmacological interventions with physical or cognitive (or both) interventions. Recently, a review was conducted by merging treatment guidelines and best practice recommendations for management of neuropathic pain into a comprehensive algorithm (Fig. 8.1).

A Cochrane review on cannabis-derived products for chronic neuropathic pain found that despite the fact that all cannabis-based products reduce pain intensity, improve sleep, and reduce psychological distress, yet more people had to stop the medications due to cannabis side effects when compared with placebo.

Treatment of cramps has been the subject of various Cochrane reviews. They found low-quality evidence that quinine (200 mg to 500 mg daily) significantly reduces cramp number and cramp days and moderate quality evidence that quinine reduces cramp intensity. There is moderate-quality evidence that with use up to 60 days, the incidence of serious adverse events is not significantly greater than for placebo in the identified trials. Reviews on magnesium supplementation or stretching of muscles showed that these interventions were not particularly helpful. Clinical practice suggests that some patients seem to benefit from these.

It is uncertain whether an endurance-based exercise programme may be useful for the treatment of spasticity in ALS, as the evidence is of very low quality. In the absence of any high-quality study on the use of drugs such as baclofen, no statement can be made about efficacy. Real-world data on the delta-9-tetrahydrocannabinol (THC):cannabidiol (CBD) oromucosal spray (THC:CBD), approved for the treatment of spasticity in multiple sclerosis, show encouraging results. However, proper RCTs are warranted to assess patients' satisfaction in relation to adverse events.

Anaesthetics Management

Malignant hyperthermia is a pharmacogenetic life-threatening complication that develops when susceptible people are exposed to volatile anaesthetics (e.g., sevoflurane, isoflurane, and desflurane), succinylcholine, or a combination of both.

The risk of death from a malignant hyperthermia reaction has declined considerably since the

Chapter 8 Management

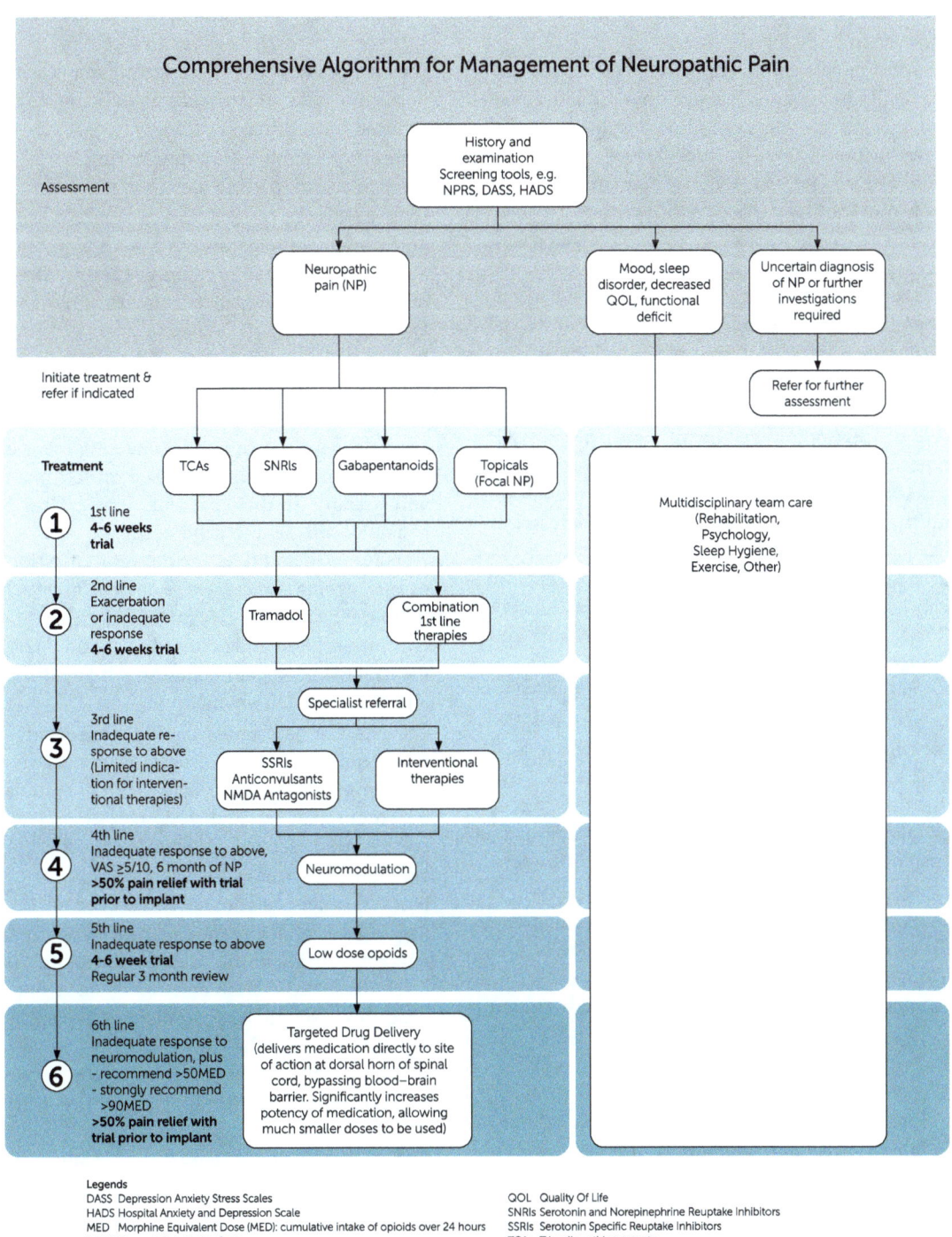

Figure 8.1 Algorithm for pain management. Adapted from *Pain Medicine*, Oxford University Press: Bates D et al. A comprehensive algorithm for management of neuropathic pain. *Pain Med* 2019;20 (Suppl 1):S2–S12), by permission.

introduction of dantrolene. The cause of this hereditary disorder is a disturbance of the calcium balance within skeletal muscle cells. The clinical picture may include generalized muscle cramping, muscle contracture, and massive rhabdomyolysis, and may ultimately lead to hypercapnia, hyperkalaemia, acute renal failure, hypoxaemia, cardiac arrhythmias, diffuse intravascular coagulation, and an uncontrolled increase in body temperature.

Most people with malignant hyperthermia susceptibility have autosomal dominant mutations in the skeletal muscle ryanodine receptor (*RYR1*) gene, encoding the principal skeletal muscle calcium release channel, RyR1. There are less common mutations in the dihydropyridine receptor gene (*CACNA1S*), encoding a voltage-gated calcium channel closely interacting with RyR1. An autosomal recessive myopathy caused by mutations in *STAC3*, encoding a key element of the excitation–contraction coupling machinery with a role in facilitating dihydropyridine receptor–RyR1 interactions, is also associated with a high risk of developing malignant hyperthermia. Of note, about 20% of malignant hyperthermia-susceptible individuals do not have the above mutations, suggesting either further genetic heterogeneity or the presence of pathogenic variants not detectable with currently applied diagnostic approaches. Therefore, absence of mutations in *RYR1*, *CACNA1S*, or *STAC3* does not rule out malignant hyperthermia susceptibility.

Patients with neuromuscular disorders (NMDs) in general are at increased risk of perioperative complications related to anaesthesia due to associated cardiorespiratory morbidity, specific risks associated with certain underlying genetic defects, or other factors. A consensus on anaesthetic management in patients with neuromuscular disorders, achieved in 2021, stated the following:

- Surgery and the associated need for sedation and/or anaesthesia pose a burden on the neuromuscular patient. They should only receive anaesthesia or sedation in the setting of a 24-h high-care facility.
- Surgery or diagnostic procedures should be performed using regional anaesthesia if possible, preferably as a single technique or alternatively in combination with general anaesthesia.
- A careful preoperative examination, multisystem evaluation, and clear communication among anaesthesiologists, surgeons, cardiologists, pneumologists, and neurologists are crucial.
- Premedication should be avoided, and if absolutely required only be used in reduced doses with concurrent pulse oximetry (SpO2) and respiratory rate monitoring.
- Patients with NMDs should be scheduled for surgery preferentially as the first case of the day, because prolonged fasting may cause hypoglycaemia, in particular in patients with reduced muscle mass.
- Continuous temperature monitoring is recommended to avoid a drop in body temperature.
- Short-acting opioids, sedatives, and hypnotic agents are preferred to minimize respiratory depression on emergence from anaesthesia.
- Depolarizing muscle relaxants (succinylcholine) should not be used in patients with a known or suspected NMD.
- Most patients with a neuromuscular disorder are more sensitive to nondepolarizing muscle relaxants owing to their reduced muscle mass and strength. In these patients, a lower dose is generally sufficient to achieve muscle relaxation. In addition, the duration of action of such agents is increased. The dose must therefore be reduced and the muscle relaxation effect monitored and adjusted (e.g., in DMD, myasthenia gravis, mitochondrial myopathies, and *RYR1*-related myopathy).
- The effect of neuromuscular blocking agents (NMBAs) should be measured by quantitative neuromuscular monitoring to prevent residual neuromuscular blockade following emergence from anaesthesia and extubation.
- When there is residual neuromuscular blockade after use of other NMBAs or sugammadex (as a specific pharmacological antagonist of rocuronium and vecuronium) is unavailable, extubation and emergence from anaesthesia should be postponed until baseline muscular strength has recovered spontaneously. In this scenario, postoperative sedation and ventilatory support are necessary.
- Volatile anaesthetics are only strictly contraindicated in patients with variants in the *RYR1* gene. Patients with variants in the *CACNA1S* and/or *STAC3* genes should be referred to a malignant hyperthermia (MH) investigation centre for advice on the risk of MH before exposure to volatile anaesthetics.
- The prolonged use of volatile anaesthetics in patients with NMDs is not recommended.
- After general anaesthesia or sedation, up to 24 h of monitoring (including electrocardiogram (ECG), SpO2, preferably

CO_2 monitoring, as well as surveillance for signs of ongoing rhabdomyolysis) may be necessary.
- Early mobilization and feeding after surgery should be pursued. Respiratory physiotherapy can improve breathing and facilitate coughing.
- Through annual review at follow-up visits, medical professionals can contribute to the improved use of medical alert cards, often provided by patient advocacy organizations. Medical alerts should be clearly visible in electronic health records (EHRs), and recommendations for essential perioperative precautions should be included in correspondence with other healthcare providers.

In addition to the general recommendations summarized above, also disease-specific pre-, intra-, and postoperative recommendations concerning six groups of NMDs (neuromuscular junction disorders, myotonic dystrophies types 1 and 2, muscle chanellopathies, muscular dystrophies, congenital myopathies, and congenital muscular dystrophies and mitochondrial and metabolic myopathies) are provided in the consensus statement.

Pregnancy

Pregnancy in women with a neuromuscular disorder deserves special attention. Patients with a neuromuscular disease should be properly counselled. Preconception counselling and an individualized multidisciplinary care plan provided by a team composed of an obstetrician, neurologist, anaesthesist, midwife, and, if necessary, a geneticist, cardiologist, or pulmonologist in women with autoimmune or genetic disorders is important. In autoimmune diseases, counselling on medication adjustment and management throughout pregnancy and in the postpartum stage is particularly recommended, as medications used not only have risks for the mother but also potential risks for the fetus. With appropriate counselling and management, maternal and fetal outcomes can be optimized in women with neuromuscular disorders.

Obstetrical Issues

Obstetrical issues are summarized in Table 8.1. A word of caution is needed, since the data have mainly been derived from questionnaires, retrospective cohort studies, and case reports.

Rhabdomyolysis during labour may be triggered by prolonged exercise/fasting in carnitine palmitoyltransferase 2 (CPT2) or very long-chain acyl-CoA dehydrogenase (VLCAD) deficiency and McArdle disease.

Increased breech presentation was observed in DM1 and LGMD, ascribed to uterine anomaly, placenta previa (DM1), fetal malformation, polyhydramnios (DM1), or preterm delivery. It was more frequently found in wheelchair-bound women and is possibly underrecognized. Increased perinatal death is found in up to 15% in DM1.

Accelerated deterioration of muscle strength has been reported during or after pregnancy in women with various neuromuscular diseases. Sometimes this is transient, albeit mostly permanent. However, it is reassuring that walking ability was maintained in nearly all women who had been ambulant before pregnancy.

Pregnancy can have a variable effect on women with MG, that is, a relapse in 30–50%, and an unpredictable remission in 30%. Pregnancy does not worsen the long-term outcome. Risk factors include respiratory failure, cholinergic crises, postpartum haemorrhage, or treatment with magnesium for eclampsia. Neonatal MG occurs in 10–20% and develops 1.5 ± 2.6 days after delivery due to transplacental transmission of anti-acetylcholine receptor (AChR) antibodies or anti-MuSK antibodies and resolves usually within 1 month.

Of note, unmasking of disease during pregnancy in DM1, DM2, and nondystrophic myotonias has been reported.

Other complications that may occur during pregnancy or labour are entrapment neuropathies (e.g., carpal tunnel syndrome, meralgia paresthetica).

Special precautions are recommended for pregnant women with a myopathy associated with a dilated cardiomyopathy, in particular if the left ventricle ejection fraction (LVEF) is below 40% and/or when heart failure symptoms are present. The third trimester, labour, and delivery are the periods with the highest risk of cardiac complications. These patients should be referred to an expert centre for close cardiac monitoring during pregnancy and delivery.

A reduced lung function during pregnancy can be a major risk factor for mother and child. There is a high aspiration risk in the third trimester and at time of delivery. However, successful pregnancies in patients with severe scoliosis and progressive respiratory compromise in SMA, nemaline myopathy,

Table 8.1 Obstetrical issues in women with a neuromuscular disorder

Disease	Decreased fertility	Increased rate of miscarriage/preterm birth	Complications during pregnancy	Increase in instrumental delivery
MG	No	Slightly increased	Preterm rupture of amniotic membranes, especially if worsening of MG during pregnancy	Increased frequency of Caesarean (C) sections
DM1	Associated with menstrual disturbances or gonadal dysfunction. More likely used reproductive technology, such as in vitro fertilization or pre-implantation genetic testing	17% (higher than age-matched average in Western countries – 13%)	Pre-eclampsia (10%); polyhydramnios (17–25%), 10-fold increase in risk of placenta previa (causes haemorrhage at delivery); preterm labour (31–50%) and delivery	An increase in C-sections due to uterine muscle abnormality
DM2			Pre-eclampsia (10%),	
SMA		Predominantly nonambulant patients	Pre-eclampsia (10%); preterm labour and delivery	
CMT		No	No preterm labour	
FSHD		No	Possibly preterm delivery, no preterm labour.	Possibly more C-sections due to abdominal muscle weakness
Pompe disease		Increased still birth rate: 3.8% (national USA mean 0.2–0.7%)		
GNE myopathy		No		Possibly
LGMDs		No		Possibly

and LGMD have been reported. There is currently no evidence-based guideline on the management of women with noninvasive ventilation and perinatal outcomes of these women and their babies.

Genetic Counselling

Genetic counselling in patients with hereditary neuromuscular disorders is performed for several reasons. First, it is used to establish or confirm the clinical diagnosis by genetic testing. If the cause is found, the risk of having an affected child and the reproductive options could be discussed, for example prenatal testing followed by possible termination of an affected pregnancy is one option and alternatively pre-implantation genetic testing (PGT) can be conducted. Sometimes an affected child is born who in retrospect has inherited the trait from a hitherto undiagnosed parent, which is not uncommon in myotonic dystrophy type 1, in which case mostly the mother is affected. Second, genetic counselling of family members and cascade testing could be performed, for example in case of myotonic dystrophy to identify family members who are at risk of sudden cardiac death in order to be able to prevent this.

There are several issues that have to be addressed:

First, it is critical to respect that some patients make clear during pretest counselling that they do not want genetic testing. The counsellor should then point out that genetic testing can always be considered in the future, and a shared decision can be made about when this will be discussed again. Second, the use of genetic tests in asymptomatic at-risk relatives in late-onset disorders, such as ALS, requires not only careful counselling but also strong psychosocial support, not only for the individuals who were found to be a carrier, but also for those who did not carry the trait since they may suffer from 'survivor's guilt'. At-risk family members may have compelling reasons for seeking presymptomatic testing: to reduce uncertainty, to plan for the future, and to make decisions about family planning. Guidelines for presymptomatic genetic testing in ALS have been tailored after protocols for Huntington disease and Alzheimer disease, which include pretest genetic counselling, also discussing the decision to learn the results and whether the disclosure should be in-person or via telephone, baseline neurological and cognitive assessment, psychological evaluation, presence of a support person, and posttest genetic counselling. Third, in accordance with an international consensus, caution is recommended in performing genetic testing in asymptomatic children at risk for neuromuscular disorders for which there is currently no treatment. Fourth, the disclosure of genetic information by an at-risk adult to their partner, before marriage or reproduction, or to family members can be a very difficult decision. Professional genetic counsellors can help their patients plan how best to disclose information to relatives or back this up by providing written information in a brief summary letter that they can pass on to their relatives.

Early reproductive carrier screening is a consideration in families with autosomal recessive or X-linked recessive diseases to enable identification of carriers so that the carriers can be informed of the possibilities and reproductive options. Carrier screening of (future) parents may take place preconceptionally. Preconception expanded carrier screening aims to identify couples with an increased risk of having a child with an autosomal recessive disorder before pregnancy, thereby enabling reproductive choices. Carrier screening programmes may be targeted at specific populations with particularly high incidences of certain recessive diseases, for example the programmes for Tay–Sachs disease in Ashkenazi Jewish communities. For Tay–Sachs disease, single-gene disease carrier screening programmes were started in 1970, and in a matter of years, the incidence of Tay–Sachs disease was reduced by more than 90% in the USA and Canada.

Transition from Paediatric Care to Adulthood Care

Due to improved therapeutic options and the expansion of care structures for children with neuromuscular diseases, more and more adolescents with severe neuromuscular disease reach adulthood. Due to increasing life expectancy, an expansion of the phenotype with new or previously subtle organ manifestations is observed. This requires multi- or rather interdisciplinary treatment that extends beyond the period of paediatric care. Since patients and their parents have often been cared for in the paediatric department until they reach adulthood – in some cases from birth – an appropriate transition into the adult medical system should be achieved, but this is often a challenge. Transition from paediatric to adult care in NMDs is a process encompassing not just physical aspects but also psychological and social ones. Family involvement is important for a successful transition of young individuals with disabilities.

Telemonitoring

Telemedicine is the use of telecommunication and information technologies to support the delivery of healthcare at a distance. Video or telephone visits can give patients real-time access to a physician without the need to travel. It received a big boost during the COVID-19 pandemic. Its potential in neuromuscular medicine has been proposed to supplement existing practices in ways that are objective, valid, and less burdensome for patients.

As mentioned above, remote monitoring of non-invasive ventilation is currently widely practised. There is also evidence that continuous remote monitoring of data reflecting disease progression in ALS patients (data regarding their well-being, body weight, and functional status) using a mobile application is well received by patients and healthcare professionals. Likewise, people with ALS who received palliative care online were generally satisfied.

Increasingly, digital health tools are used in research, for example ankle- or wrist-worn inertial sensors to monitor upper and lower motor functions in DMD, spinal muscular atrophy, and myotonic dystrophy.

Suggested Reading

Accogli G, Ferrante C, Fanizza I, et al. Neuromuscular disorders and transition from pediatric to adult care in a multidisciplinary perspective: a narrative review of the scientific evidence and current debate. *Acta Myol* 2022;41(4):188–200. doi: 10.36185/2532-1900-083. PMID: 36793653; PMCID: PMC9896595.

Bates D, Schultheis BC, Hanes MC, et al. A comprehensive algorithm for management of neuropathic pain. *Pain Med* 2019;20(Suppl 1):S2–S12. doi: 10.1093/pm/pnz075. Erratum in: Pain Med. 2023;24(2):219. PMID: 31152178; PMCID: PMC6544553.

Dangouloff T, Boemer F, Servais L. Newborn screening of neuromuscular diseases. *Neuromuscul Disord* 2021;31(10):1070–1080. doi: 10.1016/j.nmd.2021.07.008. Epub 2021 Jul 28. PMID: 34620514.

de Visser M, Oliver DJ. Palliative care in neuromuscular diseases. *Curr Opin Neurol* 2017;30(6):686-691. doi: 10.1097/WCO.0000000000000493. PMID: 28914735.

El-Tawil S, Al Musa T, Valli H, et al. Quinine for muscle cramps. *Cochrane Database Syst Rev* 2015;(4): CD005044. doi: 10.1002/14651858.CD005044.pub3. PMID: 25842375.

Fanos JH, Gronka S, Wuu J, et al. Impact of presymptomatic genetic testing for familial amyotrophic lateral sclerosis. *Genet Med* 2011;13(4):342–348. doi: 10.1097/GIM.0b013e318204d004. PMID: 21285887; PMCID: PMC4039017.

Feingold B, Mahle WT, Auerbach S, et al. SJ; American Heart Association Pediatric Heart Failure Committee of the Council on Cardiovascular Disease in the Young; Council on Clinical Cardiology; Council on Cardiovascular Radiology and Intervention; Council on Functional Genomics and Translational Biology; and Stroke Council. Management of cardiac involvement associated with neuromuscular diseases: a scientific statement from the American Heart Association. *Circulation* 2017;136(13):e200–e231. doi: 10.1161/CIR.0000000000000526. Epub 2017 Aug 24. PMID: 28838934.

Geronimo A. Remote patient monitoring in neuromuscular disease. *Muscle Nerve* 2022;66(3):233–235. doi: 10.10021/mus.27658. Epub 2022 Jun 28. PMID: 35674416.

Hawke F, Sadler SG, Katzberg HD, et al. Non-drug therapies for the secondary prevention of lower limb muscle cramps. *Cochrane Database Syst Rev* 2021;5(5): CD008496. doi: 10.1002/14651858.CD008496.pub3. PMID: 33998664; PMCID: PMC8127570.

Kaback MM. Population-based genetic screening for reproductive counseling: the Tay-Sachs disease model. *Eur J Pediatr* 2000;159 Suppl 3:S192–S195. doi: 10.1007/pl00014401. PMID: 11216898.

Moore U, Emmons SS, Rufibach L, et al. Patient reported pregnancy and birth outcomes in genetic neuromuscular diseases. *Neuromuscul Disord* 2023;33(3):241–249. doi: 10.1016/j.nmd.2022.12.013. Epub 2022 Dec 27. PMID: 36753800.

Mücke M, Phillips T, Radbruch L, Petzke F, Häuser W. Cannabis-based medicines for chronic neuropathic pain in adults. *Cochrane Database Syst Rev* 2018;3(3): CD012182. doi: 10.1002/14651858.CD012182.pub2. PMID: 29513392; PMCID: PMC6494210.

van den Bersselaar LR, Heytens L, Silva HCA, et al. European Neuromuscular Centre consensus statement on anaesthesia in patients with neuromuscular disorders. *Eur J Neurol* 2022;29(12):3486–3507. doi: 10.1111/ene.15526. Epub 2022 Sep 14. PMID: 35971866; PMCID: PMC9826444.

van den Bersselaar LR, Snoeck MMJ, Gubbels M, et al. Anaesthesia and neuromuscular disorders: what a neurologist needs to know. *Pract Neurol* 2020 Oct 27:practneurol-2020-002633. doi: 10.1136/practneurol-2020-002633. Epub ahead of print. PMID: 33109742; PMCID: PMC8172077.

van den Biggelaar RJM, Hazenberg A, Cobben NAM, et al. A randomized trial of initiation of chronic noninvasive mechanical ventilation at home vs in-hospital in patients with neuromuscular disease and thoracic cage disorder: the Dutch Homerun trial. *Chest* 2020;158(6):2493–2501. doi: 10.1016/j.chest.2020.07.007. Epub 2020 Jul 16. PMID: 32682770.

Voet NBM. Exercise in neuromuscular disorders: a promising intervention. *Acta Myol* 2019;38(4):207–214. PMID: 31970319; PMCID: PMC6955632.

Voulgaris A, Antoniadou M, Agrafiotis M, Steiropoulos P. Respiratory involvement in patients with neuromuscular diseases: a narrative review. *Pulm Med* 2019;2019:2734054. doi: 10.1155/2019/2734054. PMID: 31949952; PMCID: PMC6944960.

Zatz M, Passos-Bueno MR, Vainzof M. Neuromuscular disorders: genes, genetic counseling and therapeutic trials. *Genet Mol Biol* 2016;39(3):339–348. doi: 10.1590/1678-4685-GMB-2016-0019. PMID: 27575431; PMCID: PMC5004840.

Part II: Neuromuscular Cases

Disorders of the Anterior Horn Cell

CASE 1 — Amyotrophic Lateral Sclerosis (ALS)

Clinical History

While working is his garden, a 59-year-old man noticed pain in his neck and shoulders. He had some difficulty holding his head in an upright position and rising from a squat. The referring neurologist had performed an MRI scan of the cervical spine, which was normal. As his CK activity was moderately elevated and the EMG showed fibrillation potentials, myositis was suggested. On referral – six months after disease onset – he also mentioned difficulty climbing stairs. When walking, he experienced cramps in the calves. In recent weeks, he had developed a slurred speech and had problems fastening buttons. He had lost 10 kg (12% of his original weight). Pseudobulbar affect (forced laughter, yawning, or crying) was not mentioned at the time.

Examination

He had pseudobulbar dysarthria, marked atrophy of shoulder and arm muscles (Fig. 1.1) with widespread fasciculations, dropped head, and bent spine caused by weak neck extensor muscles (MRC grade 3–4) and paraspinal muscles. In addition, there was mild atrophy of lower leg muscles. Weakness of proximal arm muscles was more pronounced compared with distal arm weakness. He exhibited bilateral foot drop. Biceps brachii reflexes were hyperactive, knee jerks were normal, and the Achilles tendon reflexes were reduced. Plantar reflexes showed plantar flexion of the big toe. Sensation was normal. Forced vital capacity (FVC) was 80% of expected.

Diagnostic Considerations

He had a progressive disease course with clinical signs of lower motor neuron disease in the cervical, thoracic, and lumbosacral regions (muscle weakness and atrophy, fasciculations, EMG findings) and upper motor neuron signs in the bulbar and cervical region (pseudobulbar dysarthria and brisk biceps reflexes in atrophic arms). This combination of symptoms and signs and the absence of alternative

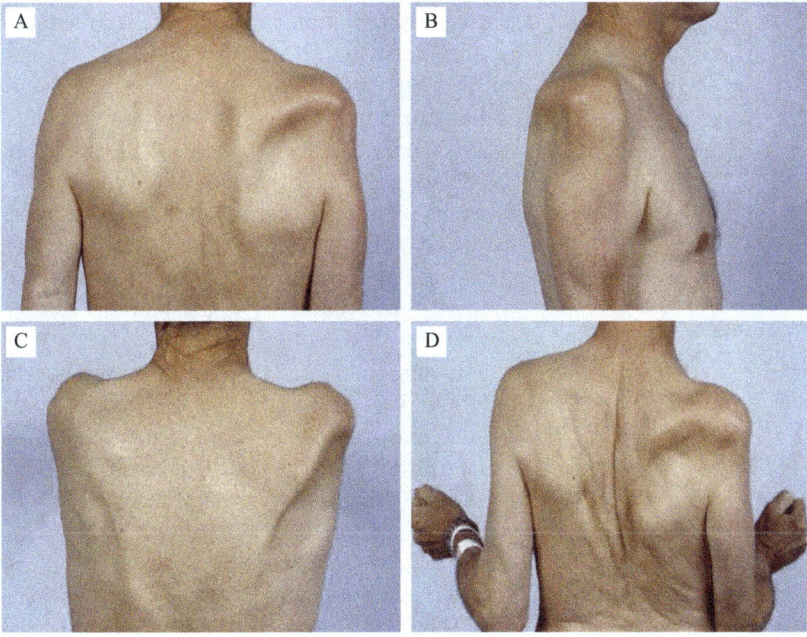

Figure 1.1 (A–D) Marked atrophy of the muscles of the right shoulder and upper arm and mild scapular winging. The supraspinatus, infraspinatus, and deltoid muscles are severely atrophic.

Table 1.1 Phenotypic types of ALS/MND spectrum

Classical ALS	M > F
Bulbar onset ~ 30%	F > M; older onset; ↓ prognosis
Flail arm, flail leg (rare)	M > F; ↑ prognosis
Upper motor neuron (pyramidal features) predominant	younger onset; ↑ prognosis
Pure lower motor neuron (progressive muscular atrophy, PMA; see **Case 3**)	M > F; younger onset; ↑ prognosis
Pure upper motor neuron (primary lateral sclerosis, PLS; see **Case 2**)	younger onset; ↑ prognosis
Extramotor involvement (cognitive/behavioural impairment)	younger onset; higher rate of bulbar-onset; ↓ prognosis; association with *C9ORF72* hexanucleotide repeat expansion which is also the most common monogenic cause of bvFTD.

F = female; M = male; ↓ prognosis = unfavourable prognostic factor; ↑ better prognosis as compared with classic ALS; bvFTD = behavioural variant of frontotemporal dementia.

diagnoses raised the suspicion of a diagnosis of amyotrophic lateral sclerosis (ALS) (Table 1.1). The following ancillary investigations were done.

Ancillary Investigations

Serum CK activity was 5 × the upper limit of normal (ULN). Thyroid function and calcium and phosphate levels were normal. Needle EMG showed widespread spontaneous muscle fibre activity and neurogenic motor unit action potentials (MUAPs) in arm, leg, and paraspinal muscles and fibrillations in the tongue. Motor nerve conduction was normal. Cognitive and behavioural screening disclosed no abnormalities. These tests were consistent with a diagnosis of ALS.

Follow-Up

He was treated with the antiglutamate drug riluzole. Eight months after onset, FVC was 52% of that expected. For some time, he had complained about increased dyspnoea when lying in a supine position. On examination, he had a decrease in FVC of more than 10 percentage points when supine compared with sitting position. This phenomenon of postural drop is caused by diaphragmatic weakness. Due to dysphagia, he had progressive weight loss. A percutaneous endoscopic gastrostomy (PEG) was performed for parenteral feeding, but he died within weeks after the procedure.

General Remarks

Amyotrophic lateral sclerosis/motor neuron disease (ALS/MND) is a progressive disease with deterioration over a period of weeks to months. ALS forms part of a spectrum that encompasses primary lateral sclerosis (PLS), progressive muscular atrophy (PMA), and ALS with or without behavioural variant (bv) of frontotemporal dementia (FTD) (Table 1.1, Fig. 1.2)). In 10–15% of cases, ALS is associated with bvFTD and 35–50% of ALS patients have or develop mild behavioural and/or cognitive changes (e.g., impairment of executive functioning and/or language impairment).

Flail arm and flail leg syndrome are also part of the MND spectrum (see **Case 3**, PMA). Incidence is higher in males as compared with females.

Symptoms and signs of ALS are due to loss of upper and lower motor neuron cells. Upper motor neuron dysfunction manifests with spasticity, weakness, brisk tendon reflexes, extensor plantar response, and often pseudobulbar affect; lower motor neuron dysfunction with atrophy, weakness, fasciculations, and decreased or absent reflexes. ALS is characterized by a mixture of signs of flaccid and spastic paralysis, frequently in the same limb or in the bulbar region. Active reflexes of weak and atrophic muscles point to combined involvement of upper and lower motor neuron cells (**Videos 1.1 and 1.2**).

Amyotrophic lateral sclerosis usually begins focally with asymmetric weakness of the limb muscles and may initially give rise to a misdiagnosis. In about one-third of the cases, there is a misdiagnosis. A foot drop suggests peroneal palsy or an L5 syndrome from a herniated lumbar disc. In about 25–30% of cases there is a bulbar onset, presenting with dysarthria, dysphagia, or dysphonia. Many patients with bulbar-onset ALS are initially referred to an ENT specialist for analysis of dysphagia and to a speech therapist for analysis and management of

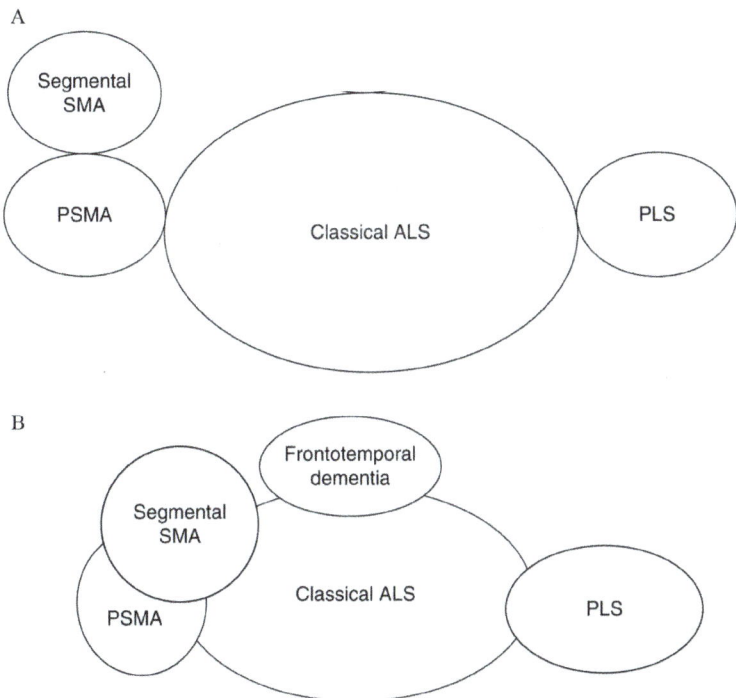

Figure 1.2 (A,B). Most patients with motor neuron disease have classic amyotrophic lateral sclerosis (ALS). Other syndromes include progressive muscular atrophy (PMA), flail arm/leg syndrome, segmental muscular atrophy (SMA), and primary lateral sclerosis (PLS) (A). Three years after diagnosis, about half of the patients with ALS will have died. Many patients with other motor neuron diseases will have developed ALS. In about 5–10%, ALS is associated with bvFTD (behavioural variant of frontotemporal dementia); 30–50% of patients with ALS have or develop cognitive and/or behavioural impairment (B).

dysarthria. However, distinction between bulbar and pseudobulbar dysarthria is unreliable. Bulbar symptoms and signs may worsen if the patient gets tired, and this may erroneously lead to a diagnosis of myasthenia gravis. Muscle weakness most commonly starts in the upper or lower limbs, more often in distal than in proximal muscles. In less than 5%, patients may present with acute respiratory failure by selective involvement of phrenic motor neurons. Vocal cord dysfunction may cause laryngospasm, stridor, and even sudden death.

There is a considerable variability in the age at onset, the site of onset, and the disease progression rate of ALS. The median age at onset is 60 years, and median time of survival is 2 to 3 years after symptom onset. Ten percent of patients survive beyond 5 years and about 5% may survive for 10 years or more. Factors associated with reduced life expectancy are the following: shorter time to referral, age > 50 years, bulbar onset, rapid deterioration of pulmonary function, and presence of cognitive/behavioural impairment (Table 1.1). Death is usually caused by respiratory insufficiency.

There is no diagnostic test for ALS. The diagnosis is made on the basis of a set of criteria, including the exclusion of mimics, some of which are treatable (Table 1.2). The El Escorial criteria for ALS, originally used for research, are applied most frequently, also in clinical practice. However, major drawbacks are the relatively low inter-rater reliability and the low sensitivity for a diagnosis of possible ALS (often PMA, which usually has a disease course resembling that of ALS, albeit somewhat less progressive). A recently proposed modification (Gold Coast criteria, Box 1.1) is more sensitive for a diagnosis of ALS without losing specificity, see also Table 4.1, p.37, and p.81.

Amyotrophic lateral sclerosis shows familial occurrence in 5–10% of patients, usually following an autosomal dominant trait, while within the much larger, apparently sporadic case population (~90%), a pathological variant will be identified in 10–20% of cases.

In monogenic disease the most frequent pathological variants are a hexanucleotide (GGGGCC) repeat expansion in *C9ORF72*, accounting for ~40%

Part II Neuromuscular Cases: Disorders of the Anterior Horn Cell

> **Box 1.1** The Gold Coast Criteria Required for the Diagnosis of ALS
>
> 1. Progressive motor impairment documented by history or repeated clinical assessment, preceded by normal motor function; AND
> 2. The presence of upper motor neuron (UMN) and lower motor neuron (LMN) dysfunction in at least one body region (with UMN and LMN dysfunction noted in the same body region* if only one body region is involved) or LMN dysfunction in at least two body regions; AND
> 3. Investigations excluding other disease processes (see Table 1.3). Evidence of LMN involvement can stem from clinical examination and/or from EMG, and evidence of UMN involvement is mainly derived from clinical examination.
>
> *Body regions are defined as bulbar, cervical, thoracic, and lumbosacral.

Table 1.2 Selected classic ALS mimic syndromes

Disease	Clinical features	Diagnostic test	Other
Cervical spondylotic myelopathy	Hyperreflexia and extensor plantar response below region with weakness and atrophy. Sensory signs. Neurogenic bladder. Slow progression (months–years).	Cervical MRI: stenosis and myelopathy. EMG: lower motor neuron signs can be found in the cervical region.	Respiration normal. Coincidental MRI abnormalities in the elderly. No firm evidence for benefit of surgery.
Inclusion body myositis (IBM)	Initial symptoms: asymmetric weakness deep finger flexor muscles, quadriceps femoris, or, less frequently, weakness of lower leg muscles, or dysphagia. Slow progression (months–years).	Muscle biopsy: endomysial cell infiltrates. Anti-cN1A a.b., Imaging forearm and thigh. EMG occasionally confusing as neurogenic MUAPs can be found.	Aspiration pneumonia may occur due to severe and often unnoticed dysphagia. Supportive treatment.
Multifocal motor neuropathy (MMN)	Asymmetric weakness and atrophy of distal arm/hand or lower leg muscles, suggesting peripheral nerve dysfunction. Fasciculation. No sensory loss. Slow progression (months–years).	Electrophysiological evidence of motor nerve conduction block.	Predominantly in men between 20 and 60 years. Good response to intravenous human immunoglobulins.
Segmental spinal muscular atrophy or Hirayama disease (if distal arms are involved)	Unilateral or asymmetric weakness and atrophy of distal arm/hand or lower leg muscles. Fasciculation. No sensory loss. Slow progression (months–years).	MRI may show atrophy of cervical spinal cord.	Supportive treatment.
Kennedy disease (X-linked recessive spinobulbar muscular atrophy)	Limb girdle weakness and atrophy. Perioral fasciculation, dysphagia, respiratory insufficiency. Sensory neuropathy, and postural tremor. Gynaecomastia in 50% of affected males. Slow progression (years).	CAG repeat expansion in androgen receptor gene.	Female carriers may have some weakness or muscle cramp–fasciculation syndrome. Supportive treatment.
Other myelopathies: (thoracic herniated disk, spinal dural arteriovenous fistula, hereditary spastic paraparesis, adrenomyelo-neuropathy)	Spastic legs. Sensory signs. No bulbar and upper limb signs. Neurogenic bladder dysfunction, incontinentia alvi. Slow progression. Acute deterioration (days–weeks) possible.	MRI of thoracic spine. MR angiography if fistula suspected. Genetic studies.	Surgical treatment (prevention of spinal cord injury); embolization (fistula).

Table 1.2 (cont.)

Disease	Clinical features	Diagnostic test	Other
Primary progressive form of spinal multiple sclerosis	Spastic legs. Disturbed propriocepsis. Neurogenic bladder. Slow progression (months–years).	MRI spinal cord and brain. Cerebrospinal fluid evidence of immunoglobulin synthesis.	Supportive treatment.
Adult onset SMA type 4	Limb girdle weakness and muscle atrophy. Finger trembling. No upper motor neuron signs. Slow progression.	Deletions of exons 7 and 8 in SMN gene.	Treatment with nusinersen (Spinraza®) – only in the occasional patient. Supportive treatment.

Table 1.3 Treatment strategies in ALS

Survival

- Antiglutamate drug riluzole — Prolongs survival with 2–3 months.
- Non-invasive ventilation (NIV) should be offered if there are symptoms, signs, or laboratory features of respiratory insufficiency, independently of bulbar function. If NIV is insufficient, invasive ventilation is an option — Prolongs survival with 3 months, may increase quality of life. Patients need to understand that ALS will continue to progress even with ventilatory support.
- Multidisciplinary care — Prolongs survival and increases quality of life.

Weight loss	Gastrostomy (PEG or RIG): stabilizes body weight and may prolong life. Insufficient evidence to suggest specific timing of gastrostomy tube placement in ALS.
Sialorrhoea	Low- to moderate-certainty evidence for the use of botulinum toxin B injections to salivary glands and moderate-certainty evidence for the use of oral dextromethorphan with quinidine for the treatment of sialorrhea. Evidence on radiotherapy versus botulinum toxin A injections, and scopolamine patches uncertain for any conclusions to be drawn.
Choking, thick mucus	N-acetylcysteine, propranolol, air stacking.
Laryngospasm (usually lasting seconds accompanied by inspiratory stridor, or audible respirations). Common causes are liquid or saliva in contact with the larynx, gastro-oesophageal reflux (GERD), smoke, strong smells, emotion, alcohol, cold bursts of air, and even spicy foods	Trigger avoidance is key. Non-pharmacological measures, e.g., rapid change to upright position of upper body, fixation of arms to stabilize the body, breathing through the nose, swallowing repetitively, and breathing with slow exhalation through lips. If frequent enough and non-pharmacological measures are ineffective, benzodiazepines bid or tid can be used. In the case of GERD, treat with anti-reflux therapy and prokinetic drugs like metoclopramide before meals and at bedtime.
Pseudobulbar signs	Dextromethorphan hydrobromide/quinidine sulfate, amitryptiline, fluvoxamine, lithium carbonate, levodopa.
Muscle cramps	Mexiletine dose of 150 mg orally twice daily. Gabapentin and tetrahydrocannabinol not shown to be effective.
Spasticity	Mild training and muscle stretching. Baclofen, tizanidine, dantrolene, and benzodiazepines reduce spasticity, but demonstrate considerable limitations in efficacy and tolerability. Delta-9-tetrahydrocannabinol (THC):cannabidiol (CBD) oromucosal spray (THC:CBD) complementary off-label treatment option.
Musculoskeletal pain can occur at any time during the course of the disease	Physiotherapy and NSAIDs.
Anxiety	Anxiolytics.

Table 1.3 (cont.)	
Depression	SSRI or amitryptiline; no clinical trials that allow a recommendation of pharmacotherapy over psychotherapy.
Breathlessness	Opioids or benzodiazepines can alleviate symptoms.
PEG = percutaneous endoscopy gastrostomy, RIG = radiologically inserted gastrostomy	

of cases of European ancestry and variants in the superoxide dismutase 1 (*SOD1*) gene accounting for ~2%. Several risk genes have been identified that are probably pathogenic only in conjunction with other genetic and environmental risk factors. It has also been shown that the co-presence of pathogenic variants in some of these genes is related to shorter survival.

There is no role for genetic testing in the diagnostic work-up for ALS. With the potential of new therapies targeting specific genetic subtypes of ALS, there may be an increasing role for genetic testing for those with a definite diagnosis. However, the complexity of genetic screening requires a framework for genetic testing and should only be performed in expertise centres after a thorough discussion on the value and potential drawbacks. Alternatively, the option of storing a DNA sample with the potential to request testing in the future is offered. Testing asymptomatic relatives of ALS patients has great potential to do harm if not carefully counselled, as is well understood from the Huntington disease experience. In these cases, involvement of specialized genetic consultants is mandatory, especially where family planning is concerned.

Breaking the bad news of ALS is a challenging task, and this should be done by a neurologist with training and expertise in ALS and with specific communication skills. The approach should be tailored to the patient's individual needs and family/carers should be involved.

Treatment mostly consists of offering symptomatic treatment. Riluzole is prescribed, albeit its effect is short lasting (2–3 months' extension of life expectancy). There are other drugs (e.g., edaravone, sodium phenylbutyrate/taurursodiol, and most recently, tofersen, an antisense oligonucleotide) for the treatment of ALS caused by variants in the *SOD1* gene. Not all of them are available in Europe.

After communication of the diagnosis, a follow-up trajectory with a multidisciplinary team should be offered, preferably starting within 2 weeks.

Multidisciplinary team-based management is provided by dedicated and well-trained professionals including a neurologist, specialized MND nurse, dietitian, physiotherapist, occupational therapist, speech and language therapist, psychologist, social worker, and a team member with palliative care expertise. The team should collaborate closely with the general practitioner and a centre for home ventilation services (Table 1.3). Telemedicine and telehealth monitoring have proven to be feasible and may be able to supplement clinic-based multidisciplinary care. All professionals should be open to discuss end-of-life care whenever this is brought forward by the patient. The discussion of their preferences and concerns about care at the end of life should take place at trigger points such as diagnosis, interventions, respiratory function changes, and other important life course events. Discussion should also include withdrawal of ventilatory support, PEG, medical aid in dying, and place of death.

Suggested Reading

Chiò A, Moglia C, Canosa A, et al. Association of copresence of pathogenic variants related to amyotrophic lateral sclerosis and prognosis. *Neurology* 2023;101(1):e83–e93. doi: 10.1212/WNL.0000000000207367. Epub 2023 May 18. PMID: 37202167; PMCID: PMC10351316.

Dharmadasa T, Scaber J, Edmond E, et al. Genetic testing in motor neurone disease. *Pract Neurol* 2022;22(2):107–116. doi: 10.1136/practneurol-2021-002989. Epub 2022 Jan 13. PMID: 35027459; PMCID: PMC8938673.

van Es MA, Hardiman O, Chio A, et al. Amyotrophic lateral sclerosis. *Lancet* 2017;390(10107):2084–2098. doi: 10.1016/S0140-6736(17)31287-4. Epub 2017 May 25. PMID: 28552366.

Govaarts R, Beeldman E, Kampelmacher MJ, et al. The frontotemporal syndrome of ALS is associated with poor survival. *J Neurol* 2016;263(12):2476–2483. doi: 10.1007/s00415-016-8290-1. Epub 2016 Sep 26. PMID: 27671483; PMCID: PMC5110703.

Van Damme P, Al-Chalabi A, Andersen PM, Chiò A, Couratier P, De Carvalho M, Hardiman O, Kuźma-Kozakiewicz M, Ludolph A, McDermott CJ, Mora JS, Petri S, Probyn K, Reviers E, Salachas F, Silani V, Tysnes OB, van den Berg LH, Villanueva G, Weber M. European Academy of Neurology (EAN) guideline on the management of amyotrophic lateral sclerosis in collaboration with European Reference Network for Neuromuscular Diseases (ERN EURO-NMD). Eur J Neurol. 2024 Jun;31(6):e16264. doi: 10.1111/ene.16264. Epub 2024 Mar 12. PMID: 38470068.

Oliver D, Radunovic A, Allen A, McDermott C. The development of the UK National Institute of Health and Care Excellence evidence-based clinical guidelines on motor neurone disease. *Amyotroph Lateral Scler Frontotemporal Degener* 2017;18 (5-6):313–323. doi: 10.1080/21678421.2017.1304558. Epub 2017 May 17. PMID: 28513234.

Shefner JM, Al-Chalabi A, Baker MR, et al. A proposal for new diagnostic criteria for ALS. *Clin Neurophysiol* 2020;131(8):1975–1978. doi: 10.1016/j.clinph .2020.04.005. Epub 2020 Apr 19. PMID: 32387049.

Primary Lateral Sclerosis (PLS)

Clinical History

At about the age of 40, the patient noticed difficulty playing tennis. He could no longer hop easily from one leg to the other. After a game, he experienced pain in both legs. At age 43, he stopped taking part in competition, and five years later had to give up playing altogether. At that time, he sometimes missed the brake and accelerator pedals of his car. Walking became increasingly difficult. Sometimes he almost fell due to weakness of his left leg, and he had to use a walking stick. From the age of 50 onwards he used a wheelchair for outdoor transportation. At 52, he could only work part-time as his dexterity decreased. Urinary continence was not an issue, but when he felt the urge, he had to rush to the toilet. His family history was not informative.

Examination

A snout reflex and a hyperactive masseter reflex could be elicited. Arm reflexes were brisk. Muscle tone of both legs was increased, and he had mild weakness of hip and knee flexors and foot extensor muscles. Knee reflexes showed a clonus, and plantar reflexes were extensor. He had a spastic gait that increased with distance. No pseudobulbar affect was detected.

Diagnostic Considerations

The slowly progressive spastic syndrome without lower motor neuron signs led to a differential diagnosis (Table 2.1, Table 2.2), including primary lateral sclerosis (PLS).

Ancillary Investigations

Previous analysis had shown no vitamin B12 deficiency, normal CSF, and normal MRI of the brain and spinal cord. EMG was normal. Normal serum (very) long-chain fatty acid ratios excluded adrenomyeloneuropathy. The most common HSP-genes were analysed and no variants were found. Therefore, a diagnosis of PLS was established.

Follow-Up

We could reassure the patient that it was highly unlikely he would develop amyotrophic lateral sclerosis (ALS), and that his life expectancy was estimated to be normal. He did, however, have to take into account the fact that his action radius would decrease further and that manual dexterity could become a problem over the years.

Table 2.1 Diagnostic criteria for primary lateral sclerosis (PLS)

The diagnosis PLS requires:

- Age ≥ 35 years
- Symptoms of progressive upper motor neuron (UMN) dysfunction for at least 2 years
- Signs of UMN dysfunction (spasticity and associated weakness, pathological hyperreflexia, Hoffman sign and extensor plantar response, pseudobulbar affect) in at least two of three regions: lower extremity, upper extremity, and bulbar.
- Sensory symptoms, lower motor neuron (LMN) involvement, or an alternative explanation for UMN involvement should be absent.
- Definite PLS is defined by the absence of significant active LMN degeneration 4 or more years from symptom onset.

Part II Neuromuscular Cases: Disorders of the Anterior Horn Cell

Table 2.2 Causes of adult-onset chronic progressive spastic paraplegia

Disease	Characteristic features
Primary progressive multiple sclerosis (MS)	1-year history of disease progression, plus two of the following criteria: (1) one or more T2 lesions characteristic of MS in one or more typical brain regions; (2) two or more T2 lesions in the spinal cord, and (3) the presence of CSF-specific oligoclonal bands.
Cervical spondylarthrotic myelopathy (**Video 2.1**)	Sensory symptoms may occur in hands. Cervical stenosis with myelopathy on MRI.
Other structural lesions: • Intra-axial or extra-axial spinal tumour • Calcified herniated thoracic disc • Arnold–Chiari malformation • Os odontoideum • Rheumatoid arthritis of the upper cervical spine	MRI shows characteristic abnormalities. Cervical lesions may have false signs suggesting abnormality at thoracic level
Vitamin B12 deficiency	Causes include gastric surgery, strict vegan diet, recreational use of nitrous oxide. Symmetric subacute paraesthesia, loss of proprioception, and progressive ataxic weakness that indicate involvement of posterior and lateral columns. Abnormal full blood cyanocobalamin (B12); increased plasma methylmalonic acid implies deficiency of functional vitamin B12. MRI may show dorsal myelopathy.
Pure hereditary spastic paraplegia (HSP)	Bilateral lower limb spasticity, hyperreflexia, and extensor plantar responses. Asymptomatic upper limb hyperreflexia without spasticity is common. Urinary symptoms are frequent. Asymptomatic, or mildly symptomatic, impairment of vibration sensation is also common. May manifest at all ages. Autosomal dominant (AD), autosomal recessive (AR), or X-linked modes of inheritance are seen, with 13–40% of cases being sporadic (i.e., with no family history). More than ~90 SPG genes have been described so far. SPG4 (*SPAST*, Spastin) is the most common AD-inherited subtype of HSP (1/3 of the HSP cases). Other common AD-inherited HSP subtypes are: SPG3A (*ATL1*, Atlastin) and SPG31 (*REEP1*). AR HSP subtypes include: SPG11 (*Spatacsin*), SPG15 (*ZFYVE26*), and SPG7 (*Paraplegin*).
Adrenomyeloneuropathy	Lower limb weakness, gait imbalance due to sensory ataxia, sphincter disturbances and impotence, slowly progressive. X-linked recessive inheritance. Onset in men 20–30 years and in women 40–50 years. Abnormal serum very long-chain fatty acid ratios. DNA analysis of the *ABCD1* gene.
Arterio-venous fistula spinal cord (mostly between T6 and L2)	Slowly progressive myelopathy and occasionally radiculopathy. On spinal MRI, multisegmental T2 hyperintensities along with associated flow voids are pathognomonic. Diagnosis can be difficult. Definitive diagnosis and localization with complete spinal angiography.
HTLV-1 infection (tropic spastic paraparesis)	Years after infection with human T-cell lymphocytotrophic virus type 1, patients may develop chronic spastic paraparesis. Endemic areas have been detected in the Caribbean, South America, sub-Saharan Africa, and Japan. Patients may have associated neuropathy.
Neurosarcoidosis	High serum and CSF ACE (not obligatory). High CSF IgG-index and oligoclonal banding. MRI of spinal cord shows myelopathy.
Krabbe disease	Brain MRI shows lesions in internal capsules. Low plasma galactocerebrosidase activity.
Copper deficiency myelopathy	Treatable cause myelopathy mimicking subacute combined degeneration due to vitamin B12 deficiency. Risk factors are previous upper gastrointestinal surgery and zinc overload.
Primary lateral sclerosis	Diagnosis by exclusion.

ACE = Angiotensin-converting enzyme; CSF = cerebrospinal fluid; HTLV1: human T-cell lymphocytotropic virus type 1.

General Remarks

Primary lateral sclerosis is a slowly progressive neurodegenerative disorder primarily affecting the adult central motor system. PLS is a diagnosis by exclusion (Table 2.2). PLS is a rare disease, representing 1–4% of all motor neuron disease (MND) patients. There is still a debate whether PLS is the extreme end of a continuum with ALS or a separate disease entity. The overlap with upper motor neuron (UMN)-predominant ALS might favour the former. A recent small autopsy case series of PLS reported that TAR DNA-binding protein 43 (TDP-43) immunoreactive pathology – which is the major pathological protein in ALS – was found within the motor cortex. However, otherwise no ALS-specific features were found on autopsy of PLS patients, such as ubiquinated cytoplasmatic inclusions or lower motor neuron (LMN) abnormalities.

In 2020, consensus diagnostic criteria were established, specifying the requirements for the diagnosis and the diagnostic certainty (Table 2.1).

Mean age at symptom onset is around 50 years, which is at least a decade earlier than non-familial ALS and a decade later than hereditary spastic paraplegia (HSP), both mimics of ALS. Symptom onset is usually in the legs, but the disease can also manifest with dysarthria, dysphagia, and pseudobulbar affect (pseudobulbar palsy) (**Video 2.2**). Spasticity and pathological reflexes are mostly bilateral and symmetrical, but rarely the patient may present with unilateral or asymmetrical UMN involvement. Three phenotypes are distinguished: the ascending paraparetic type (most frequent (70%), mostly in women), the hemiparetic phenotype (20%, Mills syndrome), and the bulbar-onset phenotype (< 10%).

Urinary urgency is commonly found in all three subtypes. Cognitive and/or behavioural impairment even up to frontotemporal dementia is a rare but well-documented clinical feature, albeit less frequent as compared to ALS.

There has been a concern that PLS might evolve in to ALS, but a recent study on 43 PLS patients showed that this is usually not the case. A significant lower level of serum neurofilament light chain (NfL) which is consistent with a slower pace of neurodegeneration is found in patients with PLS as compared to ALS. Therefore, NfL levels at disease onset are strong predictors of prognosis.

Suggested Reading

Hassan A, Mittal SO, Hu WT, et al. Natural history of 'pure' primary lateral sclerosis. *Neurology* 2021;96(17):e2231–e2238. doi: 10.1212/WNL.0000000000011771. Epub 2021 Feb 26. PMID: 33637635; PMCID: PMC8166429.

Schito P, Russo T, Domi T, et al. Clinical features and biomarkers to differentiate primary and amyotrophic lateral sclerosis in patients with an upper motor neuron syndrome. *Neurology* 2023;101(8):352–356

Shribman S, Reid E, Crosby AH, Houlden H, Warner TT. Hereditary spastic paraplegia: from diagnosis to emerging therapeutic approaches. *Lancet Neurol* 2019;18(12):1136–1146. doi: 10.1016/S1474-4422(19)30235-2. Epub 2019 Jul 31. PMID: 31377012.

Turner MR, Barohn RJ, Corcia P, et al.; Delegates of the 2nd International PLS Conference; Mitsumoto H. Primary lateral sclerosis: consensus diagnostic criteria. *J Neurol Neurosurg Psychiatry* 2020;91(4):373–377. doi: 10.1136/jnnp-2019-322541. Epub 2020 Feb 6. PMID: 32029539; PMCID: PMC7147236.

Progressive Muscular Atrophy (PMA)

Clinical History

When playing slow passages, a 55-year-old professional accordionist noticed painless cramping of the right finger flexors. Treatment with botulinum toxin for suspected dystonia had no effect. In the following months, cramps also occurred at rest, and he had to give up his profession. He also noted twitches in the limb muscles.

Examination

He had widespread fasciculations in the shoulder, chest, and abdominal wall muscles. No skeletal muscle atrophy and no muscle weakness were noted. Muscle tendon reflexes were normal and plantar responses were flexor.

Diagnostic Considerations

The combination of cramps and fasciculations may be consistent with a diagnosis of cramp-fasciculation syndrome, multifocal motor neuropathy, and preclinical stage of motor neuron disease (progressive muscular atrophy (PMA) or amyotrophic lateral sclerosis (ALS)) or segmental spinal muscular atrophy.

Ancillary Investigations

Serum CK activity was at the upper limit of normal. EMG revealed fasciculation potentials in deltoid, biceps brachii, dorsal interosseus, rectus femoris and anterior tibial muscles, but there was no spontaneous muscle fibre activity indicating denervation. Nerve conduction studies were normal. There were no conduction blocks. MRI of the neck offered no explanation.

Given the absence of overt muscle weakness, normal nerve conduction velocities, and absence of electromyographic signs of denervation and reinnervation, a diagnosis of cramp-fasciculation syndrome was established and a wait-and-see policy was recommended.

Follow-Up

Two years later, there were more fasciculations and he noticed difficulty turning a key and clipping his nails. Subsequently, dexterity of the arms decreased. On examination, he had weakness of the extensor muscles of both wrists and fingers. Otherwise there were no abnormalities. At that time, EMG showed spontaneous muscle fibre activity and 'neurogenic' motor unit action potentials, suggesting an ongoing process of denervation and reinnervation. He was subsequently diagnosed with progressive muscular atrophy (PMA).

Four years after diagnosis, walking became difficult. Expected forced vital capacity decreased from 53% to 39%. With noninvasive ventilation (NIV), daytime fatigue and sleepiness improved. Nine years after diagnosis, he developed tongue atrophy, weakness, and dysphagia. At that time, distal limb muscles were paralytic with some proximal strength preserved. Shortly afterwards, he died. Pyramidal signs were never observed.

General Remarks

Progressive muscular atrophy (PMA) is a sporadic, adult-onset, clinically isolated lower motor neuron (LMN) disease. PMA accounts for 2.5–11% of motor neuron disease (MND). PMA may evolve from segmental muscular atrophy (**Case 4**) that is characterized by weakness and atrophy restricted to one or two limbs, usually the arms, associated with hypo- or areflexia and fasciculation. Bilateral involvement of proximal arm muscles is called flail arm syndrome, neurogenic man-in-a-barrel syndrome, or brachial amyotrophic diplegia (Fig. 3.1). Flail leg syndrome is another variant of MND, a syndrome of mostly unilateral onset of distal weakness and wasting of the lower limbs, with absent lower limb tendon reflexes, slow progression, and subtle or late upper motor neuron (UMN) signs. Disease progression in flail arm or flail leg syndrome is much slower as compared with PMA. Atrophy and weakness of neck and other paraspinal muscles give rise to head drop or stooped posture ('bent spine'). PMA does not manifest with bulbar symptoms or signs at presentation.

Clinically, PMA is defined by neurological evidence of usually asymmetric LMN involvement (decreased or diminished deep tendon reflexes and muscle atrophy) of the limbs, no bulbar involvement at onset, and a lack of UMN symptoms/signs (increased jaw jerk, exaggerated tendon reflexes, Babinski sign, other pathological reflexes, pseudobulbar affect with forced crying, laughing, or yawning). Diagnosis requires clinical and electrophysiological features of LMN dysfunction in two or more different myotomal distributions (bulbar, cervical, thoracic, and lumbosacral), evidence of disease progression over time, and the exclusion of other LMN syndromes as mentioned above. PMA can be initially erroneously misdiagnosed as lumbar canal stenosis, multifocal motor neuropathy, polyneuropathy, radiculoplexopathy, or inclusion body myositis.

All patients with PMA show relentless progression. Median survival after initial weakness is about five years, compared with three years in ALS. Rapidly decreasing vital capacity (VC) is associated with poor prognosis. When PMA onset occurs in the axial muscles, the disease has a more aggressive course and more rapidly leads to noninvasive ventilation (NIV).

Corticospinal tract degeneration in the spinal cord and brainstem at autopsy has been demonstrated in about 80% of the patients with PMA. During the disease course, a proportion of patients

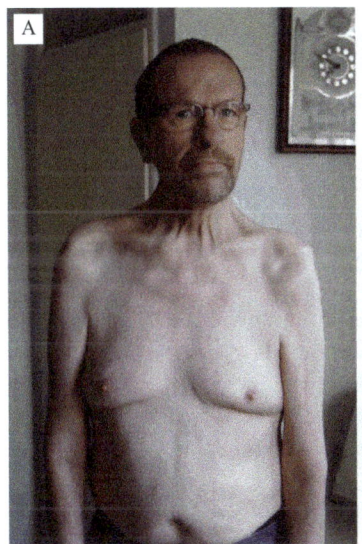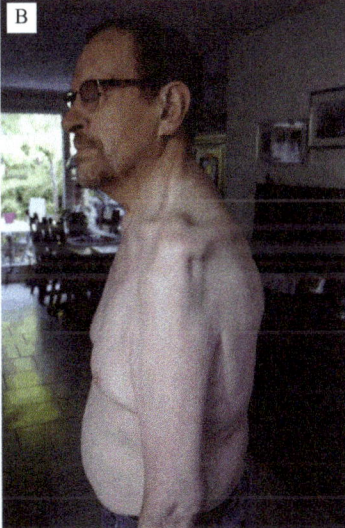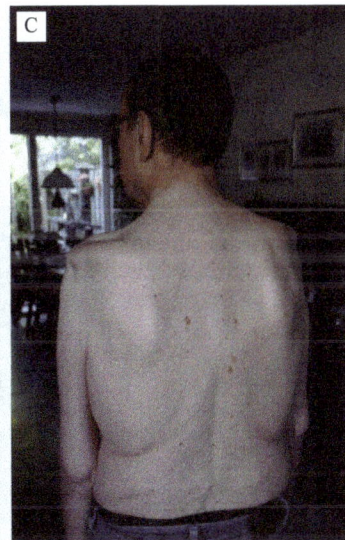

Figure 3.1 (A–C) Man-in-the-barrel or flail arm syndrome. The patient shown could no longer use the atrophic and weak muscles of both shoulders and upper arms. He retained some grip function of the hands.

(~20%) with PMA may develop pyramidal features. Additionally, magnetic resonance spectroscopy has revealed UMN involvement in more than 60% of patients with PMA, and transcranial magnetic stimulation identified UMN dysfunction in more than one-third of PMA cases, suggesting that PMA belongs to the motor neuron spectrum. In familial ALS with *SOD1* mutations, some patients have only LMN signs which is further evidence that PMA is a form of ALS/MND. Most randomized controlled therapeutic trials on ALS only recruit definite or probable ALS patients based on the revised El Escorial criteria, which categorize ALS patients into four levels of diagnostic certainty – namely, clinically definite, probable, laboratory-supported probable, and possible ALS. Since the latter pertains to PMA, these patients were never subjected to trials, potentially withholding them improvement. Recently, the Gold Coast criteria were established in which patients with isolated LMN involvement in two regions (i.e., progressive muscular atrophy (PMA)) are considered to have a form of ALS (see **Case 1**).

The principles of managing the patient with PMA do not differ from those that are applied to patients with ALS. It is not known whether the anti-glutamate drug riluzole is also effective in PMA. However, it is common practice to prescribe riluzole to PMA patients as well. As in ALS, multidisciplinary supportive treatment including Advance Care Planning is appropriate. NIV can be considered in patients with orthopnoea, a VC below 50%, or hypercapnia in order to improve daytime tiredness.

Suggested Reading

Kim WK, Liu X, Sandner J, et al. Study of 962 patients indicates progressive muscular atrophy is a form of ALS. *Neurology* 2009;73(20):1686–1692. doi: 10.1212/WNL.0b013e3181c1dea3. PMID: 19917992; PMCID: PMC2788803.

Liewluck T, Saperstein DS. Progressive muscular atrophy. *Neurol Clin* 2015;33(4):761–773. doi: 10.1016/j.ncl.2015.07.005. PMID: 26515620.

Pugdahl K, Camdessanché JP, Cengiz B, et al. Gold Coast diagnostic criteria increase sensitivity in amyotrophic lateral sclerosis. *Clin Neurophysiol* 2021;132(12):3183–3189. doi: 10.1016/j.clinph.2021.08.014. Epub 2021 Sep 8. PMID: 34544646.

Wijesekera LC, Mathers S, Talman P, et al. Natural history and clinical features of the flail arm and flail leg ALS variants. *Neurology* 2009;72(12):1087–1094. doi: 10.1212/01.wnl.0000345041.83406.a2. PMID: 19307543; PMCID: PMC2821838.

Segmental Spinal Muscular Atrophy

Clinical History

An 18-year-old man had noticed progressive painless weakness and a decrease in size of his left forearm and hand for about one year. He was not able to lift objects, and at the gym he had difficulty handling the dumbbells. He had noticed involuntary contractions not only of his forearm muscles, but also of his chest and once in his legs. Previous medical history and family history were unremarkable.

Examination

Atrophy of the left forearm and hand (Fig. 4.1A,B). MRC grade 4 weakness noted of the left-sided flexors of the wrist, fingers, mm. interossei, m. triceps brachii, and m. opponens pollicis. Normal power noted in the other limbs. Fasciculation was visible in the left forearm. Reflexes were normal and there were no sensory disturbances.

Diagnostic Considerations

Differential diagnosis includes (multifocal) motor neuropathy, entrapment neuropathy (associated with sensory symptoms), incipient progressive muscular atrophy (PMA)/amyotrophic lateral sclerosis (ALS), radiculopathy (associated with pain), syringomyelia (associated with sensory abnormalities), and neuralgic amyotrophy (associated with pain).

The pure motor involvement of the left forearm and hand may be consistent with a lesion of the skeletal muscle, the peripheral nerve, or the lower motor neuron at the cervical level. The absence of pain rules out a radicular lesion. Fasciculation is uncommon in a myopathy but may be a fortuitous phenomenon.

Ancillary Investigations

Electrophysiological examination showed a markedly reduced compound muscle action potential (CMAP) amplitude of the left ulnar nerve and the left radial nerve. Nerve conduction velocities were normal, and there was no conduction block. This made a diagnosis of multifocal motor neuropathy less likely. Concentric needle examination showed fibrillation potentials and positive sharp waves of the left extensor indicis proprius muscle and flexor carpi radialis muscle. In addition, fasciculations of the left m. interosseous I–II and signs of reinnervation of various bilateral arm muscles were found.

MRI of the cervical spinal cord was normal.

Based upon these investigations, a diagnosis of segmental spinal muscular atrophy was established.

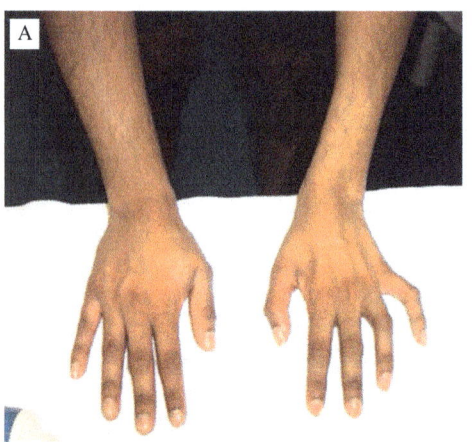
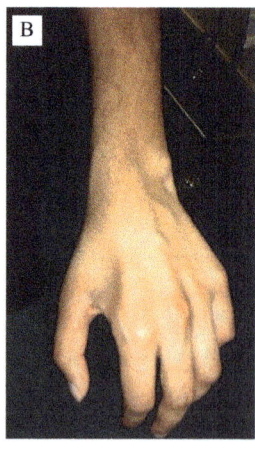

Figure 4.1 (A,B) Atrophy of the left forearm, hand, and spatium interosseum I–II; clawing of digiti 4 and 5 (A); Inability to extend the fingers (B).

Follow-Up

In the ensuing years after diagnosis, he visited the outpatient clinic a few times because of presumed progression, albeit this could not be confirmed at clinical examination. At age 37, he was again referred by his GP because there was slow but clear progression of weakness. On examination, there was severe atrophy and weakness of the left forearm and both hands and clawing of digiti 4 and 5, with MRC grade 4 weakness of most forearm muscles and MRC grade 2 of the flexors of the wrist and fingers, mm. interossei, m. opponens and adductor pollicis, and m. abductor digiti quinti. Otherwise, the musculature was normal. Sensation and reflexes were normal.

A repeat MRI showed bilateral hyperintensities at level C5–C6 at the axial T2-weighted image and hyperintensity at level C4–C6 at the sagittal T2-weighted image, which is consistent with Hirayama disease (Fig. 4.2A,B).

General Remarks

Hirayama disease or juvenile muscular atrophy of distal upper extremity or segmental/focal spinal muscular atrophy or monomelic amyotrophy presents with insidious onset of unilateral weakness and atrophy in muscles of the hand and forearm without sensory loss. In about one-third of patients, less pronounced contralateral weakness of the hand and forearm is reported. Patients experience more weakness and stiffness with cold temperatures ('cold paresis'). Initial progression over months to up to eight years is often followed by a spontaneous arrest. In the original descriptions by Hirayama, predominantly young Asian men were affected. The disease is usually sporadic. Age at onset is 15–25 years.

Chronic compression and flattening of the lower cervical spinal cord during neck flexion has been hypothesized as the pathogenetic mechanism in a number of MRI-documented cases.

Another clinical presentation is that of weakness and atrophy in muscles of the shoulder and proximal arm, which can also start unilaterally, and after years, slow progression to the contralateral shoulder occurs in most patients. This is called the 'flail arm' syndrome, which may evolve into PMA (**Case 3**).

In 'monomelic amyotrophy of lower limb' or 'wasted leg syndrome', muscle weakness and atrophy are restricted to one leg, affecting either the distal or proximal muscles. In these patients, an initially slowly progressive disease course of 1–2 years is followed by a stationary period lasting decades. This form occurs predominantly in males and is common in India.

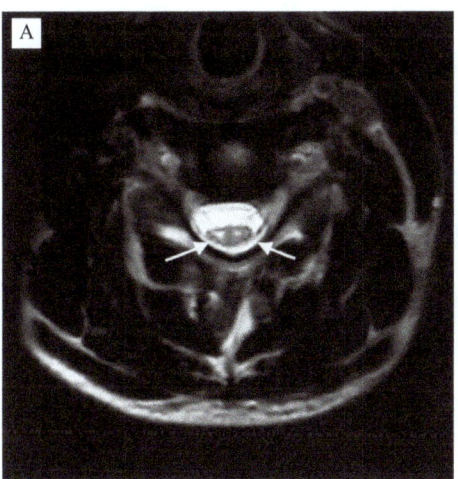 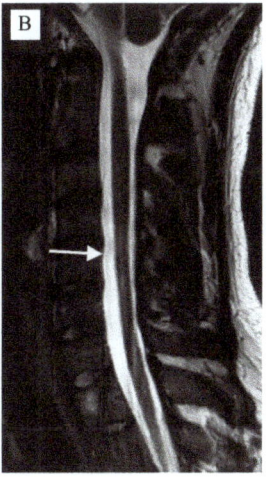

Figure 4.2 (A,B) Bilateral hyperintensities (arrows, 'snake eyes' sign) at level C5–C6 at the axial T2-weighted image (A) and hyperintensity (arrow) at level C4–C6 at the sagittal T2-weighted image (B).

Early bilateral and symmetrical weakness of distal leg muscles is usually the first manifestation of 'distal spinal muscular atrophy' (dSMA), also known as '(distal) hereditary motor neuropathy' (distal HMN) (see **Case 27**). Progression of weakness is slow and most commonly restricted to distal muscles of both legs. After many years, the hands and later the forearms are affected. Rarely, proximal muscles may also become involved.

Suggested Reading

Lay S, Gudlavalleti A, Sharma S. Hirayama disease. In *StatPearls* [Internet]. Treasure Island, FL: StatPearls Publishing; 2023 Jan–. PMID: 29763088.

Spinal and Bulbar Muscular Atrophy (SBMA; Kennedy Disease)

Clinical History

A 58-year-old man had to give up his weekly swimming club as gradually he could no longer keep up with his peers and had difficulty climbing out of the water. He had always been a keen hiker, but for the past four years had to shorten the distance. His body weight increased. Six months prior to referral he sprained his ankle after stumbling over a threshold. In the dark, he had difficulty finding his way to avoid falling. He tended to choke when drinking a cup of tea. His mother's deceased brother had become wheelchair dependent after retiring.

Examination

He was adipose with a body mass index (BMI) of 40. No gynaecomastia was observed. He had perioral fasciculation, most obvious in the mentalis muscle. The edges of his tongue were serrated and showed fasciculations. The strength of his tongue and facial muscles appeared normal. He had a postural and kinetic tremor of both arms. He had a limb girdle pattern of MRC grade 4 weakness, which affected deltoid, supraspinatus, infraspinatus, and iliopsoas muscles (**Video 5.1**). Pain sensation was normal, but vibration sensation was decreased below the knees. The Achilles tendon reflexes were absent.

Diagnostic Considerations

The combination of adult-onset limb girdle syndrome in a man, perioral fasciculation, sensory neuropathy, and positive family history with an affected male suggests a diagnosis of Kennedy disease, spinal and bulbar muscular atrophy (SBMA).

Ancillary Investigations

CK activity was 6 times the ULN. EMG showed sporadic spontaneous muscle fibre activity and long-duration giant motor unit action potentials (MUPs) in various muscles of the face and limbs. All sensory nerve action potential amplitudes were decreased. Genetic analysis revealed 51 CAG repeats in the androgen receptor gene (normal < 37).

Follow-Up

Dysphagia and limb weakness gradually progressed, but he remained ambulatory during follow-up of about 10 years.

General Remarks

Spinal and bulbar muscular atrophy (SBMA; Kennedy disease; Table 5.1) is caused by a CAG trinucleotide repeat expansion (range 39–72 repeats) in exon 1 of the androgen receptor (AR) gene on the X-chromosome. The expanded polyglutamine tract of the AR protein probably results in gain of function that is toxic to motor neurons and muscle. Kennedy disease is a predominantly motor neuronopathy and not a length-dependent axonopathy. Muscle involvement is witnessed by CK elevations up to 15 ULN.

Onset can be at any adult age, usually between 30 and 50 years, and is at younger age associated with larger repeat expansions. Anticipation, that is, earlier onset and more severe symptoms in subsequent generations due to further expansion of CAG repeat

Table 5.1 Main clinical features of spinal and bulbar muscular atrophy (SBMA, Kennedy disease)

- Wasting and weakness in proximal limb and bulbar muscles
- Dysarthria (nasal voice), dysphagia, perioral, tongue and chin (**Video 5.2**), fasciculations/twitching, laryngospasm
- Activity-induced muscle cramps, myalgia, premature exhaustion
- Postural tremor of the arms, legs, head, and voice
- Impairment of vibration sense and decreased sensory nerve action potential (SNAP) amplitude on nerve conduction testing
- Gynaecomastia, testicular atrophy, erectile dysfunction, decreased fertility, glucose intolerance

length, is not observed in SBMA. Proximal leg weakness is the presenting symptom in most cases, but weakness and wasting are usually preceded by CK elevation, muscle cramps and myalgia, increased fatigability, postural tremor of the hands, and signs of androgen insensitivity by more than 10 years. Rarely, Brugada syndrome is found by ECG testing. Female carriers are protected by their low levels of circulating testosterone but can experience muscle cramps in the calves at night and tremor, and may have mildly elevated CK activity and a neurogenic EMG. Progression is slow, much slower than in amyotrophic lateral sclerosis, which is an important mimic. Median age at loss of ambulation is 60 years. Dysphagia is present in 80% of patients, ~10 years after disease onset. More than half of patients die of respiratory infectious diseases due to aspiration, but life expectancy is nevertheless not significantly decreased. Respiratory failure is uncommon. Several pharmaceutical agents have been tested, but none have shown unequivocal efficacy in a phase III trial thus far.

Suggested Reading

Breza M, Koutsis G. Kennedy's disease (spinal and bulbar muscular atrophy): a clinically oriented review of a rare disease. *J Neurol* 2019;266(3):565–573. doi: 10.1007/s00415-018-8968-7. Epub 2018 Jul 13. PMID: 30006721.

Hashizume A, Fischbeck KH, Pennuto M, Fratta P, Katsuno M. Disease mechanism, biomarker and therapeutics for spinal and bulbar muscular atrophy (SBMA). *J Neurol Neurosurg Psychiatry* 2020;91(10):1085–1091. doi: 10.1136/jnnp-2020-322949. PMID: 32934110.

Pradat PF, Bernard E, Corcia P, et al.; French Kennedy's Disease Writing Group. The French national protocol for Kennedy's disease (SBMA): consensus diagnostic and management recommendations. *Orphanet J Rare Dis* 2020;15(1):90. doi: 10.1186/s13023-020-01366-z. PMID: 32276665; PMCID: PMC7149864.

Spinal Muscular Atrophy (SMA) Type 1

Clinical History

A three-month-old boy was seen at the outpatient clinic because of reduced spontaneous movements, which his parents had noticed for a few weeks. His legs lay to the side, he barely moved his hands, and his parents had to increasingly support his head when feeding him. For the past two weeks. drinking became slower. He also drank less and he choked daily. Coughing and crying had become weak compared with the first two months of life. Pregnancy, birth, and family history were unremarkable. He was the second child of unrelated parents and had one healthy sister who was three years old.

Examination

He was very alert and interactive. Eye movements were normal and ptosis was absent. Facial expression was normal. There was a severe generalized hypotonia with few spontaneous movements. Legs were in a froglike position and besides elbow flexion, there was no anti-gravity movement (Fig. 6.1).

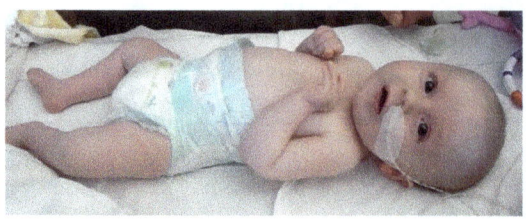

Figure 6.1 Interactive and alert child with severe hypotonia and weakness. Note the froglike position of the legs and the extended belly upon inspiration.

Weakness was distally more pronounced than proximally with absent finger extension and barely any movement of the feet, whereas the hip flexion was MRC grade 2. There was a bell-shaped chest. Inspiration was accompanied by intercostal retractions and marked abdominal extension. There was a severe head lag and the tongue showed fasciculations. Tendon reflexes were absent.

Diagnostic Considerations

Progressive muscle weakness in a formerly healthy baby has a very limited differential diagnosis. Spinal muscular atrophy is the most frequent condition within this differential diagnosis, although extremely rare cases of dermatomyositis, autoimmune myasthenia gravis, and botulism have been described at this age. The fasciculations of the tongue are a clear indicator of motor neuron involvement. Genetic analysis of the *SMN* gene is indicated and now part of newborn screening in many countries because of the possibility of DNA- and RNA-targeted therapies. The involvement of the lower motor neuron can also be confirmed instantly by EMG in case genetic diagnostics are perceived to take too much time.

Ancillary Investigations

Needle EMG of the rectus femoris muscle performed on the same day showed electrical activity during rest in the form of fibrillations and positive sharp waves, and a very poor recruitment pattern. These findings are compatible with denervation and thus involvement of the lower motor neuron. Quantitative PCR revealed a homozygous deletion of exons 7 and 8 of the survival motor neuron (*SMN*)1 gene, which confirmed the diagnosis of spinal muscular atrophy (SMA) type 1.

Follow-Up

The patient presented before RNA modification or gene therapy had reached the clinical stage of development. The unfavourable prognosis was carefully discussed with the parents. A multidisciplinary team consisting of a paediatric neurologist, pediatrician, nurse specialist, social worker, general practitioner, dietitian, and a representative of the home-care nursing team was involved to accommodate the parents' wish to provide palliative care at home. Tube feeding was initiated for both feeding and future medication use as part of palliative care planning. This plan included scenarios in case symptoms such as dyspnea, discomfort, restlessness, or nausea should occur. It provided dosing schemes for, among others, morphine, lorazepam, and ondansetron to be applied by the general practitioner. A childcare worker was involved to support the sister. After three days, all materials and medicines were provided at home and the patient was discharged. Two weeks later morphine treatment was initiated because of dyspnea. The child passed away quietly three days later. Follow-up was done by the paediatric neurologist and social worker. Parents expressed that they valued the support they had during the palliative phase. They were subsequently referred to the clinical geneticist for counselling.

General Remarks

SMA is one of the most severe neuromuscular conditions in children. It is caused by a dysfunction of the SMN protein, essential for motor neuron survival due to mutations in the *SMN1* gene on chromosome 5q. In approximately 95% of cases, this mutation is a homozygous deletion as described in this case, and both parents are asymptomatic carriers, which is essential for counselling. The incidence of this carriership is estimated between 1:45 and 1:100 in different populations. The deletion is tested using targeted multiplex ligation-dependent probe amplification (MLPA) or qPCR, and is not detected by whole exome sequencing currently.

The classic phenotypes and nomenclatures of SMA are based on age at onset and on specific motor milestones being reached in the untreated patient. Children with an onset before six months who will not develop independent sitting are classified as type 1, also known as Werdnig–Hoffman disease, the most prevalent phenotype. Type 2 is defined for children with an onset between 6 and

18 months who reach independent sitting, but not walking. Those who can walk at some point in the development are classified as type 3 (see **Case 7**). SMA type 0 with an onset at birth and type 4 in adults are more rare. It is important to realize that the variability of symptoms in SMA is in fact part of a continuous disease spectrum. The phenotypical variation is related to, although not fully explained by, the number of copies of the *SNM2* gene. This *SMN2* gene produces small quantities of functional SMN1 protein and thus ameliorates the phenotype. *SNM2* differs from *SNM1* by a single nucleotide, leading to a deletion of exon 7 in the majority of mRNA copies that produce a dysfunctional protein.

The clinical phenotype is hallmarked by progressive and generalized weakness and muscle atrophy with sparing of the extraocular muscles. Facial muscles are affected in the very severe type 0. Cognitive development is normal. Breathing pattern in type 1 is hallmarked by increased belly movements upon inspiration due to relative sparing of the diaphragm, which is opposite to a paradoxical breathing where the abdomen is retracted with inspiration in case of severe diaphragmatic weakness. In untreated cases, the prognosis of especially type 1 is unfavourable and in case of supportive care only, most children die before the age of one.

In recent years, a therapeutical land shift has occurred with the approval of three new treatments. The RNA-modifying compound nusinersen, which is administered intrathecally repeatedly, and the oral small molecule risdiplam both increase the amount of functional SMN protein derived from the *SMN2* gene by enhancing the inclusion of exon 7 in the mRNA. DNA modification is done with onasemnogene abeparvovec, a single intravenous adeno-associated virus (AAV)-mediated transfer of the *SNM1* gene (see also the general remarks in **Case 7**). Clinical trials have shown not only increased survival, but also the achievement of motor milestones, never observed in untreated children, such as independent sitting and walking in SMA type 1. It was also shown that earlier treatment improves the outcome. This is compatible with the fact that the loss of motor neurons begins before birth and is considered to be irreversible. It has led to the inclusion of SMA in the newborn screening programme of many countries, and thus the introduction of a new clinical entity, that is, presymptomatic SMA. Disease duration and the clinical status at onset of treatment are important predictors of the treatment response. In severe cases, DNA and/or RNA modification may not reduce disability, and thus lead to a more chronic neuromuscular condition. The reflection on the perceived risk–benefit balance includes the burden of lifelong treatment in case of RNA modification, especially in case of intrathecal dosing, and the risks of gene therapy, which are higher in older children as dosing is proportional to body weight.

Palliative care in severe SMA patients thus remains an important aspect of their management if the new therapies are not available or deemed not to be in the best interest of the child. It is directed towards any sign or symptom that indicates distress in the child, and considers specific needs and wishes from both the child and their families. Advance Care Planning should be initiated as soon as possible after the diagnosis and is not restricted to end-of-life care. Objectives should be defined together with the caregivers and, if possible, the child. This requires a multidisciplinary approach and includes not only pharmacological treatments, but also psychological and social support with the primary goal being to optimize quality of life.

Suggested Reading

Baranello G, Darras BT, Day JW, et al.; FIREFISH Working Group. Risdiplam in type 1 spinal muscular atrophy. *N Engl J Med* 2021;384(10):915–923. doi: 10.1056/NEJMoa2009965. Epub 2021 Feb 24. PMID: 33626251.

Finkel RS, Mercuri E, Darras BT, et al.; ENDEAR Study Group. Nusinersen versus sham control in infantile-onset spinal muscular atrophy. *N Engl J Med* 2017;377(18):1723–1732. doi: 10.1056/NEJMoa1702752. PMID: 29091570.

Finkel RS, Mercuri E, Meyer OH, et al.; SMA Care Group. Diagnosis and management of spinal muscular atrophy: part 2: pulmonary and acute care; medications, supplements and immunizations; other organ systems; and ethics. *Neuromuscul Disord* 2018;28(3):197–207. doi: 10.1016/j.nmd.2017.11.004. Epub 2017 Nov 23. PMID: 29305137.

Kirschner J, Butoianu N, Goemans N, et al. European ad-hoc consensus statement on gene replacement therapy for spinal muscular atrophy. *Eur J Paediatr Neurol* 2020;28:38–43. doi: 10.1016/j.

ejpn.2020.07.001. Epub 2020 Jul 9. PMID: 32763124; PMCID: PMC7347351.

Mendell JR, Al-Zaidy S, Shell R, et al. Single-dose gene-replacement therapy for spinal muscular atrophy. *N Engl J Med* 2017;377(18):1713–1722. doi: 10.1056/NEJMoa1706198. PMID: 29091557.

Mercuri E, Finkel RS, Muntoni F, et al.; SMA Care Group. Diagnosis and management of spinal muscular atrophy: part 1: recommendations for diagnosis, rehabilitation, orthopedic and nutritional care. *Neuromuscul Disord* 2018;28(2):103–115. doi: 10.1016/j.nmd.2017.11.005. Epub 2017 Nov 23. PMID: 29290580.

Spinal Muscular Atrophy (SMA) Type 3

Renske Wadman

Clinical History

A 27-year-old woman consulted the neurology clinic because of progressive muscle weakness in legs and arms. She noticed increasing difficulty in walking, with a maximum walking time of 15 minutes when there was a slight upwards slope, climbing stairs, and lifting heavy things. She had more and more frequent falls in which it felt like her legs suddenly could not bear her weight anymore. Once she fell, she wasn't able to get up from the floor without help. At the time of referral, she also experienced problems rising from a sitting position. She also mentioned problems with repeated movements due to fatigability, for example, when she walked or was cleaning out the dishwasher.

In retrospect, she remembered that she had had a 'typical' walk from the age of five and had never been able to run. A subtle tremor of her fingers was already present in kindergarten. Her medical history was otherwise unremarkable. She had two healthy siblings.

Examination

There was atrophy of the deltoids and quadriceps muscles, and she had a slight tremor (also called polyminimyoclonus) and apparent hypermobility of her fingers. There were no visible fasciculations in tongue or limbs. She had symmetric severe weakness (MRC grade 3) of the quadriceps, gluteus, and iliopsoas muscles, and symmetric moderate weakness (MRC grade 4) of deltoids and triceps brachii muscles. The triceps and knee reflexes were absent. Sensation was normal. There were no joint contractures, but she had a subtle S-curve scoliosis. She wasn't able to get up from a chair without help and hyperextending her legs. Walking showed a waddling gait.

Diagnostic Considerations

The gradual onset of proximal muscle weakness pointed to a genetic disease. In particular, the pronounced weakness in quadriceps and triceps muscles, and only mildly increased CK (see below) made spinal muscular atrophy (SMA) a diagnostic possibility. The absence of fasciculations did not argue against this diagnosis. Fasciculations can be found in the tongue, but are not present in every patient. Since SMA is now a treatable disease, it should be excluded in every patient with slowly progressive proximal muscle weakness and CK < 10 × ULN. With the confirmation of a homozygous deletion of the *SMN1* gene the diagnosis of SMA would be confirmed.

Multiplex ligation-dependent probe amplification (MLPA) and quantitative PCR can detect deletions in the *SMN1* gene. Exome sequencing is (for now) not able to detect deletions of the *SMN1* gene and a genetic diagnosis of SMA will be missed. In case of a heterozygous deletion and clinical suspicion of SMA, sequence analysis of the persistent allele should be done to detect a mutation. It was decided to perform SMN1 gene analysis first, and in case of a negative result, to proceed with gene panel analysis to diagnose late-onset Pompe disease (also treatable), and limb girdle muscular dystrophies, among others.

Ancillary Investigations

Serum CK activity was elevated (598 U/L, 2–3 × ULN). MLPA) showed a homozygous deletion of the *SMN1* gene (exons 7 and 8), with 4 copies of *SMN2*. Next-generation sequencing panel analysis showed no other variants or mutations.

Follow-Up

After confirmation of the *SMN1* gene deletion, we established the diagnosis of SMA type 3 based upon on the highest achieved motor milestone in our patient, i.e., independent walking. Additional analysis of respiratory function showed no clinical signs of nocturnal hypoventilation and no abnormalities in vital capacity. She and her family were referred to a geneticist for counselling. Her parents and younger sister were confirmed carriers, her brother was not.

Based on the reimbursement criteria of her country, in the absence of contra-indications and after informed consent, we started the patient on nusinersen treatment, an intrathecal *SMN2* antisense oligonucleotide. She started (per protocol) with a loading dose of four lumbar intrathecal injections (each 12 mg nusinersen) within two months. Afterwards she got maintenance dosing of 12 mg nusinersen intrathecally every four months. She did not experience any side effects, apart from uncomplicated postdural puncture headache after the third injection. She maintained the ability to walk during the first year of treatment.

In addition, she started with pyridostigmine 30 mg 3 times a day with good effects on her fatigability symptoms.

General Remarks

Spinal muscular atrophy (SMA) is one of the most severe hereditary diseases of childhood, and causes severe disabilities, also in later-onset phenotypes. It is caused by the loss of function of the *SMN1* gene, leading to a lack of functional SMN protein. Reduced levels of SMN protein primarily causes motor neuron degeneration, but also results in changes in the structure and function of the neuromuscular junction and muscles.

The *SMN2* gene, almost identical to *SMN1* and present in 1–5 copies, produces very small amounts of functional SMN protein. The *SMN2* copy number correlates with disease severity, but cannot predict the SMA phenotype in the individual patient.

There is a large variability in disease severity of SMA (Table 7.1). Disease severity in symptomatic patients is classified according to the age at onset and highest achieved motor milestone. In case of discrepancy, the latter defines the SMA types. The SMA type reflects the functional

Table 7.1 Classifying features of spinal muscular atrophy types 0–4

SMA type	Highest achieved motor milestone	Age at onset	*SMN2* copies*	Percentage of total SMA (incidence)	Life expectancy without *SMN*-targeting treatments
0	None; contractures, weakness, and/or respiratory insufficiency	Pre- or neonatal	1	< 1%	Days–weeks, dependence on respiratory support
1	Never able to sit unsupported	0–6 months	2	50%	Median 6–13 months
2	Sits unsupported, but never walks without assistance	6–18 months	3	30%	Shortened, depending on respiratory co-morbidity
3	Walks unsupported	> 18 months	3–4	20%	Normal
4	Walks unsupported	> 18 years	4–5	< 1%	Normal

*<i>SMN2</i> copy number that is most frequently reported in the particular SMA type. *SMN2* copy number is correlated with disease severity, e.g., SMA type, but cannot predict SMA type with certainty in the individual patient

abilities at time of disease onset, but also gives information on disease course according to comorbidities such as scoliosis, respiratory problems and bulbar symptoms.

The pattern of weakness in SMA includes proximal and axial muscles, in particular the deltoid, triceps, hamstrings, quadriceps, and intercostal muscles. Facial muscles and diaphragm are relatively spared. The SMA type 1 phenotype is described in Case 6. Children with SMA type 2 learn to sit independently. Most will need respiratory and bulbar support and spinal surgery in their (late) teenage years. Patients with SMA type 3 learn to walk independently, but most will lose this ability later in life. Timing of losing ambulation is correlated with age of first symptoms. Patients with SMA type 3 with onset in childhood have the risk of developing symptoms of hypoventilation and/or swallowing problems, and some will need spinal surgery because of severe scoliosis. Patients with SMA type 4 develop proximal muscle weakness after the age of 18 years. They will not develop bulbar or respiratory symptoms. Muscle weakness is progressive in patients with SMA types 2, 3, and 4 at all ages and disease stages. Cognitive development is normal in SMA type 2, 3, and 4.

The majority of patients with SMA types 2, 3, and 4 complain of fatigability, which means they are unable to perform repetitive tasks with the persistent effort or muscle strength.

In SMA there is no clinically manifest cardiac dysfunction.

With the introduction of SMA in the newborn screening programmes, a new phenotype has emerged: presymptomatic SMA. These children have genetically confirmed SMA by a homozygous deletion of *SMN1*. Prediction of the clinical phenotype is limited due to the wide range of clinical variability per *SMN2* copy number. It is important to realize that most newborn screening programmes only detect the homozygous deletion of *SMN1*, which accounts for 95% of the SMA population. Patients with a heterozygous deletion and a pathogenic variant in the other allele are therefore not detected by these programmes.

Recently, three *SMN*-gene targeting therapies have been introduced in the treatment of SMA. These therapies include the intravenous AAV9-vector-based *SMN1*-replacement therapy 'onasemnogene abeparvovec' and two *SMN2* splice modulators, the intrathecal antisense oligonucleotide (ASO) 'nusinersen' and the oral small molecule 'risdiplam'. All three therapies have shown to alter survival and motor function in infants with SMA type 1. *SMN2* splice modulators have also proven their efficacy on motor function in children and (young) adults with SMA types 2 and 3.

Treatment effects of *SMN* targeting therapies are best in patients with shorter disease duration before starting treatment, or when started presymptomatically. Diagnostic and therapeutic delays need be avoided by means of rapid analysis of the *SMN* locus and subsequent start of therapy.

Due to the extremely high costs of each of these three therapies, reimbursement is limited and differs per country.

Next to the motor neuron degeneration, there is neuromuscular junction dysfunction with apparent fatigability in patients with SMA. Treatment with pyridostigmine is a proven symptomatic treatment to improve fatigability in patients with SMA types 2, 3, and 4.

Apart from therapeutic interventions, supportive management is still equally important. Management of patients with SMA is multidisciplinary, and can include rehabilitation, respiratory care, bulbar support, assessment of scoliosis and/or contractures, genetic counselling and/or family planning, and palliative care.

Suggested Reading

Mercuri E, Finkel RS, Muntoni F, et al.; SMA Care Group. Diagnosis and management of spinal muscular atrophy: part 1: Recommendations for diagnosis, rehabilitation, orthopedic and nutritional care. *Neuromuscul Disord* 2018;28(2):103–115. doi: 10.1016/j.nmd.2017.11.005. Epub 2017 Nov 23. PMID: 29290580.

Mercuri E, Darras BT, Chiriboga CA, et al.; CHERISH Study Group. Nusinersen versus sham control in later-onset spinal muscular atrophy. *N Engl J Med* 2018;378(7):625–635. doi: 10.1056/NEJMoa1710504. PMID: 29443664.

Oskoui M, Day JW, Deconinck N, et al.; SUNFISH Working Group. Two-year efficacy and safety of risdiplam in patients with type 2 or non-ambulant type 3 spinal muscular atrophy (SMA). *J Neurol* 2023;270(5):2531–2546. doi: 10.1007/s00415-023-11560-1. Epub 2023 Feb 3. Erratum in: J Neurol.

2023 Apr 18;: PMID: 36735057; PMCID: PMC9897618.

Stam M, Wijngaarde CA, Bartels B, et al. Randomized double-blind placebo-controlled crossover trial with pyridostigmine in spinal muscular atrophy types 2-4. *Brain Commun* 2022;5(1):fcac324. doi: 10.1093/braincomms/fcac324. PMID: 36632180; PMCID: PMC9825780.

Wijngaarde CA, Stam M, Otto LAM, et al. Muscle strength and motor function in adolescents and adults with spinal muscular atrophy. *Neurology* 2020;95(14):e1988–e1998. doi: 10.1212/WNL.0000000000010540. Epub 2020 Jul 30. PMID: 32732299.

Postpolio Syndrome (PPS); Poliomyelitis Anterior Acuta, West Nile Virus Poliomyelitis, Acute Flaccid Weakness in Children

Clinical History

A 63-year-old woman was referred because of decreased strength of her right leg manifesting with buckling of the knee for the past five years. Sometimes this led to falls, which made her feel insecure while walking. She experienced some aching in her right heel and in her right knee after long walks. She was able to walk for two hours. She and her husband loved to walk in the mountains, and during those hikes she used a cane. The previous history is relevant because at age 5 years she had suffered from poliomyelitis anterior acuta, which had affected both legs. She had a partial recovery in the sense that she regained normal strength of her left leg and was left with residual weakness of her right leg. She underwent surgery at age 10 years (ankle arthrodesis on the right and epiphysiodesis of the left leg).

She has always been very active and has worked as a speech therapist until retirement at age 62 years.

Examination

The patient had atrophy of the thighs and lower legs, right more than left. The right leg was 3 cm shorter than the left. She had a hypermobile right hip, valgus deformity of the right knee, which was instable, and a thoracic scoliosis. The pelvic girdle and proximal leg muscles were MRC grade 3 to 4 on the right and grade 4 to 5 on the left. The anterior tibial muscle on the right was almost paralytic (grade 1) and normal on the left; the calf muscle was grade 3 on the right and showed normal strength on the left. There were no fasciculations. Knee and Achilles tendon jerks were negative on the right and reduced on the left. She had a Trendelenburg gait due to weakness of her right-sided hip abductors and a genu recurvatum of the right leg. Sensation was normal.

Diagnostic Considerations

The patient had signs of lower motor neuron disease (atrophy and weakness, no sensory abnormalities, and reduced to absent reflexes). She fulfilled the diagnostic criteria of postpolio syndrome (Table 8.1). She had had paralytic poliomyelitis with a history of an acute paralytic illness and signs of residual weakness, subsequently partial functional recovery, followed by an interval (≥ 15 years) of stable neurological function. Gradual onset of progressive and persistent muscle weakness and abnormal fatigability with muscle atrophy and muscle weakness on clinical examination were consistent with a diagnosis of postpolio syndrome. There was no other neurological, orthopaedic, or medical explanation for her gradually developing symptoms.

Ancillary Investigations

A whole-body MRI showed that nearly all muscles of the right pelvic girdle region, thigh, and lower leg were replaced by fat, and there were also abnormalities in the left-sided thigh and calf muscles (Fig. 8.1A–C).

Follow-Up

Over the ensuing eight years, walking became more insecure with an increased tendency to falling, leading to a fracture of her pelvis at

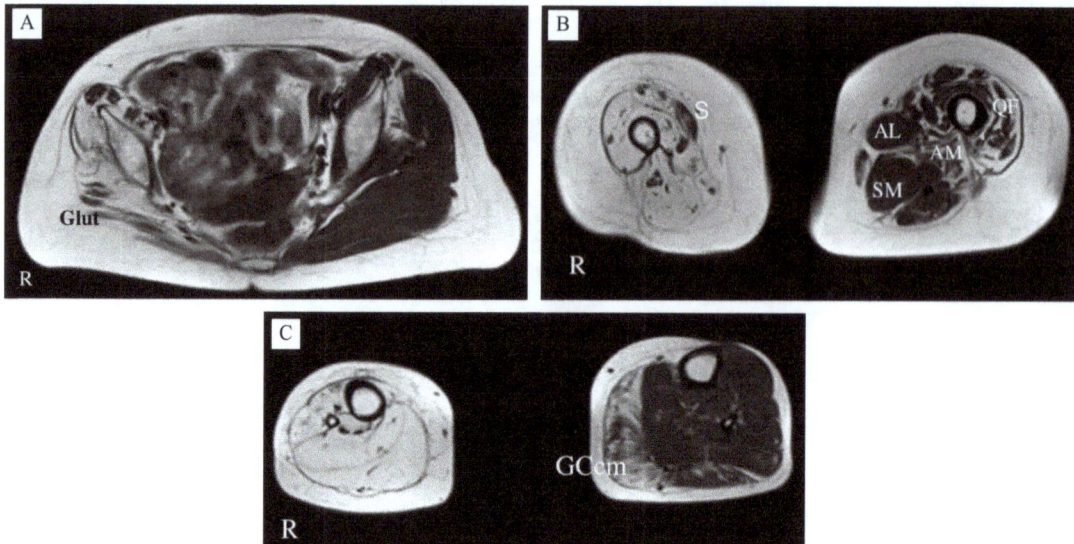

Figure 8.1 (A–C) (A) In the right (R) leg, at the pelvic level, the gluteal (Glut) muscles are completely replaced by fat. (B) Only part of the right sartorius (S) muscle is preserved in the right leg. There are also severe abnormalities of the left leg, in particular of the quadriceps femoris (QF) and the adductor magnus (AM) muscle. The adductor longus (AL) and semimembranosus (SM) muscles are hypertrophic, which has to be considered as a compensatory mechanism. (C) In the lower legs, all right-sided muscles are replaced by fat, as is the left caput mediale of the gastrocnemius muscle (GCcm).

age 70 years. Since then, she increasingly used a walker.

General Remarks

Several years after acute paralytic poliomyelitis, many polio survivors experience new or increased muscle weakness and atrophy in muscles that had been affected during polio and had partly or completely recovered. Following the acute phase, axonal sprouting takes place, reinnervating the muscles of the affected regions and leading to enlarged and thus vulnerable motor units. Overuse of functioning muscle units is thought to induce detrimental structural alterations at the level of the sprouting nerve terminals. However, there are numerous other pathophysiological explanations, so the exact etiology of postpolio syndrome (PPS) remains elusive.

In addition to muscle weakness, fatigue, myalgia, joint pain, and cold intolerance can be experienced. Usually, progression is slow. Some patients complain about rapid decline, albeit that may be attributed to progression of weakness in patients who were left with severe sequalae and had so far just managed to remain ambulatory, but due to the deterioration in strength lost ambulation.

Criteria for PPS were established in the early 1990s and were later refined (Table 8.1). PPS has been reported in 15–80% of all polio survivors depending on the criteria applied and the population studied. To reach a diagnosis, medical history taking and clinical examination usually suffice. If there is any doubt about a history of polio, EMG may be helpful in demonstrating lower motor neuron involvement. Usually, signs of reinnervation prevail, spontaneous muscle fibre activity being minimal or absent. EMG and muscle biopsy evidence of ongoing denervation do not distinguish between stable patients with prior paralytic poliomyelitis and patients with PPS. Imaging of the skeletal muscles may be useful, as asymmetric involvement of limbs in which muscles are partially or completely replaced by fat indicates a past history of polio. Muscle imaging is also helpful in showing the extent of muscle damage.

Acute polio is largely spinal, involving the limbs and respiratory and axial muscles; these are the muscles that show increased or new weakness. If the bulbar muscles were primarily involved during acute polio, PPS may manifest in those muscles, for example with dysphagia, hoarseness, or even laryngospasm and stridor.

Table 8.1 Diagnostic criteria for postpolio syndrome (PPS)

- Prior paralytic poliomyelitis with evidence of motor neuron loss, as confirmed by a history of the acute paralytic illness, signs of residual weakness, and atrophy of muscles on neurological examination or signs of denervation on EMG
- Period of partial or complete functional recovery after acute paralytic poliomyelitis, followed by an interval (≥ 15 years) of stable neurological function
- Gradual or sudden onset of progressive and persistent muscle weakness or abnormal fatigability (i.e., decreased endurance), with or without generalized fatigue, muscle atrophy, or muscle and joint pain. Sudden onset may follow a period of inactivity, trauma, or surgery. Less frequent symptoms attributed to PPS include new difficulties with swallowing or breathing.
- Symptoms and signs persisting for at least 1 year
- No other neurological, orthopaedic, or medical explanation

It is of utmost importance to exclude additional, in principle treatable, conditions in patients with PPS. We have encountered patients who have had polio with residual sequelae and who developed other disorders such as entrapment neuropathy, especially in individuals using crutches.

Referral to a multidisciplinary rehabilitation team is recommended. There is no evidence so far for beneficial effects of any treatment.

Polio is caused by an infection with an enterovirus that is asymptomatic or associated with flu-like symptoms in 95% of cases, but may give rise to a paralytic illness in 5% of infected patients. Administration of vaccines (oral polio vaccine (OPV) or inactivated polio vaccine (IPV)) has almost eradicated the wild poliovirus. Only a few cases of wild poliovirus type 1 have been reported in Asia and Africa. However, there is another form of polio – with a clinical picture that resembles that of wild poliovirus – that can spread within communities: circulating vaccine-derived poliovirus (cVDPV) mutated from the live weakened virus in OPV. While cVDPVs are rare, an increasing number of cases have been reported in recent years due to low immunization rates within communities, in particular in Africa, but recently also in New York, which calls for strengthening polio surveillance systems and ensuring high vaccination coverage.

A polio-like syndrome may be caused by the West Nile virus (WNV), a mosquito-borne arbovirus from the *Flaviviridae* family. The infection is commonly found in Africa, the Middle East, Japan, North America, and Europe. A few cases have been reported in the Netherlands, but these infections were contracted abroad, albeit recently a patient may have contracted the virus due to a bite of a local mosquito carrying WNV. In 60–80% of cases, WNV infections are asymptomatic. In less than 1%, there are neurological complications including meningitis, encephalitis, and poliomyelitis or a combination. WNV-poliomyelitis typically manifests with asymmetrical muscle weakness within 48 hours after the appearance of general signs of infection. Initially, there is a rapid increase of flaccid paresis, which may remain stable or progress to tetraparesis, bulbar weakness, respiratory insufficiency, and eventually death. As in poliomyelitis anterior acuta, there may be long-term sequelae (muscle weakness, fatigue, myalgia). Diagnosis is made by testing of serum or cerebrospinal fluid to detect WNV-specific IgM antibodies.

Since 2012, a distinct syndrome of acute flaccid paralysis with anterior myelitis has been reported, predominantly in children. Outbreaks of this potentially life-threatening polio-like syndrome very likely caused by a nonpolio enterovirus (D68), termed acute flaccid myelitis (AFM), occurs worldwide and has to be distinguished from myriad other causes of acute flaccid paralysis, since there is no sensitive or specific diagnostic test for AFM (inability to isolate enterovirus D68 by PCR or culture from the cerebrospinal fluid of patients with AFM).

Suggested Reading

Koopman FS, Beelen A, Gilhus NE, de Visser M, Nollet F. Treatment for postpolio syndrome. *Cochrane Database Syst Rev* 2015;(5):CD007818. doi: 10.1002/14651858.CD007818.pub3. PMID: 25984923.

Li Hi Shing S, Chipika RH, Finegan E, et al. Post-polio syndrome: more than just a lower motor neuron disease. *Front Neurol* 2019;10:773. doi: 10.3389/fneur.2019.00773. PMID: 31379723; PMCID: PMC6646725.

Murphy OC, Messacar K, Benson L, et al.; AFM working group. Acute flaccid myelitis: cause, diagnosis, and management. *Lancet* 2021;397(10271):334–346. doi: 10.1016/S0140-6736(20)32723-9. Epub 2020 Dec 23. PMID: 33357469; PMCID: PMC7909727.

Patel H, Sander B, Nelder MP. Long-term sequelae of West Nile virus-related illness: a systematic review. *Lancet Infect Dis* 2015;15(8):951–959. doi: 10.1016/S1473-3099(15)00134-6. Epub 2015 Jul 7. PMID: 26163373.

Peripheral Neuropathies

Guillain–Barré Syndrome (GBS) and Miller–Fisher Syndrome (MFS)

Clinical History

A 20-year-old previously healthy man suddenly noticed that he was unable to run. The next day he could not climb the stairs and lost strength in his arms. He was admitted to hospital, and over the next hours he progressively lost muscle power in his arms and legs. Swallowing was progressively impaired, and he noticed minor tingling in both hands and feet. He had had a minor upper respiratory tract infection a week prior to admission.

Examination

The patient was slightly short of breath and could barely walk. Cranial nerve examination showed bilateral facial weakness. There was a severe symmetric paresis of both arms and legs (proximal MRC grade 4, other muscle groups grade 3). There were sensory disturbances of both hands and distally from his knees. He had an areflexia and normal plantar reflexes. The modified Erasmus GBS Respiratory Insufficiency Score (mEGRIS) can be used to estimate the risk of requiring mechanical ventilation. It requires four clinical factors to estimate that risk at any time during the first two months from disease onset. The risk of requiring mechanical ventilation is greater in patients with rapid disease progression, bulbar palsy, and weaker (lower MRC scores) neck flexion and bilateral hip flexion. mEGRIS in the patient was 5, indicating a chance of about 40–80% of developing respiratory failure requiring artificial ventilation.

Diagnostic Considerations

The diagnosis of Guillain–Barré syndrome (GBS) was made at hospital admission. The patient had predominantly weakness, but as there also were sensory disturbances, and the evolution of weakness was typical of GBS, other disorders with rapidly progressive muscle weakness such as myasthenia gravis and myositis were excluded or considered to be extremely unlikely. CSF examination can be helpful in GBS, especially if there is doubt about the diagnosis. It usually shows an increased protein level, but this can be absent, especially in the first week after onset of disease. A CSF cellular reaction (especially when > 50 cells/μL) points to another cause, such as leptomeningeal malignancy or an infectious polyradiculitis (e.g., Lyme disease).

Ancillary Investigations

Standard blood tests were normal. CSF examination showed a slightly increased total protein level (0.6 g/L) without an increase in white blood cells. EMG performed one week after onset of weakness showed extremely low compound muscle action potentials and nonrecordable sensory action potentials, compatible with a severe motor and sensory axonal polyneuropathy.

Follow-Up

Treatment with intravenous immunoglobulin (IVIg) (dosage 0.4 g/kg body weight for five consecutive days) was immediately started. When discussing the diagnosis with the patient, we told him that it was likely that he would need ventilatory support for some time, but that the paralysis would be transient and muscle power would return. Within a few hours, swallowing became more difficult, and weakness progressed. Vital capacity decreased to 1.2 litres (24% of predicted). He needed artificial ventilation within 24 hours after admission to hospital. Fortunately, he could be weaned from the ventilator after eight days and improved further. He was discharged to a rehabilitation centre and made a complete recovery within three months.

General Remarks

Guillain–Barré Syndrome (GBS)

The diagnosis of typical GBS is often rather straightforward (Table 9.1), but it is important to note that GBS can have various phenotypes (Fig. 9.1).

Most patients (about 70%) have had an infection (often diarrhoea or an upper respiratory

Table 9.1 Diagnostic criteria for motor-sensory or motor GBS

Features required

- Progressive bilateral weakness of arms and legs (weakness may start in legs)
- Tendon reflexes absent or decreased in affected limbs
- Progressive worsening ≤ 4 weeks (only applies if duration of worsening is known)

Features that strongly support diagnosis

- Relative symmetry
- Relatively mild/absent sensory symptoms and signs
- Cranial nerve involvement (especially bilateral facial palsy)
- Autonomic dysfunction
- Respiratory insufficiency (due to muscle weakness)
- Pain (muscular/radicular in back or limb)
- May have history of infection (< 6 weeks, possibly also surgery)

Laboratory findings that support diagnosis

- *CSF*: protein level often increased; normal protein level does not rule out diagnosis
- *EMG:* nerve conduction studies compatible with polyneuropathy (especially if features of demyelination are present), but may be normal during first days of disease
- *Blood* tests: typically normal
- GQ1b antibodies often present, especially in MFS

Findings that cast doubt on the diagnosis

- Marked asymmetric weakness
- Severe respiratory dysfunction at onset with mild limb weakness
- Predominant sensory signs at onset (paraesthesias often occur) with mild weakness
- Fever at onset
- Sensory level, or extensor plantar responses
- Hyper-reflexia/clonus (initial hyper-reflexia does not exclude GBS)
- Bladder/bowel dysfunction (does not exclude GBS)
- Abdominal pain or vomiting
- Alteration of consciousness
- CSF: mono- or polymorphonuclear cells > 50×10^6/L
- No further worsening after 24 h
- Relatively slow worsening with mild weakness

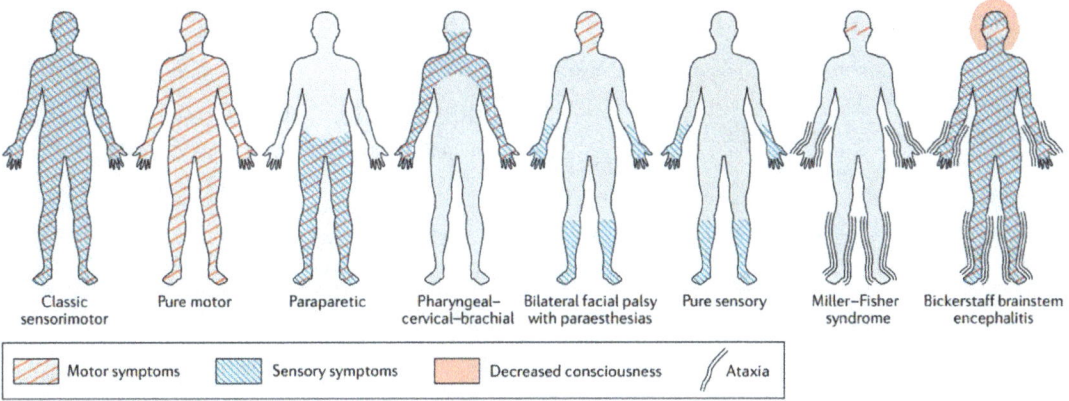

Figure 9.1 From: Leonhard et al. Nat Rev Neurol 2019;15:671–683, with permission. Frequencies of Guillain-Barré Syndrome (GBS) variants: sensimotor 61%, pure motor 23%, Miller Fisher syndrome (or MFS-GBS overlap) 10%, other variants all about 1%. (Based upon Doets A, Verboon C, van den Berg B et al. Brain 2018;141:2866–2877).

infection) one to three weeks prior to the onset of weakness. These infections may elicit GBS in susceptible persons, in some cases through a mechanism of cross-reacting antibodies with GM1-like structures present on peripheral nerves. Patients may have sensory disturbances and cranial muscle weakness (facial palsy, ophthalmoplegia, or swallowing difficulties). Weakness is progressive over maximal four weeks (by definition), but most patients have reached their maximal level of weakness within two weeks. About 20–25% of GBS patients need artificial ventilation for some time. After the progressive phase, there is a stationary phase generally ranging from weeks to months, after which recovery starts. Other causes of rapidly progressive weakness (such as myasthenia gravis, myositis, neuromyelitis, leptomeningeal metastasis or infection, severe metabolic or electrolyte disorders) need to be ruled out or be made unlikely. CSF examination is helpful, especially to rule out an increased number of white blood cells. EMG examination is useful, especially when there is doubt about the diagnosis and if it is not clear that weakness is due to a polyneuropathy. Nerve conduction studies in patients with GBS often show demyelination – acute inflammatory demyelinating polyneuropathy (AIDP) – but may also indicate signs of axonal degeneration – acute motor axonal neuropathy (AMAN) or acute motor and sensory axonal neuropathy (AMSAN). Although nerve conduction studies can make a distinction between AIDP and AMAN, this currently does not lead to another treatment.

Miller–Fisher Syndrome (MFS)

Miller–Fisher syndrome (MFS) is a cranial nerve variant of GBS (**Video 9.1**). These patients have a combination of ophthalmoplegia, ataxia, and areflexia. The course of disease is otherwise compatible with that of GBS. A combination of symptoms compatible with MFS and GBS also occurs – MFS–GBS overlap syndrome.

Treatment and Prognosis

Proper medical care that includes regular measurements of the forced vital capacity or single breath counting is essential to prevent emergency intubation. The mEGRIS is a simple clinical prognostic scale that can be used at presentation to predict the chance of requiring artificial ventilation. It is also advised to regularly check for swallowing difficulties and autonomic failure (blood pressure, heart rhythm disturbances, ileus). Treatment with intravenous immunoglobulin (IVIg) or with plasma exchange (PE) should be started within the first two weeks after onset of weakness in any case in patients who are unable to walk. The treatment schedule of IVIg is 0.4 g/kg body weight for five days, for PE usually four to five plasma exchanges in one to two weeks are given. Mainly for practical reasons, IVIg is the preferred treatment. Despite IVIg treatment, patients with GBS may further deteriorate. Repeating a course of IVIg in GBS patients with a poor prognosis (and very likely also in patients who keep deteriorating) is not effective and induces more severe side effects (SID–GBS trial). However, IVIg should be given again in the 10% of GBS patients who initially improve or stabilize after IVIg and then deteriorate again (treatment-related fluctuation). About 20% of GBS patients are still unable to walk unaided after half a year. The modified Erasmus Outcome Score (mEGOS) can be used early in the course of disease to estimate the risk of being unable to walk unaided after 4 and 26 weeks. This risk is increased in older patients, those with preceding diarrhoea, and those with a higher GBS disability score or severe limb weakness at hospital admission.

Pain can precede the onset of weakness and – like fatigue – can remain present for years. GBS currently is often still a severe disease. The results of new therapeutic trials like those using complement blockers or an agent that rapidly cleaves IgG (including pathogenic antibodies) are eagerly awaited.

Suggested Reading

Doets AY, Lingsma HF, Walgaard C, et al.; IGOS Consortium. Predicting outcome in Guillain-Barré syndrome: international validation of the modified Erasmus GBS Outcome Score. *Neurology* 2022;98(5): e518–e532. doi: 10.1212/WNL.0000000000013139. Epub 2021 Dec 22. PMID: 34937789; PMCID: PMC8826467.

Doets AY, Walgaard C, Lingsma HF, et al.; IGOS Consortium. International validation of the Erasmus Guillain-Barré Syndrome Respiratory Insufficiency Score. *Ann Neurol* 2022;91(4):521–531. doi: 10.1002/ana.26312. Epub 2022 Feb 21. PMID: 35106830; PMCID: PMC9306880.

van Doorn PA, Van den Bergh PYK, Hadden RDM et al. European Academy of Neurology/Peripheral Nerve

Society Guideline on diagnosis and treatment of Guillain-Barré syndrome. *Eur J Neurol.* 2023 Dec;30 (12):3646–3674. doi: 10.1111/ene.16073. Epub 2023 Oct 10. PMID: 37814552; J Peripher Nerv Syst. 2023 Dec;28(4):535–563. doi: 10.1111/jns.12594. Epub ahead of print 2023 Oct 10 PMID: 37814552

Leonhard SE, Mandarakas MR, Gondim FAA, et al. Diagnosis and management of Guillain-Barré syndrome in ten steps. *Nat Rev Neurol* 2019;15 (11):671–683. doi: 10.1038/s41582-019-0250-9. Epub 2019 Sep 20. PMID: 31541214; PMCID: PMC6821638.

Walgaard C, Jacobs BC, Lingsma HF, et al.; Dutch GBS Study Group. Second intravenous immunoglobulin dose in patients with Guillain-Barré syndrome with poor prognosis (SID-GBS): a double-blind, randomised, placebo-controlled trial. *Lancet Neurol* 2021;20(4):275–283. doi: 10.1016/S1474-4422(20) 30494-4. Epub 2021 Mar 17. PMID: 33743237.

Walgaard C, Lingsma HF, Ruts L, et al. Early recognition of poor prognosis in Guillain-Barré syndrome. *Neurology* 2011;76(11):968–975. doi: 10.1212/ WNL.0b013e3182104407. PMID: 21403108; PMCID: PMC3059137.

Willison HJ, Jacobs BC, van Doorn PA. Guillain-Barré syndrome. *Lancet.* 2016 Aug 13;388(10045):717–727. doi: 10.1016/S0140-6736(16)00339-1. Epub 2016 Mar 2. PMID: 26948435.

Chronic Inflammatory Demyelinating Polyneuropathy (CIDP)

Clinical History

A previously healthy, very active 68-year-old man, who usually cycled over 100 km several times a week, noticed progressive tingling in his feet and lower legs that increased over several weeks. This was followed by progressive weakness in the arms and legs exceeding a period of eight weeks. After three months of progression, weakness became so severe that he could not even walk without help. He did not use drugs or drink alcohol.

Examination

General examination revealed no abnormalities. There were no cranial nerve abnormalities. There was symmetric proximal and distal weakness of the arms (MRC grade 4) and proximal weakness of the legs (MRC grade 3), which was slightly worse compared with the weakness in his lower legs and feet (both MRC grade 4). Touch and pain sense were diminished distally from the elbows and knees. Vibration sense had disappeared up to the level of the hips. Tendon reflexes were absent.

Diagnostic Considerations

Both history and neurological examination were compatible with typical chronic inflammatory demyelinating polyneuropathy (CIDP) (Table 10.1). The differential diagnosis of CIDP, however,

Table 10.1 Clinical criteria for CIDP

Typical CIDP

All of the following:
- Progressive or relapsing, symmetric, proximal, and distal muscle weakness of upper and lower limbs, and sensory involvement of at least two limbs
- Developing over at least 8 weeks
- Absent or reduced tendon reflexes in all limbs

CIDP variants

One of the following, but otherwise as in typical CIDP (tendon reflexes may be normal in unaffected limbs):
- Distal CIDP: distal sensory loss and muscle weakness predominantly in lower limbs
- Multifocal CIDP: sensory loss and muscle weakness in a multifocal pattern, usually asymmetric, upper limb predominant, in more than one limb
- Focal CIDP: sensory loss and muscle weakness in only one limb
- Motor CIDP: motor symptoms and signs without sensory involvement
- Sensory CIDP: sensory symptoms and signs without motor involvement

is broad (Table 10.2). It is especially important to check for the presence of a monoclonal protein, as that could indicate diagnosis other than for CIDP. If an IgM monoclonal protein is found, it is important to check also for the presence of antibodies against myelin-associated glycoprotein (MAG), which if present is compatible with an IgM-anti-MAG neuropathy and not with the diagnosis of CIDP.

Table 10.2 Differential diagnosis of typical CIDP (in alphabetical order, non-exhaustive)

AL amyloidosis, hereditary transthyretin (TTR) amyloidosis

Chronic ataxic neuropathy, ophthalmoplegia, M-protein, cold agglutinins, disialosyl antibodies

Guillain–Barré syndrome

Hepatic neuropathy

HIV-related neuropathy

Multiple myeloma

Osteosclerotic myeloma

POEMS syndrome

Uremic neuropathy

Vitamin B12 deficiency (e.g., nitrous oxide poisoning)

Autoimmune nodopathy

Ancillary Investigations

Routine serological examination revealed no abnormalities; no monoclonal protein was found.

EMG clearly showed features of a motor and sensory demyelinating polyneuropathy, compatible with CIDP. Abnormalities included slow motor and sensory nerve conduction velocities, increased distal motor latencies, and nerve conduction blocks. Compound muscle action potentials of the motor nerves clearly showed temporal dispersion. CSF examination revealed a mildly elevated total protein (0.7 g/L), without cells.

Follow-Up

The diagnosis typical CIDP was based upon the following findings:
- Symmetric proximal and distal weakness of the limbs
- Progression over at least eight weeks
- EMG features compatible with a demyelinating polyneuropathy
- Routine blood examination, including screening for a monoclonal protein, was normal

The patient was treated with intravenous immunoglobulins (IVIg) at a dose of 0.4 g/kg body weight for five consecutive days (induction course). Muscle strength improved within a week. However, a few weeks later, he deteriorated again. IVIg maintenance treatment was started (0.4 g/kg body weight once every three weeks). Within three months, the patient was able to perform all daily activities including cycling. In general, muscle strength in between the IVIg infusions was relatively stable and he did not notice a clear deterioration in the days just prior to the next IVIg infusion (no end of dose deterioration). Over the years there were a few periods with deterioration (cause unknown), which responded very well to a temporary increase of the IVIg dosage or by shortening of the interval between the IVIg infusions. Fifteen years later, after regular attempts (about once every six months) to reduce the IVIg dosage it appeared that there was an objective increase in muscle weakness indicating that he still needed maintenance treatment.

General Remarks

Diagnosis

CIDP can be divided into typical CIDP and in five CIDP variants (multifocal, focal, distal, motor, or sensory CIDP) (Table 10.1, Fig. 10.1, **Video 10.1**). Most often, patients have typical CIDP with symmetric proximal and distal weakness and sensory disturbances, absent or reduced tendon reflexes, and a progressive phase exceeding 8 weeks. The levels of diagnostic certainty are CIDP and possible CIDP, which mainly depends on the abnormalities found with nerve conduction studies. CSF total protein may be increased and can be helpful to increase the level of the diagnostic certainty, especially in cases with inconclusive nerve conduction studies. However, if clinical examination and EMG show features compatible with demyelination, it is usually not required to perform a lumbar puncture. In case of doubt, nerve ultrasound or MRI can be helpful to increase the diagnostic certainty.

Treatment and Prognosis

Intravenous immunoglobulin (IVIg) and corticosteroids are proven effective induction and maintenance treatments for CIDP. Plasma exchange is recommended if IVIg and corticosteroids are ineffective. Subcutaneous immunoglobulin can also be used as maintenance treatment. In CIDP, there is usually progression over a period of at least eight weeks. However, about 10–15% of patients have a relatively rapid progressive course of disease, which may initially resemble GBS. This condition is called acute-onset CIDP and should be treated as for CIDP.

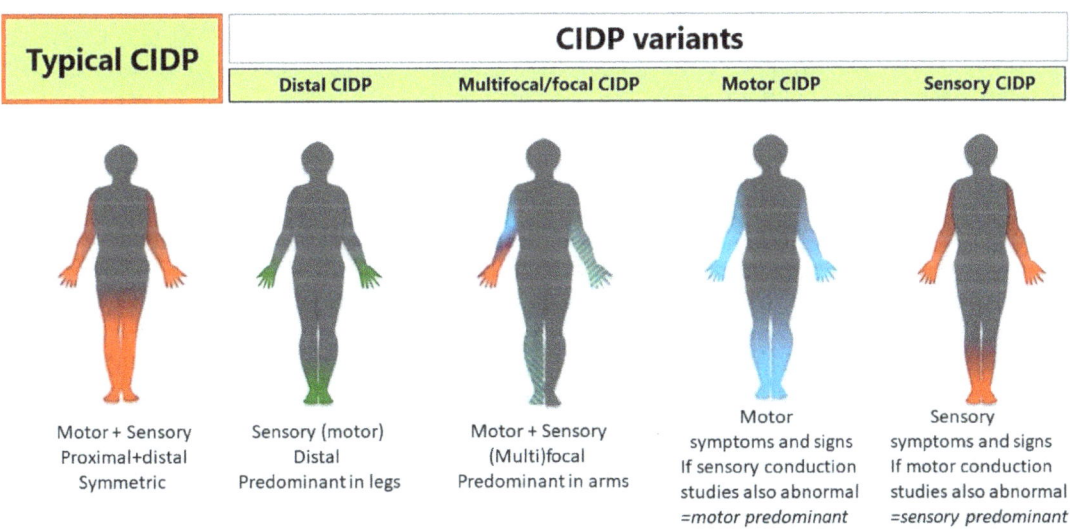

Figure 10.1 Distribution of weakness and sensory disturbances in typical CIDP and in CIDP variants. Based upon Van den Bergh PYK et al., *J Peripher Nerv Syst* 2021;26:242–268, with permission.

The diagnosis of CIDP can be difficult, but the disease is treatable, and most patients have a good prognosis. Treatment is required for months to years.

Suggested Reading

Adrichem ME, Lucke IM, Vrancken AFJE, et al. Withdrawal of intravenous immunoglobulin in chronic inflammatory demyelinating polyradiculoneuropathy. Brain 2022;145(5):1641-1652. doi: 10.1093/brain/awac054. PMID: 35139161; PMCID: PMC9166547.

Van den Bergh PYK, van Doorn PA, Hadden RDM, et al. European Academy of Neurology/Peripheral Nerve Society guideline on diagnosis and treatment of chronic inflammatory demyelinating polyradiculoneuropathy: report of a joint Task Force-Second revision. *J Peripher Nerv Syst*. 2021 Sep;26(3):242–268. doi: 10.1111/jns.12455. Epub 2021 Jul 30. Erratum in: J Peripher Nerv Syst 2022;27 (1):94. Erratum in: Eur J Neurol. 2022 Apr;29 (4):1288. PMID: 34085743.Bottom of Form

Oaklander AL, Lunn MP, Hughes RA, et al. Treatments for chronic inflammatory demyelinating polyradiculoneuropathy (CIDP): an overview of systematic reviews. *Cochrane Database Syst Rev* 2017;1(1):CD010369. doi: 10.1002/14651858.CD010369.pub2. PMID: 28084646; PMCID: PMC5468847.

IgM Anti-MAG Polyneuropathy

Clinical History

A 62-year-old man reported slowly progressive symptoms over a period of two years. He could no longer walk steadily and developed numb feelings on the soles of both feet and a tremor of both hands. He was not known to have diabetes and ate a healthy, balanced diet, drank one glass of alcohol a day, and had not been treated with neurotoxic medication.

Examination

He had a stocking-and-glove sensory loss with a marked postural and kinetic tremor of both hands.

Vibration sense was absent at his knees and more distally. Position sense was impaired at the toes. He had weakness (MRC grade 4) of the dorsiflexors of the feet. Reflexes at the legs were absent. Tandem walking was impossible. He had moderate signs of ataxia when conducting the knee–heel test.

Diagnostic Considerations

Slowly developing symmetric distal sensory and motor symptoms and absent reflexes of the legs are compatible with a length-dependent sensory-motor polyneuropathy. In general, the combination of signs and symptoms may indicate which causes or risk factors for polyneuropathy are more likely than others. The absence of needles and pins, and pain, in the presence of vibration and position sense disturbances with a tremor and ataxia make, for example, diabetes as a cause of this sensory-motor polyneuropathy less likely than, for example, vitamin B12 deficiency, or a paraprotein-associated polyneuropathy, especially in the presence of antibodies against myelin-associated glycoprotein (MAG). The slowly progressive course, relative mild weakness, and the rarity of the disease made an autoimmune nodopathy with antibodies against NF155, Caspr1, or Contactin 1 (all paranodal antigens) less likely.

Ancillary Investigations

Routine blood analysis, including glucose, Hb1Ac, ESR, gamma-GT, creatinine, vitamins B1, B6, B12, folic acid, and TSH, was normal. The patient had a serum IgM-kappa monoclonal protein that was so low that it could not be quantified. Total serum IgM (2.5 g/L), IgG, and IgA were all within normal limits. Because of the presence of an IgM paraprotein, anti-MAG antibodies were determined. These antibodies were clearly positive using a standard anti-MAG ELISA. Nerve conduction studies showed markedly increased distal motor latencies and slowing of motor nerve conduction (median and ulnar nerves 38–42 m/s) in the lower arms, compatible with peripheral nerve demyelination (Fig. 11.1). Amplitudes of sensory nerve action potentials were small, compatible with axonal degeneration. The haematologist conducted bone marrow analysis, which showed 15–20% IgM and

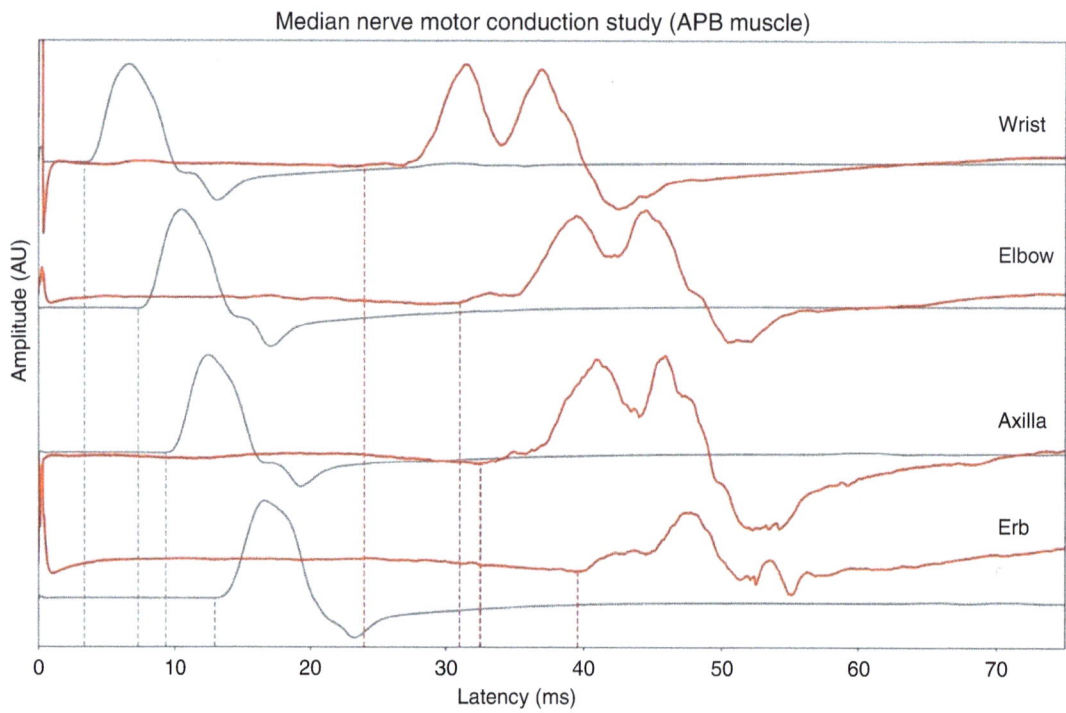

Figure 11.1 Median nerve motor conduction studies (abductor pollicis brevis muscle) after stimulation at the level of the wrist, elbow, axilla, and Erb.
In the patient with anti-MAG neuropathy delayed distal motor latencies and additionally abnormal compound action potentials, indicative of a demyelinating polyneuropathy. Courtesy Dr. Robert van den Berg.
GREY: normal control; RED: patient with IgM MGUS and anti-MAG antibodies.

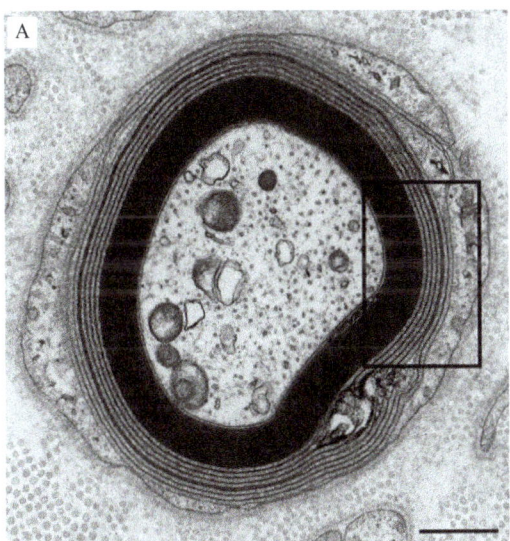 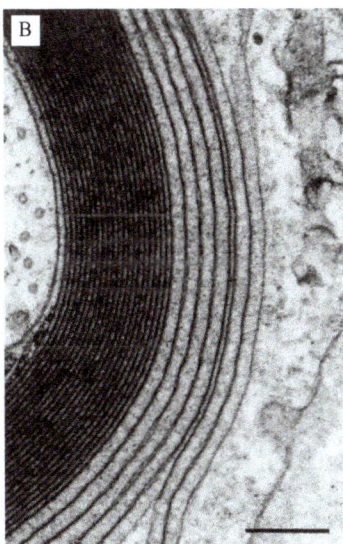

Figure 11.2 Patient with polyneuropathy and MGUS with anti-MAG antibodies. Widely spaced myelin, defined as two or more wraps of myelin with a regularly separated intraperiod line and an intact major dense line, is observed in the outer layers of the myelin lamellae. From Sommer C et al., *J Peripher Nerv Syst* 2021;26:S21–41, with permission.

kappa light chain positive B lymphocytes (normally absent). Plasma cell involvement of the bone marrow was 3%.

Follow-Up

The haematologist diagnosed an IgM monoclonal gammopathy of undetermined significance (MGUS). Because of the low malignancy grade and the absence of systemic B-symptoms (temperature > 38°C, night sweats, and weight loss > 10% over six months), treatment was not indicated from a haematological point of view. We concluded that the (motor) sensory ataxic IgM anti-MAG neuropathy likely caused his increasing walking disability. Because the patient slightly deteriorated over the next six months, he was twice treated with rituximab (anti-CD20 monoclonal antibody), which showed clinical benefit (especially his balance was better six months after initiating treatment). Further follow-up showed stable disability without an increase of the M-protein, and five years after initial complaints the patient could still walk without help.

General Remarks

The prevalence of chronic polyneuropathy in general increases with age, ranging from 1.2% (50–60 years of age) to 13.2% (> 80 years of age). Patients with a chronic polyneuropathy need to be screened for the presence of a range of possible risk factors such as diabetes, vitamin deficiencies, and a serum monoclonal protein. If a monoclonal protein is found, this requires further investigation, which is usually conducted by a haematologist. Paraproteins (or monoclonal gammopathies) are monoclonal immunoglobulins secreted by clonally expanded cells within the B-cell lineage. Monoclonal gammopathies associated with neurological manifestations include MGUS, multiple myeloma, lymphoplasmacytic lymphomas, Waldenström macroglobulinaemia, and less frequently non-Hodgkin lymphoma and other lymphoproliferative disorders. Anti-MAG antibodies are typically associated with an IgM monoclonal gammopathy and not with an IgG or IgA monoclonal gammopathy. Anti-MAG antibodies can be found in about half of the patients with chronic polyneuropathy associated with an IgM monoclonal gammopathy.

Characteristics of MGUS

- Monoclonal (M)-protein or an abnormal free light chain (FLC) ratio in peripheral blood.
- Serum monoclonal protein < 30 g/L, and for an individual to be diagnosed with light chain MGUS, the free light chain kappa/lambda ratio has to be abnormal.
- Clonal bone marrow plasma cells < 10%

Table 11.1 Various diseases associated with a monoclonal gammopathy and a polyneuropathy (non-exhaustive)

Diagnosis	Clinical features	EMG	Lab tests	Associated malignancy
IgM anti-MAG	Distal sensory-motor polyneuropathy, ataxia, tremor	Demyelinating Prolonged distal latencies	Anti-MAG	Waldenström, B-cell lymphoma
IgM anti-MAG-negative	Variable, can be compatible with CIDP	Demyelinating	Anti-MAG neg	Waldenström, B-cell lymphoma, MGUS
Cryoglobulinaemic vasculitis	Polyneuropathy or mononeuritis. Pain, rash, arthritis. Symptoms can be worse with low temperature	Axonal (demyelinating)	Cryoglobulinaemia	Non-Hodgkin B-cell lymphoma, chronic infections (usually hepatitis C), MGUS
POEMS	Polyneuropathy, sclerotic bone lesions, organomegaly, endocrinopathy, skin changes	Demyelinating (axonal)	VEGF, immune-fixation, Free lambda light chains. Mostly IgG or IgA M-protein	Osteosclerotic myeloma
Neurolymphomatosis	Asymmetry, cranial nerves, (multiple) mononeuropathy, pain. Sometimes CNS symptoms	Axonal or demyelinating	CSF: monoclonal cells nerve biopsy: lymphoma/monoclonal cells	B-cell lymphoma, Waldenström
AL amyloidosis	Polyneuropathy, rapidly progressive, pain, dys-autonomia, bilateral CTS. Multi-organ disease (especially heart)	Axonal	Free lambda light chains. Mostly IgG or IgA. Biopsy (amyloid)	Plasma cell disorder
Bing–Neel	Polyneuropathy, headache, CNS symptoms, visual loss	Axonal	CSF: increased cells, somatic MYD88 mutation MRI: meningeal enhancement	Waldenström, lymphoplasmacytic lymphoma, IgM MGUS

- Clinical work-up must be negative for evidence of end-organ damage from plasma cell dyscrasia, such as hypercalcaemia, anaemia, renal failure, lymphadenopathy, hepatosplenomegaly, one or more lytic bone lesions (skeletal radiography, CT, or PET-CT).

If a patient has a monoclonal protein and the abnormalities exceed the laboratory levels compatible with MGUS and/or has abnormalities in the clinical workup (see above), the diagnosis would be smouldering myeloma, multiple myeloma, or another haematological disease. If MGUS is diagnosed, patients must be regularly monitored (in case of an IgG paraprotein usually every two years, in case of an IgM paraprotein usually every year) for a progressive haematological disease, in particular myeloma (11% lifelong risk), macroglobulinemia (IgM), other lympho-proliferative disorders, or light chain amyloidosis (AL amyloidosis). IgM monoclonal gammopathy is associated with a range of neurological symptoms, including polyneuropathy (Table 11.1).

Both the prevalence of chronic axonal polyneuropathy (in general) and of an IgG or IgM MGUS increase with age. Therefore, the presence of an IgG or IgM MGUS can also be coincidental, especially in older patients with a mild chronic axonal neuropathy when no other cause is identified. A causal relationship is more likely in young patients, if the polyneuropathy is rapidly progressive, or if the patient with an IgM MGUS has a distal symmetric

Table 11.2 Main features of MGUS polyneuropathy

- Symmetric sensory > motor polyneuropathy
- Distal > proximal (length-dependent polyneuropathy)
- Slow progression
- MGUS

If IgM MGUS:

- Anti-MAG antibodies in half of the cases
- Gnostic sensory signs / ataxia often present
- Nerve conduction studies showing increased distal motor latency

sensorimotor polyneuropathy with ataxia, a postural and kinetic tremor, increased motor distal latency times (nerve conduction studies) in the presence of anti-MAG antibodies (Table 11.2).

EMG in most of these patients shows signs of demyelination (especially increased distal motor latency times) (Fig. 11.1), whereas pure axonal features are found in a minority of patients. Nerve biopsies in these patients (usually not needed since anti-MAG antibody assays are widely available) show widening of myelin lamellae (Fig. 11.2). As MAG is located at the paranode, loss of the function – probably due to the presence of MAG antibodies – is likely associated with widening of myelin lamellae and dysfunction of nerve conduction.

As anti-MAG antibodies (with levels clearly above the standard test cut-off value) are virtually only found in the context of an IgM-MGUS or an IgM lymphoplasmacytic lymphoma, its presence is considered incompatible with the diagnosis of chronic inflammatory demyelinating polyneuropathy (CIDP).

Treatment

Evidence-based treatment strategies for IgM MGUS-associated neuropathies are largely lacking. Therapies that have been evaluated in relatively small series include intravenous immunoglobulins (IVIg), plasma exchange, corticosteroids, interferon-alpha, chlorambucil, fludarabine, cyclophosphamide and prednisone, and rituximab (anti-CD20 treatment). In a Cochrane review (Lunn & Nobile-Orazio, 2016) it was concluded that there is inadequate reliable evidence from trials of immunotherapies in anti-MAG paraproteinaemic neuropathy to form an evidence-based conclusion supporting any particular immunotherapy treatment. IVIg has a statistically but probably not clinically significant benefit in the short term. However, a meta-analysis of two trials and more recent studies evaluating the effect of rituximab provides (low-level) evidence of a benefit of this drug in these patients.

Despite the absence of evidence from large RCTs, rituximab currently is often used in patients with an IgM anti-MAG-related polyneuropathy. Some individuals can have benefit from rituximab as it may stabilize or improve neurological function. If effective, the effect usually starts after three to six months and may last for two to three years. New and larger trials evaluating the effect of immunotherapy including rituximab in patients with IgM anti-MAG-related polyneuropathy are awaited.

Suggested Reading

Carroll AS, Lunn MPT. Paraproteinaemic neuropathy: MGUS and beyond. *Pract Neurol* 2021;21(6):492–503. doi: 10.1136/practneurol-2020-002837. Epub 2021 Jul 19. PMID: 34282034.

Chaganti S, Hannaford A, Vucic S. Rituximab in chronic immune mediated neuropathies: a systematic review. *Neuromuscul Disord* 2022;32(8):621–627. doi: 10.1016/j.nmd.2022.05.013. Epub 2022 May 24. PMID: 35672205.

Lunn MP, Nobile-Orazio E. Immunotherapy for IgM anti-myelin-associated glycoprotein paraprotein-associated peripheral neuropathies. *Cochrane Database Syst Rev* 2016;10(10):CD002827. doi: 10.1002/14651858.CD002827.pub4. PMID: 27701752; PMCID: PMC6457998.

Parisi M, Dogliotti I, Clerico M, et al. Efficacy of rituximab in anti-myelin-associated glycoprotein demyelinating polyneuropathy: Clinical, hematological and neurophysiological correlations during 2 years of follow-up. *Eur J Neurol* 2022;29(12):3611–3622. doi: 10.1111/ene.15553. Epub 2022 Sep 25. PMID: 36083713; PMCID: PMC9825860.

Sommer C, Carroll AS, Koike H, et al. Nerve biopsy in acquired neuropathies. *J Peripher Nerv Syst* 2021;26 Suppl 2:S21–S41. doi: 10.1111/jns.12464. Epub 2021 Sep 14. PMID: 34523188.

Taams NE, Drenthen J, Hanewinckel R, Ikram MA, van Doorn PA. Prevalence and risk factor profiles for chronic axonal polyneuropathy in the general population. *Neurology* 2022:10.1212/WNL.0000000000201168. doi: 10.1212/WNL.0000000000201168. Epub ahead of print. PMID: 36008153.

Vallat JM, Duchesne M, Corcia P, et al. The wide spectrum of pathophysiologic mechanisms of paraproteinemic neuropathy. *Neurology* 2021;96(5):214–225. doi: 10.1212/WNL.0000000000011324. Epub 2020 Dec 4. PMID: 33277411.

CASE 12 Polyneuropathy, Organomegaly, Endocrine Manifestations, Monoclonal Protein, and Skin Changes (POEMS) Syndrome

Clinical History

A 49-year-old man noticed a diminished sensation in his feet. Two months later, climbing stairs became difficult due to proximal muscle weakness of his legs. Over the next three months, sensory disturbances and both proximal and distal weakness progressed in arms and legs requiring the use of a walker or a wheelchair. Besides COPD, he was previously in a healthy condition. Based upon ancillary investigations, he was initially diagnosed with chronic inflammatory demyelinating polyneuropathy (CIDP), had received a course of intravenous Ig (IVIg), and was subsequently treated with high-dose corticosteroids (60 mg/day). He did not smoke or use drugs such as nitric oxide.

Examination

We examined the patient, about eight months after onset of symptoms, when he was wheelchair-bound. General examination revealed clear atrophy of the lower arms and hand muscles as well as the proximal muscles of the legs. There was erythema of part of the hands and knuckles (Fig. 12.1). His hands and feet were very cold and sweaty. Cranial nerves revealed no abnormalities. Arms: proximal muscle weakness MRC grade 4, wrist extensors MRC grade 2, intrinsic hand muscles 3, grip force was almost absent. Legs: proximal and knee extensors grade 4, dorsiflexors and extensors feet grade 0. Sensory examination: hyperpathy of both hands. Legs: diminished sensation for pain and touch distally up to halfway the lower legs. Position sense was impaired distally of his knees. Vibration sense was almost absent distally from the hips. Areflexia with flexor response was observed. He was able to rise from a chair, to stand, and to make a transfer to his wheelchair. Walking was impossible without help.

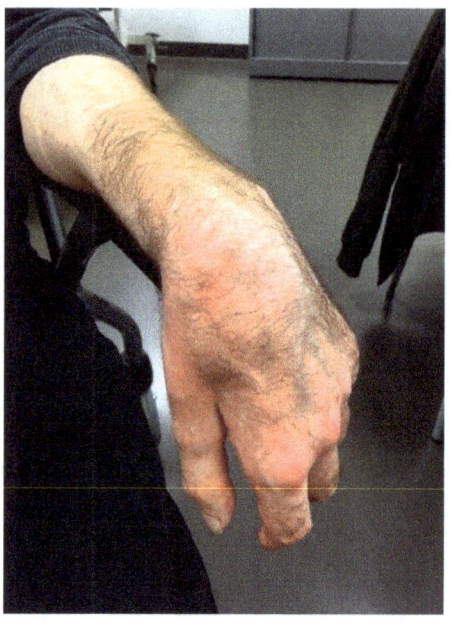

Figure 12.1 Atrophy of forearm and dorsal interosseal I muscle and discolouration of the hand in the described patient.

Diagnostic Considerations

Based on the symmetric proximal and distal weakness and sensory disturbances for a period of over two months, CIDP was considered. EMG examination showed a demyelinating polyneuropathy, which had been the reason to start IVIg (on referral, it was reported that there had been no response) and subsequently corticosteroids 60 mg/day. When we first examined the patient, weakness and especially the severe atrophy of both the intrinsic hand muscles and forearms was strikingly present (Fig. 12.1). Erythema on the knuckles of the fingers suggested Gottron sign, but other skin features of dermatomyositis were absent. Especially the severe atrophy of his forearms was considered disproportional for a diagnosis of CIDP. This was one of the reasons that we considered a haematological abnormality, in particular POEMS (polyneuropathy, organomegaly, endocrinopathy, monoclonal protein, and skin changes) syndrome, or another diagnosis related to the presence of a paraprotein, in particular multiple myeloma or amyloidosis. Other types of malignancy were also considered, but most of these are not associated with a demyelinating polyneuropathy. In patients suspected to have CIDP, often in the presence of ataxia, who do not improve after conventional treatment, an autoimmune nodopathy should also be considered. In these patients, testing of antibodies against paranodal antigens (neurofascin 155, Caspr 1, and Contactin 1) should be performed. Because there was severe atrophy that developed over a few months, motor neuron disease could be considered, but this is not compatible with the severe sensory abnormalities. The patient did not use drugs (especially no amiodarone, see **Case 24**) known to be associated with a demyelinating polyneuropathy.

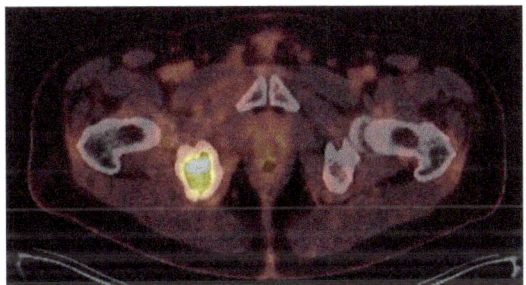

Figure 12.2 PET-CT showing increased uptake (highlight) in the acetabulum (plasmacytoma).

Ancillary Investigations

Glucose 12.5 mmol/L; HbA1c 34 (26–42 mmol/mol), CK 40 U/L (< 171), IgA 1.84, IgG 13.3; IgM 0.86 (normal). IgG-L M(para)-protein (8 g/L), free-ratio kappa/lambda ratio: 1.19 (0.26–1.65). Vascular endothelial growth factor (VEGF) 92.000 pg/mL (0.016–0.786). Hormones: testosterone: 5.8 (10–30 nmol/L); TSH, cortisol, LH, oestradiol, growth hormone, and prolactin: no abnormalities. Normal CSF: 2 mononuclear cells, total protein 1.45 g/L.

EMG: No or low sensory nerve action potentials (SNAPs), sensory nerve conduction velocity ulnar nerve 34 m/s. Motor nerve conduction velocities of ulnar and median nerves 24–40 m/s. In two nerves increased motor distal latencies and motor nerve conduction blocks were found. These results were compatible with the EAN/PNS criteria for CIDP.

Bone marrow: 3% plasma cells, no amyloid. CT-abdomen: no liver or splenomegaly. PET-CT: osteosclerotic plasmacytoma, no muscle abnormalities (Fig. 12.2).

Follow-Up

Based on the combination of abnormalities, that is, EMG showing a demyelinating polyneuropathy, the presence of an IgG-L M-protein, a sclerotic bone lesion, the erythema, the presence of highly increased VEGF, and low testosterone compatible with hypogonadism, the diagnosis POEMS was made. The patient initially was treated with a combination of corticosteroids and lenalenomide, and with local radiotherapy. This resulted in improvement of the strength of wrist extensors and proximal leg muscles. IgG-L paraprotein decreased to 2 g/L, and the abnormalities on the PET-CT improved. A few months later he received autologous stem cell transplantation. This all went very well, and the patient made a remarkable improvement within months. Muscle force in his hands almost completely normalized, but distal weakness in the feet persisted. With the use of ankle-foot orthoses he could walk relatively well.

General Remarks

POEMS syndrome is a rare clonal plasma cell disorder characterized by multi-systemic features. Although the acronym stands for polyneuropathy, organomegaly, endocrinopathy, monoclonal gammopathy, and skin changes, not all of these symptoms need to be present.

A polyneuropathy (most often demyelinating) and a monoclonal paraprotein (about 90% of cases are lambda light chain restricted) are requirements, and additionally there are other major and minor criteria (Table 12.1, Fig. 12.3). More than 90% of patients have cutaneous manifestations, which may include hyperpigmentation, haemangioma, skin thickening, and hypertrichosis. These skin changes may be restricted to the hands and fingers (acrocyanosis, white nails). Endocrinopathy can be an important part of the syndrome; however, diabetes and thyroid disease alone are insufficient because they are quite common. Hence, tests for other endocrine abnormalities (hypogonadism, abnormal adrenal function, and calcium metabolism) are required. VEGF level reflects disease activity, which is helpful for the diagnosis and evaluation of treatment response. VEGF is a cytokine produced by plasma cells that increases vascular permeability and causes a capillary leak syndrome, leading to pleural effusion, ascites, peripheral oedema, and in some patients also papilloedema. It has been

Part II Neuromuscular Cases: Peripheral Neuropathies

Table 12.1 Diagnostic criteria for POEMS syndrome

Mandatory major criteria (both required)
- Polyneuropathy, typically conduction slowing ('demyelinating')
- Monoclonal plasma cell disorder, typically lambda light chain restricted

Other major criteria (one required)
- Sclerotic bone lesions
- Elevated VEGF (typically plasma levels > 200 pg/mL)
- Castleman disease (lymph node hyperplasia in chest or abdomen, actually in any area of the body where lymph nodes are found)

Minor criteria (one required)
- Organomegaly (splenomegaly, hepatomegaly, lymphadenopathy)
- Extravascular volume overload (peripheral oedema, ascites, pleural effusions)
- Endocrinopathy (adrenal, pituitary dysfunction, hypogonadism, parathyroid)*
- Skin changes (hyperpigmentation, hypertrichosis, glomeruloid haemangioma, plethora, acrocyanosis, flushing, white nails)
- Papilloedema
- Thrombocytosis or polycythaemia

* Given the frequent occurrence of thyroid dysfunction and diabetes mellitus, these conditions alone are not diagnostic of POEMS syndrome.

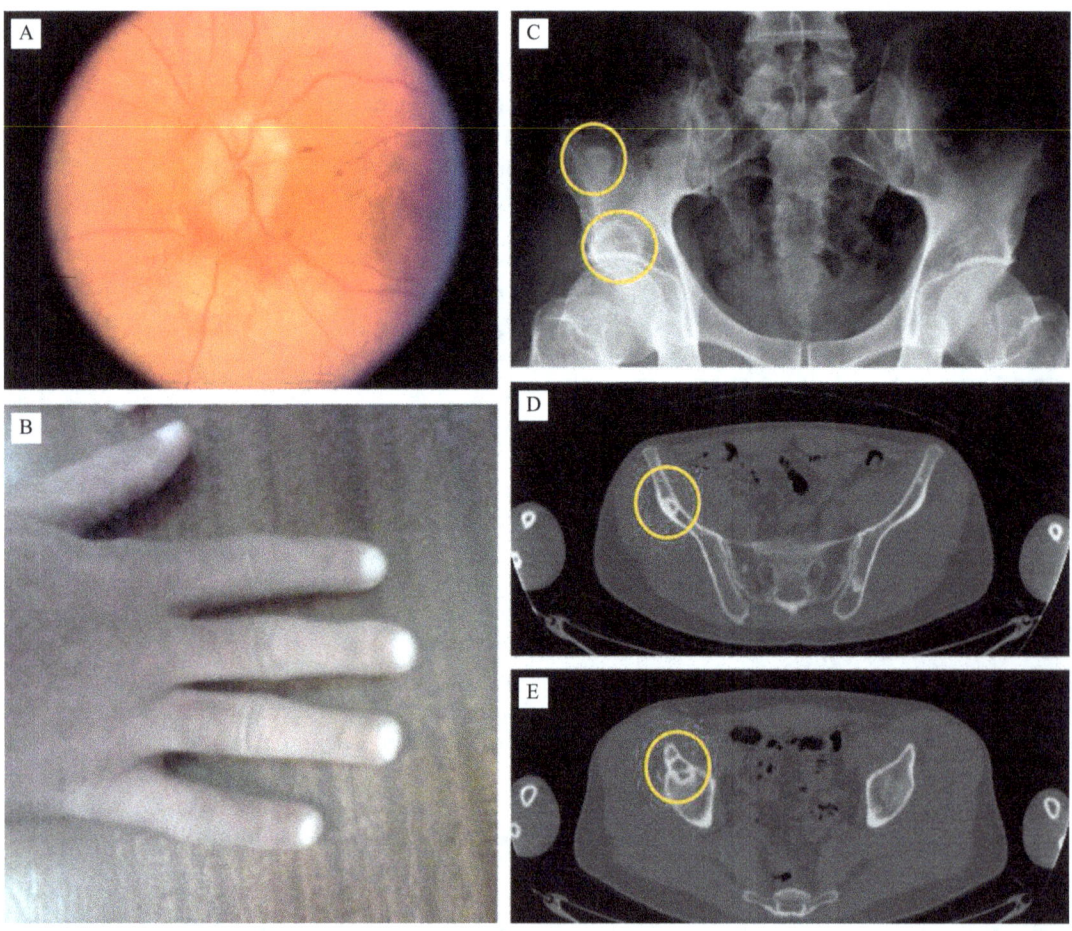

Figure 12.3 (A–E) Manifestations of POEMS syndrome. Optic disc oedema (A). Skin changes including white nails and cyanosis (B). Mixed lytic osteosclerotic bone lesions on plain radiograph (C) and CT scan (D and E). From Dispenzieri A, Am *J Hematol* 2019;94:812–827, with permission.

reported that a VEGF cut-off limit of 200 pg/mL has a sensitivity of 68% and specificity of 95%, whereas a cut-off of 1,920 pg/mL gives a sensitivity of 73.3% and a specificity of 97.6%. The diagnosis POEMS can be difficult but should always be in the differential diagnosis, especially when a CIDP is considered in a patient with lambda light chain monoclonal gammopathy, and if there is no fast response after IVIg or corticosteroids.

Treatment and Prognosis

Early diagnosis and active treatment targeted to the monoclonal protein can result in a good recovery. However, symptoms may also persist. The prognosis is particularly poor when treatment is delayed. There are several treatment options. Conventional agents such as corticosteroids and melphalan are considered an effective and safe combination. Radiotherapy can be effective in patients with localized lesions. The anti-myeloma agents lenalidomide, thalidomide, and bortezomib have shown good outcomes for POEMS syndrome, but these are not effective in all patients, and large-scale studies with long-term follow-up are required. Autologous hematopoietic stem cell transplantation is another option for high-risk transplant-eligible patients.

Suggested Reading

Bou Zerdan M, George TI, Bunting ST, Chaulagain CP. Recent advances in the treatment and supportive care of POEMS syndrome. *J Clin Med* 2022;11(23):7011. doi: 10.3390/jcm11237011. PMID: 36498588; PMCID: PMC9741379.

Dispenzieri A. POEMS syndrome: 2019 update on diagnosis, risk-stratification, and management. *Am J Hematol* 2019;94(7):812–827. doi: 10.1002/ajh.25495. Epub 2019 May 23. PMID: 31012139.

D'Sa S, Khwaja J, Keddie S, et al. Comprehensive diagnosis and management of POEMS syndrome. *Hemasphere* 2022;6(11):e796. doi: 10.1097/HS9.0000000000000796. PMID: 36340912; PMCID: PMC9624442.

Khouri J, Nakashima M, Wong S. Update on the diagnosis and treatment of POEMS (polyneuropathy, organomegaly, endocrinopathy, monoclonal gammopathy, and skin changes) syndrome: a review. *JAMA Oncol* 2021;7(9):1383–1391. doi: 10.1001/jamaoncol.2021.0586. PMID: 34081097.

Kim YR. Update on the POEMS syndrome. *Blood Res* 2022;57(S1):27–31. doi: 10.5045/br.2022.2022001. PMID: 35483922; PMCID: PMC9057663.

Vasculitic Neuropathy

Clinical History

A 53-year-old man developed a left-sided foot drop and a painful sensation on the ventral side of the foot and outer part of the lower leg. Two weeks later, the same symptoms also developed on the right side. In addition, he noticed progressive numbness of his lower legs. Three weeks later, he noticed weakness of his right hand, and was unable to spread his fingers. He had no other symptoms, and his medical history was not informative. He did not recall a tick bite or erythema migrans, or any pulmonary abnormality, and had not visited tropical countries. He does not sit with crossed legs.

Examination

Six weeks after disease onset, walking was impaired due to bilateral drop foot. Cranial nerves were normal. He had no atrophy of the arms or hands. Sensory innervation in the area of the ulnar nerve on the right side and the peroneal nerve on both sides was impaired. There was atrophy of the anterior tibial muscles. He was unable to stand on his heels and could barely stand on his toes. Several muscle groups were paretic, predominantly the interossei, hamstrings, peroneal, anterior and posterior tibial muscles, and the triceps surae (MRC grade 4). Pain, touch, and vibration senses were impaired in the feet. Achilles tendon reflexes were absent. Provocative tests for radiculopathy tests

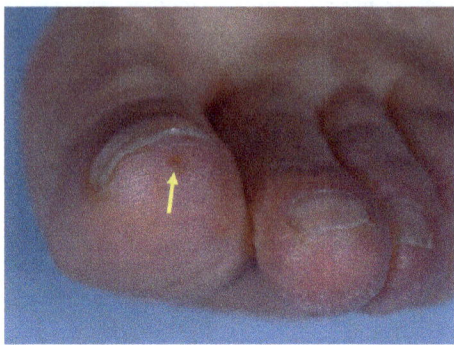

Figure 13.1 Skin lesion (arrow) suggestive of vasculitis in the described patient.

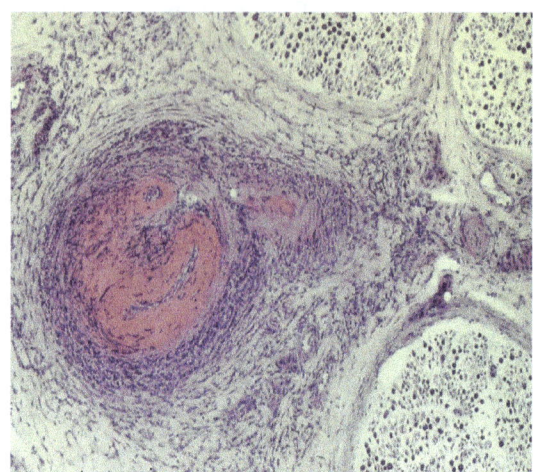

Figure 13.2 Sural nerve biopsy showing necrotizing vasculitis with fibrinoid necrosis of the vascular wall with inflammatory cell infiltrate and occlusion of the lumen (H&E stain).

were negative. Clinical examination of the skin revealed signs suggestive of vasculitis (Fig. 13.1).

Diagnostic Considerations

Painful multifocal peripheral nerve involvement and the presence of skin lesions were suggestive for a vasculitis. Serological abnormalities indicating a systemic vasculitis would be helpful for the diagnosis. Multifocal chronic inflammatory demyelinating polyneuropathy (CIDP) can progress rapidly. Therefore, electrodiagnostic testing should focus on demyelinating abnormalities. There were no other features suggesting chronic inflammation, such as sarcoidosis. The absence of a history of a tick bite, erythema migrans, or radicular symptoms made Lyme disease unlikely; however, serological testing and cerebrospinal examination should be considered. Although there were no clinical signs suggestive of diabetes, systemic disease, or (haematological) malignancy, serological examination should be conducted to screen for these diseases. The rapid development of signs and symptoms is not compatible with leprosy as a cause of this multifocal neuropathy. The painful rapidly progressive multifocal neuropathy with skin changes in the absence of signs indicating one the above-mentioned diseases suggested a predominantly nonsystemic vasculitis, which can be diagnosed in a sural nerve biopsy.

Ancillary Investigations

C-reactive protein (CRP) was 11 (normal < 10); the number of eosinophilic granulocytes was slightly raised. Glucose and HbA1c were normal. Anti-nuclear antibodies (ANA) 1:160 (normally: negative). Anti-neutrophil cytoplasmic autoantibodies (ANCA), SS-A, and SS-B were negative. There was no monoclonal protein; liver enzymes and creatinine levels were normal. Serological testing for syphilis and Lyme disease was negative. Motor nerve action potentials of the right-sided ulnar nerve and both tibial and peroneal nerves were decreased, compatible with axonal degeneration. Sensory nerve action potentials of the right-sided ulnar nerve were decreased, and the sural nerve action potentials were absent. Motor nerve conduction studies of the ulnar, median, and radial nerve did not show signs of demyelination (no motor nerve conduction blocks, no nerve conduction slowing or increased distal latency times).

Cerebral spinal fluid analysis revealed a slightly elevated protein content, 0.5 g/L (normal < 0.45), and a mild pleiocytosis of 8×10^6 lymphocytes/L (normal < 4), without malignant cells.

A sural nerve biopsy showed signs of vasculitis with fibrinoid necrosis of the vascular wall (Fig. 13.2).

Follow-Up

The patient was diagnosed with a vasculitic neuropathy. Treatment with corticosteroids 60 mg/day was started. Pain decreased and sensory abnormalities improved. Weakness did not progress further and tended to improve over the next few months.

To establish whether muscle strength eventually improves warrants a longer treatment duration and observation period.

General Remarks

Most patients with vasculitis have systemic features either as a manifestation of primary systemic vasculitis such as polyarteritis nodosa (PAN), eosinophilic granulomatosis with polyangiitis (EGPA), microscopic polyangiitis (MPA), or a systemic vasculitis secondary to underlying connective tissue disease, cryoglobulinaemia, drug exposure, viral infection, or paraneoplastic syndrome (Table 13.1).

Vasculitis, however, may also be confined to the peripheral nervous system. In the latter group, low titres of ANA and slightly elevated levels of CRP or ESR can be found. Nonsystemic vasculitic neuropathy is a rare disease that usually has a subacute onset with progressive sensory or sensorimotor deficits. Asymmetry, pain, and weakness are other key features (Table 13.2). However, not all patients with a peripheral nerve vasculitis have clear asymmetric features over time, and some may only present with painful symmetric involvement resembling a polyneuropathy.

The diagnosis of nonsystemic vasculitis can only be made by excluding other causes, for example by the absence of clinical signs of systemic vasculitis, or clearly positive ANA, ANCA, or SS-A/SS-B. If the diagnosis cannot be made based on serological tests, a nerve biopsy may be indicated. Most often a sural nerve biopsy will be conducted. To increase the sensitivity to find a vasculitis (not only a perivascular infiltrate) in nerve and/or muscle we usually try to do a combined sural nerve and a peroneal muscle biopsy via one incision.

High-dose corticosteroids (60 mg/day or 1 mg/kg/day) are the mainstay of treatment for vasculitis. In severe cases, treatment can be initiated with high-dose methylprednisolone (IV), and especially in systemic vasculitis, a combination with pulse cyclophosphamide or rituximab can be considered. The best treatment for the nonsystemic form has yet to be established. In addition to corticosteroids, cytotoxic drugs (such as azathioprine) are often co-administrated to act as a more potent combination, or to reduce the corticosteroid dosage especially when there is a fear of side effects when using long-term high-dose

Table 13.2 Main features of a peripheral nerve vasculitis

- Usually asymmetric motor and sensory involvement
- Peroneal/fibular and ulnar nerve(s) are frequently involved
- Often (but not always) painful
- Progressive in weeks to months
- Most often systemic disease and/or associated with other disorders
- Lab: CRP, ANA, ANCA not increased in isolated peripheral nerve vasculitis
- EMG: usually multifocal abnormalities, no signs of demyelination
- If no clinical or laboratory abnormalities indicating a systemic vasculitis are found, consider sural nerve biopsy

Table 13.1 Classification of vasculitis associated with neuropathy

Primary systemic vasculitis

Microscopic polyangiitis, granulomatosis with polyangiitis (previously Wegener granulomatosis), eosinophilic granulomatosis with polyangiitis (previously Churg–Strauss syndrome), cryoglobulinaemia (non-HCV), Henoch–Schönlein purpura, PAN, giant cell arteritis

Secondary systemic vasculitis

Associated with one of the following:

Connective tissue disorders: rheumatoid arthritis, systemic lupus erythematosus
Sjogren syndrome, systemic sclerosis, dermatomyositis, mixed connective tissue disease
Other disorders: sarcoidosis, Behçet disease, inflammatory bowel disease
Infection (such as HBV, HCV, HIV, CMV, leprosy, Lyme disease, HTLV-1)
Drugs or malignancy

Nonsystemic vasculitis

- Nonsystemic vasculitic neuropathy
- Diabetic radiculoplexus neuropathy
- Localized cutaneous/neuropathic vasculitis: cutaneous PAN

corticosteroids. Rehabilitation care such as ankle-foot orthoses and physiotherapy is often indicated.

Systemic vasculitis may have a very severe and even lethal disease course. The prognosis regarding the neuropathy varies. In nonsystemic vasculitis, the progression is generally slower than in systemic vasculitis and the prognosis is better. Patients with nonsystemic vasculitis may recover completely. However, steroid treatment may be required for a long period. Long-term follow-up studies show that most patients can walk without assistance and are independent as far as activities of daily living are concerned.

Suggested Reading

Collins MP, Dyck PJB, Hadden RDM. Update on classification, epidemiology, clinical phenotype and imaging of the nonsystemic vasculitic neuropathies. *Curr Opin Neurol* 2019;32(5):684–695. doi: 10.1097/WCO.0000000000000727. PMID: 31313704.

Gwathmey KG, Tracy JA, Dyck PJB. Peripheral nerve vasculitis: classification and disease associations. *Neurol Clin* 2019;37(2):303–333. doi: 10.1016/j.ncl.2019.01.013. Epub 2019 Mar 18. PMID: 30952411.

Koike H, Nishi R, Ohyama K, et al. ANCA-associated vasculitic neuropathies: a review. *Neurol Ther* 2022;11(1):21–38. doi: 10.1007/s40120-021-00315-7. Epub 2022 Jan 19. PMID: 35044596; PMCID: PMC8857368.

Small-Fibre Neuropathy (SFN)

Clinical History

A 48-year-old man had complained about the painful soles of his feet for several months. This pain was present constantly but increased on touch and when walking. He was a marathon runner but could no longer train or walk properly because of the pain. He did not report weakness, sensory disturbances, discoloration of his feet, or swelling of his joints. Otherwise, he was healthy. He was not known to have diabetes mellitus or any other chronic disorder, such as sarcoidosis, which can cause a painful neuropathy. There were no cardiovascular or intestinal complaints, and no symptoms of autonomic dysfunction. Symptoms that could suggest malignancy were absent. He did not use any medication, had not been treated with any neurotoxic drug earlier, did not smoke, and drank only very limited amounts of alcohol. There was no family history of neurological disorders.

Examination

Neurological examination was normal. In particular, the tendon reflexes were normal and there were no sensory disturbances, except for the fact that touching the soles of his feet was extremely painful. On inspection, his feet looked normal. No discolorations of the skin nor abnormalities of the joints or tendons were observed. He did not show clinical signs of autonomic dysfunction, such as abnormal sweating, and a test for orthostatic hypotension was negative.

Diagnostic Considerations

The clinical symptoms, in combination with a normal neurological examination with the exception of hyperpathia of the soles of his feet, suggested the presence of small-fibre neuropathy (SFN) (Table 14.1). Electrophysiological studies are useful to assess whether the symptoms of SFN are part of a

Table 14.1 Symptoms suggesting SFN

Sensory symptoms
- Pain (burning sensation, tingling, shooting painful cold sensation, pins and needles)
- Dysesthesia (distorted sensitivity to a stimulus)
- Allodynia (abnormal pain due to a stimulus that does not normally provoke pain)
- Hypesthesia to heat, cold, and pinprick

Autonomic symptoms
- Hypo/anhidrosis, hyperhydrosis, sicca syndrome
- Gastrointestinal symptoms (constipation, diarrhoea, early or slow gastric emptying)
- Urinary incontinence or retention, erectile dysfunction
- Disorders of accommodation
- Orthostatic hypotension

Table 14.2 Diseases associated with SFN

Metabolic	Diabetes mellitus, hypothyroidism, hypertriglyceridemia, uraemia, vitamin B12 deficiency
Toxic	Alcohol, drugs (nitrofurantoin, chemotherapy, antiretroviral agents), vitamin B6 intoxication
Immune-mediated	Sarcoidosis, Sjögren syndrome, Guillain–Barré syndrome, paraneoplastic, scleroderma, systemic lupus erythematosus, vasculitis, paraprotein-related cryoglobulinaemia, primary amyloidosis
Infections	HIV, hepatitis C virus, influenza, leprosy, Lyme disease, sepsis/critical illness
Genetic	Hereditary amyloidosis (hATTR), hereditary sensory and autonomic neuropathy (HSAN), Fabry disease, variants of genes for the voltage-gated sodium channel, mainly *SCN9A* and *COL6A5*
Idiopathic (I-SFN)	No cause yet identified

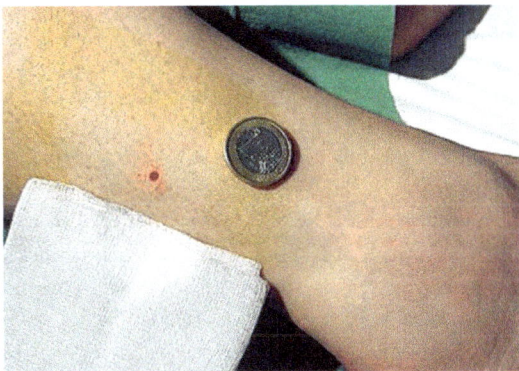

Figure 14.1 Skin biopsy taken at the ankle. Note the small size of the biopsy compared with the 1 euro coin.

polyneuropathy. As SFN can also be a feature of a systemic disease such as in diabetes/prediabetes, sarcoidosis, or Sjögren disease (Table 14.2), it is also useful to conduct serological or other laboratory studies. Vitamin B6 intoxication and B12 deficiency can cause SFN. Some other diseases that may cause painful feet, such as arthritis (painful, local swelling), or erythromelalgia (episodic, located at the toes, soles, dorsum, or the entire foot, becomes red or violaceous, hot, painful, sometimes with swelling), were considered unlikely.

Ancillary Investigations

Routine laboratory examination revealed no abnormalities, in particular ESR and HbA1c were normal, and there were no signs of liver or kidney dysfunction. There was no indication of sarcoidosis (no symptoms, ESR normal, s-IL2 R (CD25) was not increased) or Sjögren disease (SS-A and SS-B were negative). Vitamin B6 and B12 levels were normal. He had no monoclonal protein and TSH was normal. Nerve conduction studies were normal. Detailed quantitative sensory testing was not available in our centre. Other diseases associated with SFN were excluded, or considered unlikely (see Table 14.2). As SFN was considered, a skin biopsy was taken (Fig. 14.1). This biopsy showed a reduced intra-epidermal nerve fibre density (IENFD), compatible with the diagnosis of definite SFN. Genetic testing for sodium channel (*SCN9A*, *SCN10A*, *SCN11A*) variants was not performed.

Follow-Up

We did not identify a cause of SFN in this patient and during the next five years no other disease known to be related to SFN was diagnosed. The patient was treated with several drugs for painful neuropathy with limited success.

General Remarks

The clinical presentation of SFN is dominated by pain or autonomic disturbances (see Table 14.1). Pain in SFN is most frequently described as burning, shooting, or prickling. Dysautonomic features may include dry eyes or mouth, orthostatic dizziness, bowel and micturition disturbances, accommodation problems, impotence, flushes, and palpitations. SFN typically presents in a length-dependent fashion, often first affecting the feet. More rarely, the clinical presentation is characterized by non-length-dependent, focal, or multifocal symptoms. An autonomic phenotype also occurs. Pure (isolated) SFN does not show abnormalities in motor and large sensory nerve fibre function at neurological examination and nerve conduction studies (NCS).

The term 'small-fibre neuropathy' is used when there is structural injury selectively affecting small-diameter sensory and/or autonomic axons (thinly myelinated Aδ and unmyelinated C fibres). SFN complicates many diseases but can also be an isolated disorder (see Table 14.2). Especially from a (differential) diagnostic perspective, it is important to differentiate isolated (or pure) SFN from disorders associated with large-fibre neuropathies that often have tactile, vibration, and position sense abnormalities and reduced tendon reflexes. Nerve conduction studies (NCS) show abnormalities in patients with large-fibre neuropathies, whereas these are normal in isolated SFN. Many patients with large-fibre neuropathy additionally may have small nerve fibre involvement (nonisolated SFN).

SFN involvement is suggested initially by history taking and physical examination (see Table 14.1). However, the diagnosis of SFN can be difficult as clinical symptoms can be vague and NCS are normal in isolated SFN. Therefore, additional investigations are required to definitely diagnose SFN (Table 14.3). Functional neurophysiological testing, including testing of autonomic function, with, for example, heat sensitivity testing or quantitative sensory testing, can provide diagnostic information indicating SFN. In particular, measurement of IENFD in a skin biopsy has significantly improved the diagnostics of SFN (Figs. 14.2 and 14.3). It has been found that a skin biopsy taken at the ankle has a sensitivity of 58–90% in patients suggested as having SFN, with a specificity of 95% (largely dependent upon the selection of patients and controls), and is considered the gold standard for the diagnosis. Taking a skin biopsy is relatively easy and the procedure is relatively harmless. However, there is a practical disadvantage of using skin biopsies as a routine diagnostic tool, because determination of IENFD is a time-consuming and a technically dedicated

Table 14.3 Grading the diagnosis of SFN

Possible SFN

Length-dependent symptoms and/or clinical signs of small-fibre damage

Probable SFN

Length-dependent symptoms, clinical signs of small-fibre damage, and normal sural nerve conduction studies

Definite SFN

Length-dependent symptoms, clinical signs of small-fibre damage, normal sural nerve conduction studies, and reduced IENFD at the ankle and/or abnormal thermal threshold

From: Tesfaye S et al. *Diabetes Care* 2010;33:2285–2293.

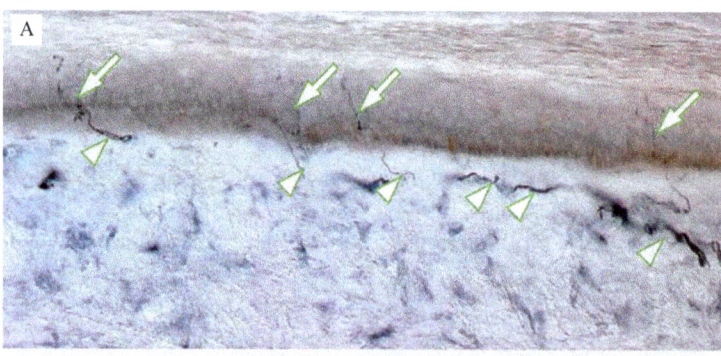
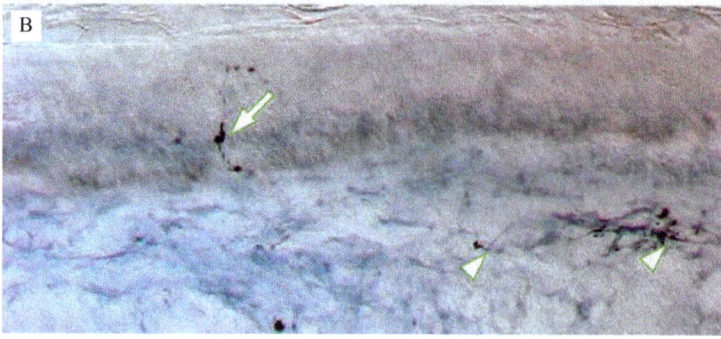

Figure 14.2 (A,B) Intra-epidermal nerve fibre density (IENFD). Healthy control: normal density of intra-epidermal nerve fibres (stained black, arrows) (A). Reduced number of intra-epidermal nerve fibres in a patient with diabetic neuropathy (B). From Sommer C, Lauria G, Skin biopsy in the management of peripheral neuropathy. *Lancet Neurol* 2007;6:632–642, with permission.

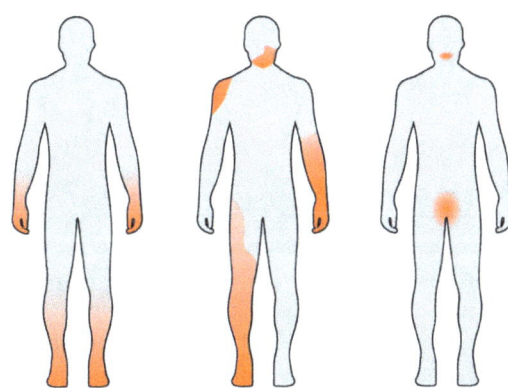

Length-dependent   Non-length-dependent   Atypical/focal

Figure 14.3 Small-fibre neuropathy can have different clinical presentations. The typical pattern of a length-dependent polyneuropathy includes pinprick and thermal sensory loss as well as evoked or spontaneous pain in a stocking-glove distribution. Some patients complain of patchy or diffuse distribution of symptoms in a non-length-dependent manner. Focal involvement as in burning mouth syndrome or vulvodynia can occur also. From Devigili et al., *Expert Rev Neurother* 2020;23:1–14, with permission.

procedure that is only available in some laboratories.

There are many different conditions associated with SFN (see Table 14.2). Still, the cause remains unknown in about 50% of cases. An important advance is the finding that 25–30% of cases initially labelled as idiopathic SFN are in fact associated with gain-of-function variants of the voltage-gated sodium channels Nav1.7, Nav1.8, and Nav1.9 (encoded by the genes *SCN9A*, *SCN10A*, and *SCN11A*). These sodium channels are present on dorsal roots and sympathetic ganglions and on their small-diameter peripheral axons. Gain-of-function variants can make these sodium channels hyperexcitable, leading to neuronal and length-dependent axonal degeneration and to clinical signs of a painful SFN.

Management of small-fibre neuropathy depends on the underlying cause and on concurrent treatment of neuropathic pain. There is no neuroprotective therapy available. Pain due to SFN is often difficult to treat. If pain persists after treatment of the underlying cause (if known), treatment with antidepressants (such as amitriptyline), anticonvulsants (such as pregabalin, lacosamide, topiramate, sodium valproate, or carbamazepine), opioids, topical therapies with capsaicin, or nonpharmacological treatments (e.g., cooling the extremities or transcutaneous electrical nerve stimulation (TENS)) can be tried. In patients with *SCN9A* variants, nonselective sodium channel blockers (e.g., carbamazepine, lidocaine, or mexiletine) could be tried. There is no best practice for pain treatment in SFN, and most data are derived from studies that include patients with combined mixed neuropathic pain syndromes. A randomized placebo-controlled study indicated that treatment with intravenous immunoglobulin (IVIg) is not effective in idiopathic SFN (Geerts et al., 2021). Additional controlled trials studying the effect of pharmacological treatment of pain due to SFN are urgently needed.

Suggested Reading

Chan ACY, Kumar S, Tan G, et al. Expanding the genetic causes of small-fiber neuropathy: SCN genes and beyond. *Muscle Nerve* 2023;67(4):259–271. doi: 10.1002/mus.27752. Epub 2022 Nov 30. PMID: 36448457.

Devigili G, Cazzato D, Lauria G. Clinical diagnosis and management of small fiber neuropathy: an update on best practice. *Expert Rev Neurother* 2020;20(9):967–980. doi: 10.1080/14737175.2020.1794825. Epub 2020 Jul 23. PMID: 32654574.

Geerts M, de Greef BTA, Sopacua M, et al. Intravenous immunoglobulin therapy in patients with painful idiopathic small fiber neuropathy. *Neurology* 2021;96(20):e2534–e2545. doi: 10.1212/WNL.0000000000011919. Epub 2021 Mar 25. PMID: 33766992; PMCID: PMC8205474.

Hoeijmakers JGJ, Merkies ISJ, Faber CG. Small fiber neuropathies: expanding their etiologies. *Curr Opin Neurol* 2022;35(5):545–552. doi: 10.1097/WCO.0000000000001103. Epub 2022 Aug 11. PMID: 35950732.

Sopacua M, Hoeijmakers JGJ, Merkies ISJ, et al. Small-fiber neuropathy: expanding the clinical pain universe. *J Peripher Nerv Syst* 2019;24(1):19–33. doi: 10.1111/jns.12298. Epub 2019 Jan 8. PMID: 30569495.

Terkelsen AJ, Karlsson P, Lauria G, et al. The diagnostic challenge of small fibre neuropathy: clinical presentations, evaluations, and causes. *Lancet Neurol* 2017;16(11):934–944. doi: 10.1016/S1474-4422(17)30329-0. Erratum in: Lancet Neurol. 2017 Dec;16(12):954. PMID: 29029847.

Case 15: Sensory Neuronopathy (SNN, Ganglionopathy)

Clinical History

A 73-year-old-woman noticed pain in her right lower leg and thigh and left foot. After a few weeks of physiotherapy, she gradually developed tingling in her feet and a 'plastic' sensation in the soles of her feet. A few weeks later, her feet became completely numb, and she noticed painful tingling in her hands and around her left knee. Because of the tingling in her hands, she could barely use a fork and knife. Walking became difficult due to the dull feelings in her legs. Several drugs against painful neuropathy did not help. For years she had smoked two packs of cigarettes a week. A total of 50 pack-years was estimated.

Examination

The cranial nerves were normal. Pain and tactile sense were impaired in her hands and absent in her feet just above the ankles. The position sense of the big toe was absent, but the vibration sense appeared normal. She demonstrated sensory ataxia with the knee–heel test. There was minor bilateral weakness of the extensor hallucis longus muscle. Knee tendon reflexes were markedly reduced, Achilles tendon reflexes were absent. She had a broad-based gait. While standing with eyes closed, she had impressive positive Romberg sign.

Diagnostic Considerations

The subacute onset of painful multifocal/asymmetric sensory neuropathy and sensory ataxia in a patient with a 50 pack-year history of smoking suggested a paraneoplastic sensory neuronopathy (SNN). Some other considerations were Sjögren syndrome; a sensory ataxic variant of chronic inflammatory demyelinating polyneuropathy (CIDP); pyridoxine intoxication; herpes zoster dorsal root ganglia infection; and some more chronic conditions like chronic ataxic neuropathy, ophthalmoplegia, immunoglobulin M (IgM) paraprotein, cold agglutinins, and disialosyl antibodies (CANOMAD); syphilis; and chronic immune sensory polyradiculoneuropathy (CISP).

Ancillary Investigations

Routine laboratory analysis did not reveal abnormalities. EMG showed normal motor and sensory conduction velocities, but sensory nerve action potentials (SNAPs) were slightly decreased. A CT scan of the thorax revealed a tumour in the right lung. Pathological examination on a lung biopsy demonstrated a small-cell lung carcinoma (SCLC). Serum anti-Hu antibodies were strongly positive.

Follow-Up

The patient was diagnosed with subacute paraneoplastic sensory neuronopathy. She received systemic chemotherapy and chest radiotherapy. She reached remission of SCLC and reported less sensory disturbances. During this period, neurological examination did not clearly change.

General Remarks

Sensory Neuronopathies (SNN) (Ganglionopathies)

Sensory neuronopathies (SNN) or ganglionopathies are a rare and heterogeneous spectrum of acquired and genetic disorders caused by selective, primary degeneration of dorsal root ganglia (DRG) and their central and peripheral projections. DRG vascularization is dense and has a unique characteristic not found anywhere else in the peripheral nervous system (PNS), as capillaries in DRG are fenestrated, forming a loose blood–nerve interface. As a consequence, DRG exhibit a high permeability to many molecules such as blood-derived immune cells, antibodies, viruses, or toxic components (Fig. 15.1). Some conditions specifically or predominantly affect subgroups of neurons, resulting in either a predominantly ataxic or a painful neuropathy.

Inflammatory damage to DRG and their projections often results in a multifocal pattern of sensory deficits and is sometimes accompanied by motor symptoms due to additional involvement

Case 15 Sensory Neuronopathy (SNN, Ganglionopathy)

Table 15.1 Diagnostic criteria for sensory neuronopathy (SNN)

(a) Ataxia in the lower or upper limbs at onset or full development of the neuropathy	3.1
(b) Asymmetric distribution of sensory loss at onset or full development of the neuropathy	1.7
(c) Sensory loss not restricted to the lower limbs at full development	2.0
(d) At least one SAP absent or three SAP < 30% of the lower limit of normal in the upper limbs, not explained by entrapment neuropathy	2.8
(e) Fewer than two nerves with abnormal motor NCS in the lower limbs	3.1
	Total score 0–12.7

- Possible SNN if total score > 6.5
- Probable SNN if total score > 6.5 and if the initial work-up does not show biological perturbations or ENMG findings (conduction blocks, temporal dispersion) excluding SNN. Or if the patient has one of the following disorders: onconeural antibodies or a cancer within 5 years, cisplatin treatment, or Sjögren syndrome. Or MRI shows a high signal in the posterior column of the spinal cord.
- Definite SNN if DRG degeneration is pathologically demonstrated, but DRG biopsy is not recommended.

DRG = dorsal root ganglia; ENMG = electroneuromyographic study; NCS = nerve conduction studies; SAP = sensory action potential.

Shortened version of: Graus et al., Updated diagnostic criteria for paraneoplastic neurologic syndromes, *Neurol Neuroimmunol Neuroinflamm* 2021;8:e1014. doi: 10.1212

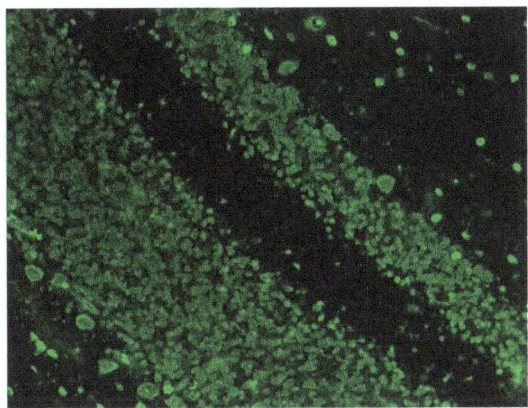

Figure 15.1 Immunofluorescent staining of dorsal root ganglia, by the presence of anti-Hu antibodies. Courtesy Dr. S. Veenbergen.

of motor nerve roots of peripheral nerves. This is in contrast with the usual length-dependent pattern found in most polyneuropathies

Patients with SNN – regardless of aetiology – have a non-length-dependent involvement of all sensory modalities, which is clinically predominated by sensory ataxia. There is a patchy and asymmetric sensory deficit, with reduced or absent tendon reflexes, and there is no weakness. Knee–heel and/or finger–nose test are usually clearly impaired, and patients have difficulty with an attempt to stand or to walk with closed eyes. Painful paraesthesias or dysesthesias may occur. Diagnostic criteria based upon the clinical and electrophysiological work-up can be helpful in making the diagnosis of SNN in patients with a clinically pure sensory neuropathy (Table 15.1).

Paraneoplastic SNN

A paraneoplastic origin should be in particular considered if there is a subacute evolution in combination with severe pain, increased number of cells in the CSF, or when there is additional motor involvement. The most frequent antibody found in paraneoplastic SNN is anti-Hu, followed by CV2/CRMP5 and amphiphysin (Table 15.2). SNN can occur at any point during the course of cancer, even during or after chemotherapy or after radiation. SNN is mostly associated with small-cell lung carcinoma (SCLC), whereas other tumours (lung adenocarcinoma, breast, prostate) are far less frequently associated with SNN. In a patient with onconeural antibodies in whom the initial work-up for cancer is negative, malignancy screening should be repeated after three months and every six months for four years after disease onset.

The prognosis of tumour-related SNN depends upon the type of tumour. If the neuropathy directly precedes the symptoms of the tumour, the prognosis may be better because of a combination of early detection and treatment of the malignancy.

Table 15.2 High-risk antibodies (> 70% associated with cancer) for paraneoplastic sensory neuronopathy (SNN)

Antibody	Neurological phenotype	Frequency of cancer	Usual tumours
Hu	SNN, chronic GI pseudo-obstruction, EM, and LE	85%	SCLC ≫ NSCLC, neuroendocrine tumours, neuroblastoma
CV2/CRMP5	SNN and EM	80%	SCLC and thymoma
PCA2	Sensorimotor neuropathy, rapidly progressive cerebellar syndrome, EM	80%	SCLC, NSCLC, and breast cancer
Amphiphysin	SNN, polyradiculoneuropathy, EM, SPS	80%	SCLC and breast cancer

CRMP5 = collapsin response-mediator protein 5; EM = encephalomyelitis; GI= gastrointestinal; LE = limbic encephalitis; NSCLC = non-small-cell lung cancer; PCA = Purkinje cell antibody; SCLC = small-cell lung cancer; SNN = sensory neuronopathy; SPS = stiff-person syndrome.

From: Graus et al., Updated diagnostic criteria for paraneoplastic neurologic syndromes, *Neurol Neuroimmunol Neuroinflamm* 2021;8:e1014. doi: 10.1212

Suggested Reading

Amato AA, Ropper AH. Sensory ganglionopathy. *i* 2020;383(17):1657–1662. doi: 10.1056/NEJMra2023935. PMID: 33085862.

Antoine JC. Sensory neuronopathies, diagnostic criteria and causes. *Curr Opin Neurol* 2022;35(5):553–561. doi: 10.1097/WCO.0000000000001105. Epub 2022 Aug 11. PMID: 35950727.

Camdessanché JP, Jousserand G, Ferraud K, et al. The pattern and diagnostic criteria of sensory neuronopathy: a case-control study. *Brain* 2009;132:1723–1733. doi: 10.1093/brain/awp136. Epub 2009 Jun 8. PMID: 19506068; PMCID: PMC2702838.

Fargeot G, Echaniz-Laguna A. Sensory neuronopathies: new genes, new antibodies and new concepts. *J Neurol Neurosurg Psychiatry* 2021;jnnp-2020-325536. doi: 10.1136/jnnp-2020-325536. Epub ahead of print. PMID: 33563795.

Graus F, Vogrig A, Muñiz-Castrillo S, et al. Updated diagnostic criteria for paraneoplastic neurologic syndromes. *Neurol Neuroimmunol Neuroinflamm* 2021;8(4):e1014. doi: 10.1212/NXI.0000000000001014. PMID: 34006622; PMCID: PMC8237398.

Titulaer MJ, Soffietti R, Dalmau J, et al.; European Federation of Neurological Societies.Screening for tumours in paraneoplastic syndromes: report of an EFNS task force. *Eur J Neurol* 2011;18(1):19–e3. doi: 10.1111/j.1468-1331.2010.03220.x. Epub 2010 Sep 29. PMID: 20880069; PMCID: PMC3086523.

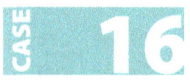

Wartenberg Migrant Sensory Neuropathy

Clinical History

A 64-year-old man's complaints had begun four years earlier with a burning pain at the glans of the penis, which lasted for several days, and was followed by a numb feeling that resolved after a few weeks. Some months later, there was an electric shock-like sensation at the side of his right lower leg, soon followed by numbness in that affected skin area. Over the ensuing years, there was a repeating pattern of a short-lasting sharp, burning pain, often during only one day, which evolved into a numb feeling that most of the time resolved completely in weeks to months. Several body parts had been affected in this way: the upper left leg, the fingers of his right hand, one by one, and the chest. Lately this had also occurred on his right cheek. The frequency of the attacks had not changed over the years. There had never been any weakness or any symptoms indicating autonomic dysfunction, apart from a dry mouth. He did not recall having made any sudden stretching movements prior to the onset of any attack. He was otherwise healthy, without weight loss or other systemic symptoms. He did not feel functionally disabled.

Examination

There was a 'half-numb' feeling at the touch of some body parts that had been affected. Otherwise, the neurological examination was normal, including a full examination of the sensation, and tendon reflexes.

Diagnostic Considerations

The clinical history is very typical for Wartenberg migrant sensory neuropathy. We considered a nonsystemic vasculitic neuropathy less likely because of the lack of motor involvement and the lack of progression. In hereditary neuropathy with liability to pressure palsy, there are usually sensory disturbances that can be attributed to entrapment of large nerves. There was no preceding pain. Because of the remitting and relapsing disease course, we further considered a pure sensory form of chronic inflammatory demyelinating neuropathy, but the pattern of sudden neuropathic pain followed by sensory loss is not typical for this disease. Sensory neuronopathies such as may occur in Sjögren syndrome or in cancer were considered even less likely because of the intermittent nature of the complaints and the absence of progression over many years.

Ancillary Investigations

Because the alternative diagnoses were very unlikely we did not perform laboratory investigations, nerve conduction studies, or nerve ultrasound studies. We also refrained from performing a sural nerve biopsy since the finding of vasculitis (see below) would not alter our wait-and-see policy.

Follow-Up

We explained to the patient that Wartenberg migratory sensory neuropathy is a chronic disorder that in general does not get worse over time. As for pain medication, he had experienced that paracetamol and NSAIDs did not relieve the pain. Besides, the attacks were not perceived severe enough to justify the daily use of medication against neuropathic pain, and in addition, he was also reluctant to use a drug that could affect his cognition.

General Remarks

Wartenberg migrant sensory neuropathy is characterized by a typical history of multifocal attacks that start with a sudden-onset stabbing or burning sensation in the distribution of a small cutaneous nerve, lasting one or a few days (Table 16.1). This is followed by a loss of sensation that resolves completely or partially in weeks to months. All cutaneous nerves can be affected, including the trigeminal nerve. Wartenberg neuropathy remains a clinical diagnosis. There are no ancillary investigations to confirm the diagnosis. Laboratory studies are normal. Sensory nerve action potentials may be absent or small in affected nerves. High-resolution ultrasound can show enlargement of multiple nerves even if clinical testing and nerve conduction studies are normal.

In the long run, a minority of patients are completely asymptomatic. In about half of the patients, some numbness remains. In some patients, there is persistent pain. The attack frequency is variable, usually not more than twice a year.

The cause is not known. About half of the patients recall that abrupt stretching of the affected body part, for example overextending the foot or flexing the wrist, precedes the onset of an episode. In the other patients, without mechanical triggers, the disorder is considered a form of nonsystemic vasculitis but findings in sural nerve biopsies have been inconclusive.

Table 16.1 Main clinical features of Wartenberg migrant sensory neuropathy

- Age at onset 30–60 years
- Multifocal sensory impairment in the distribution of small cutaneous nerves, completely or partially resolving in weeks–months, preceded by short-lasting burning pain
- Mechanical trigger (e.g., abrupt stretching) in 50% of patients
- Attack rate varies, usually no more than two episodes per year
- Limited impact on daily life
- In general. no progression to polyneuropathy

Because of the relatively benign course, treatment other than medication if there is persistent burdensome pain is not advocated.

Suggested Reading

Collins MP, Hadden RD. The nonsystemic vasculitic neuropathies. *Nat Rev Neurol* 2017;13(5):302–316. doi: 10.1038/nrneurol.2017.42. PMID: 28447661.

Herraets IJT, Goedee HS, Telleman JA, et al. High-resolution ultrasound in patients with Wartenberg's migrant sensory neuritis, a case-control study. *Clin Neurophysiol* 2018;129(1):232–237. doi: 10.1016/j.clinph.2017.10.040. Epub 2017 Nov 21. PMID: 29202391.

Stork AC, van der Meulen MF, van der Pol WL, et al. Wartenberg's migrant sensory neuritis: a prospective follow-up study. *J Neurol* 2010;257(8):1344–1348. doi: 10.1007/s00415-010-5530-7. Epub 2010 Mar 31. PMID: 20354714; PMCID: PMC2910306.

CASE 17 Multifocal Motor Neuropathy (MMN)

Clinical History

A 50-year-old man was initially seen by a rheumatologist because he had crooked fingers on the left hand and painful cramps. No rheumatological abnormalities were found. In the next three years, he developed severe atrophy and weakness of the left hand, and could not hold a glass of water. There were no sensory complaints. His GP considered motor neuron disease.

Examination

When we investigated the patient, he already had clear atrophy of the left first dorsal interosseous and thenar muscles (Fig. 17.1). Fasciculations were found in the left triceps and in the right calf muscles. There was weakness of the following muscles: extensor pollicis (MRC grade 3); first dorsal interosseous (4); flexor pollicis (0); abductor pollicis brevis (2); opponens pollicis (4); deep and superficial flexors of the second and third fingers (4), all on the left. He had bilateral weakness of the calf muscle, MRC grade 4. Sensation was normal. Tendon reflexes were low in the arms and absent in the legs. Plantar responses were flexor. He could rise from a chair without difficulty, could stand on his heels, but not on tiptoes.

Diagnostic Considerations

The combination of slowly gradual progressive multifocal motor weakness without sensory disturbances was clinically compatible with motor neuron disease, segmental spinal muscular atrophy, multifocal motor chronic inflammatory demyelinating polyneuropathy (CIDP), and multifocal motor neuropathy (MMN) (Tables 17.1 and 17.2).

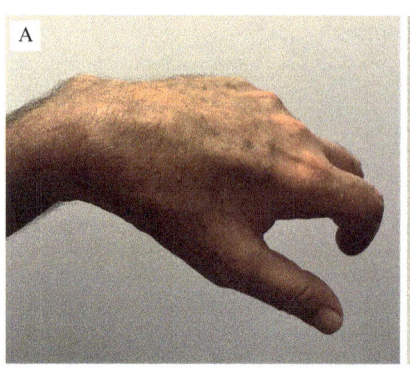
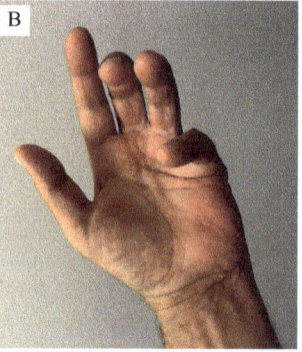

Figure 17.1 Patient with MMN: atrophy, weakness, and functional loss of the hands, without sensory disturbances and in the presence of multifocal motor nerve conduction blocks (nerve conduction studies), due to involvement of multiple motor nerves (ulnar, radial, and median nerve).

Table 17.1 Diagnostic criteria for multifocal motor neuropathy (MMN), based on the criteria proposed by the European Federation of Neurological Societies/Peripheral Nerve Society (EFNS/PNS), 2010, and by Vlam et al., 2011

A. Clinical criteria

The two core criteria for MMN (both must be present)

- Slowly progressive or stepwise progressive, focal, asymmetric limb weakness, that is, motor involvement in the motor nerve distribution of at least two nerves, for more than one month. If symptoms and signs are present only in the distribution of one nerve, only a possible diagnosis can be made.
- No objective sensory abnormalities except for minor vibration sense abnormalities in the lower limbs.

Supportive clinical criteria

- Predominant upper limb involvement
- Decreased or absent tendon reflexes in the affected limb
- Absence of cranial nerve involvement
- Cramps and fasciculations in the affected limb
- Response in terms of reduction of disability or increase in muscle strength to immunomodulatory treatment

Clinical exclusion criteria

- Upper motor neuron signs
- Marked bulbar involvement
- Sensory impairment more marked than minor vibration loss in the lower limbs
- Diffuse symmetric weakness during the initial weeks

B. Electrophysiological criteria

(1) Definite motor nerve conduction block* present in at least one motor nerve

(2) Probable motor nerve conduction blocks* in at least two nerves

(3) Normal sensory nerve conduction in upper limb segments with conduction blocks and normal SNAP amplitudes

Proposed level of certainty

Definite MMN: combination of clinical criteria AND electrophysiological criteria 1 and 3

Probable MMN: combination of clinical criteria AND electrophysiological criteria 2 and 3

Possible MMM: combination of clinical criteria AND laboratory findings AND nerve conduction studies (not meeting 1 or 2), showing demyelination in the absence of sensory abnormalities

The diagnosis of MMN is more likely when the following laboratory findings are present.

C. Supportive laboratory findings

- High-titre IgM anti-GM1 antibodies
- MRI abnormalities on T2-weighted MRI of brachial plexus
- CSF protein < 1g/L

SNAP = sensory nerve action potential.
* Conduction block(s) must be found at sites different from common entrapment or compression sites

---

Motor neuron disease usually has a faster rate of progression. This especially is the case in amyotrophic lateral sclerosis (ALS), in which patients additionally have upper motor neuron signs. Atrophy and weakness in progressive muscular atrophy (PMA) is usually more generalized, and relatively rapidly progressive, but somewhat slower than in most patients with ALS, and may resemble the patient's clinical picture. Other diagnoses that need to be considered: multifocal CIDP, previously also known as Lewis–Sumner syndrome or multifocal acquired demyelinating sensory and motor neuropathy (MADSAM), but these patients mostly have sensory disturbances as well. Hereditary neuropathy with liability to pressure palsies (HNPP) usually has conduction blocks at sites of entrapment, prolonged distal motor latencies, and some slowing of sensory and motor nerve conduction. In inclusion body myositis (IBM), there is characteristically asymmetric weakness of the deep finger flexors, but not of other hand muscles until much later in the disease course. Mononeuritis multiplex due to vasculitis is usually painful, includes sensory loss, and has a stepwise progressive course. Nerve conduction studies are essential to make a distinction between these various conditions and MMN.

Table 17.2 Differential diagnosis of multifocal motor neuropathy (MMN)*

	Multifocal motor neuropathy (MMN)	Motor neuron disease (MND)	Segmental or focal spinal muscular atrophy (SMA)	Chronic inflammatory demyelinating polyneuropathy (CIDP)	Multifocal CIDP
Weakness	Asymmetric	Asymmetric	Asymmetric	Symmetric	Asymmetric
Sensory involvement	No	No	No	Yes	Often
Course	Slowly progressive	Rapidly progressive (ALS)	Slowly progressive	Progressive or relapsing	Progressive or relapsing
CSF protein	Normal	Normal	Normal	Often increased	Can be increased
IgM-GM1 antibodies	Often present	No	No	No	No
EMG (nerve conduction studies)	Multifocal motor conduction blocks (CBs)	No CBs	No CBs	Signs of demyelination, often with CBs	Multifocal motor and sensory CBs
Nerve US/MRI increased signal	Asymmetric	No	May be abnormal	Symmetric	Symmetric/ asymmetric
Response to IVIg	Yes	No	No	Yes	Yes
Long term IVIg required	Yes	Not applicable	Not applicable	Sometimes	Sometimes
Response to cortico-steroids	No	No	No	Yes	Yes

ALS = amyotrophic lateral sclerosis; CB = conduction block; IVIg = intravenous immunoglobulins.
* This table does not list inclusion body myositis (IBM) and hereditary neuropathy with liability to pressure palsies (HNPP).

Ancillary Investigations

An EMG showed proximal conduction blocks in the left median and ulnar nerves, and the left tibial nerve. Sensory nerve conduction was normal. Laboratory investigation revealed normal CK and no IgM anti-GM1 antibodies.

Follow-Up

The EMG findings of two or even three motor nerve conduction blocks are compatible with the diagnosis of multifocal motor neuropathy (MMN) and not with PMA, segmental SMA, ALS, or IBM. The late onset, a negative family history, as well as the absence of a history of pressure palsies, and of conduction blocks over nerve compression sites excluded HNPP. The other differential diagnoses were ruled out based upon the clinical likelihood in combination with the EMG findings (Table 17.2). The patient was treated with a five-day course of intravenous immunoglobulins (IVIg) (0.4.g/kg/day) leading to clear improvement. He could again hold a glass of water and muscle cramps largely disappeared. The foot drop virtually disappeared as well. He required intermittent IVIg infusions, on average in a dosage of 40 g every 3 weeks to maintain a relatively good clinical condition. Attempts to reduce the dosage or frequency of IVIg infusions during a treatment period of 10 years failed.

General Remarks

MMN is a rare condition that was first described some 40 years ago. It is a pure motor neuropathy

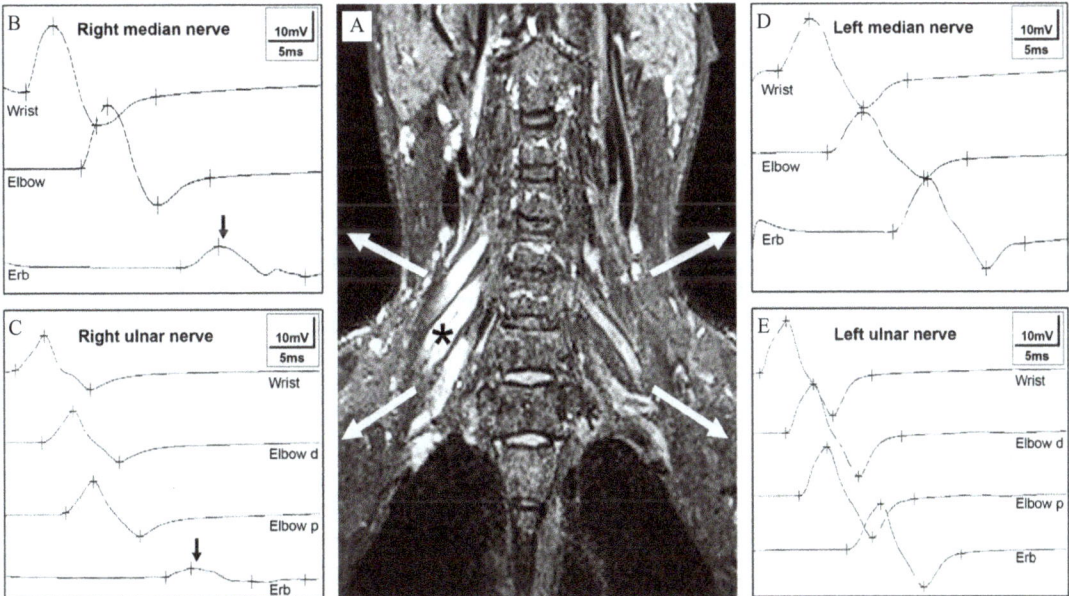

Figure 17.2 (A–E) MRI showing asymmetrical thickening of nerve trunks and corresponding motor nerve conduction blocks. MRI of the brachial plexus in multifocal motor neuropathy (A). Coronal short tau inversion recovery (STIR) MRI demonstrates diffuse enlargement and abnormally high signals at the level of the trunks in the right brachial plexus (asterisk). Electrodiagnostic studies reveal partial conduction block in the right median and ulnar nerves, localized between the elbow and Erb's point (B,C; black arrows). No blocks are observed in the left median and ulnar nerves (D,E). From Echaniz-Laguna A, Dietemann JL, Neurological picture. Seeing the blocks: MRI of the brachial plexus in multifocal motor neuropathy. *J Neurol Neurosurg Psychiatry* 2011;82:728, with permission.

with slowly progressive weakness of distal limb muscles and electrophysiological conduction blocks (CBs) outside nerve compression sites (ulnar groove, carpal tunnel, and peroneal/fibular head). The mean age at onset is 40 years (range 20–70 years). Onset in childhood or in adults over 70 years of age is rare. Onset is mostly in a hand, but patients may present with a foot drop. The weak muscles initially belong to the innervation area of a single peripheral nerve, and later may evolve to a more diffuse pattern. Cramps and fasciculations occur frequently in affected muscles. Initially, atrophy is not prominent, but is usually present at presentation, as there is often a referral delay. Sensation is normal. Reflexes in affected limbs can be absent or present, but are not pathologically increased as in ALS. In general, nerve conduction studies are required to diagnose MMN. If not diagnostic, nerve ultrasound or MRI of the brachial plexus or proximal median nerve can be helpful if it shows an increased nerve diameter or hypertrophy of multiple nerves. Nerve ultrasound seems more sensitive than MRI. These findings, however, are not specific to MMN, as this can also be found in other inflammatory neuropathies, such as CIDP. One study showed a combination of thickened cervicobrachial nerve roots and motor nerve conduction blocks (Fig. 17.2). The exact specificity of these imaging techniques, however, is still not fully known, as nerve hypertrophy has also been found in some patients with ALS and even in healthy controls. CSF examination is not helpful. High titres of serum IgM anti-GM1 antibodies can be found in about 40% of MMN cases. Other laboratory investigations that may help to diagnose MMN are currently not known.

MMN is hypothesized to be an immune-mediated disorder in which autoantibodies, B cells, and complement activation play a role. Without treatment, severe weakness and atrophy develop, leading to serious disability. When patients are diagnosed at a very late stage, MMN mimics severe PMA with preserved respiration. IVIg is an effective treatment for MMN. IVIg, however, is an expensive treatment and patients with MMN generally require continuation of maintenance treatment (e.g., once every three to four weeks) to avoid reappearance of muscle weakness. Therefore, IVIg should be initiated especially in MMN patients who experience weakness and disability. It is important to realize that despite the positive effects of IVIg maintenance treatment, the disease is not cured. Some patients may experience slow progression of weakness and atrophy after several years of treatment, which is likely due to secondary axonal degeneration. Surprisingly, some other immune-modulating therapies, notably corticosteroids, are ineffective. Whether anti-CD20 therapy (rituximab) or monoclonal antibodies preventing complement activation are successful requires further investigation.

Suggested Reading

Joint Task Force of the EFNS and the PNS. European Federation of Neurological Societies/Peripheral Nerve Society guideline on management of multifocal motor neuropathy. Report of a joint task force of the European Federation of Neurological Societies and the Peripheral Nerve Society – first revision. *J Peripher Nerv Syst* 2010;15(4):295–301. doi: 10.1111/j.1529-8027.2010.00290.x. PMID: 21199100.

Keddie S, Eftimov F, van den Berg LH, et al. Immunoglobulin for multifocal motor neuropathy. *Cochrane Database Syst Rev* 2022;1(1):CD004429. doi: 10.1002/14651858.CD004429.pub3. PMID: 35015296; PMCID: PMC8751207.

Oudeman J, Eftimov F, Strijkers GJ, et al. Diagnostic accuracy of MRI and ultrasound in chronic immune-mediated neuropathies. *Neurology* 2020;94(1):e62–e74. doi: 10.1212/WNL.0000000000008697. Epub 2019 Dec 11. PMID: 31827006.

Telleman JA, Herraets IJ, Goedee HS, van Asseldonk JT, Visser LH. Ultrasound scanning in the diagnosis of peripheral neuropathies. *Pract Neurol* 2021;21(3):186–195. doi: 10.1136/practneurol-2020-002645. Epub 2021 Feb 4. PMID: 33541914.

Vlam L, van der Pol WL, Cats EA, et al. Multifocal motor neuropathy: diagnosis, pathogenesis and treatment strategies. *Nat Rev Neurol* 2011;8(1):48–58. doi: 10.1038/nrneurol.2011.175. PMID: 22105211.

Yeh WZ, Dyck PJ, van den Berg LH, Kiernan MC, Taylor BV. Multifocal motor neuropathy: controversies and priorities. *J Neurol Neurosurg Psychiatry* 2020;91(2):140–148. doi: 10.1136/jnnp-2019-321532. Epub 2019 Sep 11. PMID: 31511307.

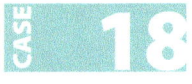

Peripheral Nerve Hyperexcitability Syndromes: Morvan Syndrome

Clinical History

A 58-year-old previously healthy man had complaints of fluctuating drooping eyelids and weakness of neck extensors, arms, and legs. He almost continuously experienced double vision. Following a diagnosis of myasthenia gravis and improvement with pyridostigmine, he noticed twitches and spasms of muscles virtually all over his body. This became severe, he did not sleep well, was restless, and almost continuously felt the urge to move and walk around. His wife mentioned that he also behaved differently. Initially, a pyridostigmine intoxication was considered, but lowering the dose did not help. Additionally, some autonomic features (constipation, erectile dysfunction) appeared.

Examination

We examined the patient three months after onset of symptoms and found a fluctuating right-sided ptosis, external ophthalmoparesis, and weakness of neck extensors, arms, and legs (all compatible with myasthenia gravis). Additional radiological examination revealed a thymoma. Half a year after thymomectomy, we noted widespread and gross abnormal muscle movements (cramps, fasciculations, gross muscle twitches) most pronounced in arms and legs, but also in all other parts of the body.

Diagnostic Considerations

Initially, myasthenia gravis with thymoma was diagnosed. Because of the widespread spontaneous muscle activity (despite reduction of pyridostigmine), autonomic disturbances, restless activity,

Table 18.1 Peripheral nerve hyperexcitability syndromes and selected related acquired disorders

Disorder	Neuromuscular features	Autonomic dysfunction	EMG	Central nervous system signs	Auto-antibodies
Cramp-fasciculation syndrome	Cramp and fasciculations	–	Fasciculations	–	Rarely CASPR2, LGI1
Isaacs syndrome	Cramp and fasciculations, painful stiffness	(+)	Neuro-myotonia, myokymia	–	CASPR2 > LGI1
Morvan syndrome	Cramp and fasciculations, painful stiffness	+	Neuro-myotonia, myokymia	Encephalo-pathy	CASPR2, LGI1
Limbic encephalitis	–	–	Normal	Encephalo-pathy	LGI1 > CASPR2, adverse outcome
Stiff person syndrome	Axial painful rigidity and spasms	–	Continuous motor unit activity	Hyperreflexia, triggered spasms	GAD65
Rippling muscle disease	Rippling, mounding, percussion-induced rapid contractions	–	Electrically silent	–	AChR and/or striated muscle

behavioural changes, and insomnia, we considered Morvan syndrome.

Ancillary Investigations

Antibodies against acetylcholine receptors (AChR): photoreceptor outer segments (pos) (> 20 nmol/L), antibodies against muscle-specific kinase (MuSK), and striated muscle were negative. Anti-CASPR2 and anti-LGI1 antibodies were positive. Repetitive nerve stimulation confirmed the neuromuscular transmission dysfunction; Needle EMG showed widespread fasciculation potentials, myokymic discharges, and multiplets.

Follow-Up

When the diagnosis of Morvan syndrome was made, based on the combination of symptoms, including central nervous system symptoms in the presence of CASPR2 and LGI1 antibodies, treatment was intensified with a combination of high-dose corticosteroids, azathioprine, and plasma exchange. The patient made a reasonably good recovery. The widespread muscle overactivity completely disappeared, but fluctuating myasthenic symptoms remained.

General Remarks

The peripheral nerve hyperexcitability syndromes (Table 18.1) form a spectrum including cramp-fasciculation syndrome, Isaacs syndrome, and Morvan syndrome, and are characterized by muscle stiffness, cramps, and muscle twitches with abnormal electrical activity on needle EMG.

Cramp-Fasciculation Syndrome

Cramp-fasciculation syndrome is considered a benign condition because it does not involve muscle weakness and does not evolve into progressive muscular atrophy or amyotrophic lateral sclerosis. However, cramps are very painful, and the muscle twitching may be worrying. Symptoms and signs are most prominent in the calves but may extend to most other parts of the body. Fasciculations and cramps can be seen on neurological examination, but there are no other abnormalities such as muscle weakness or atrophy. Needle electromyography shows fasciculation potentials and normal motor unit action potentials. Low-frequency repetitive nerve stimulations often shows after-discharges, which additionally confirms the diagnosis, but is not required to make the diagnosis. Membrane-stabilizing drugs such as carbamazepine (200–

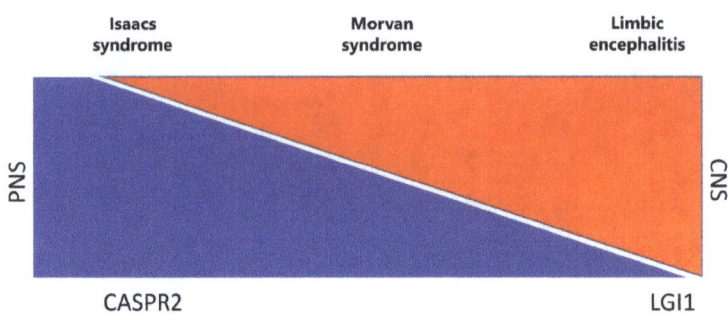

Figure 18.1 Spectrum of peripheral nerve hyperexcitability syndromes, limbic encephalitis, and antibodies against CASPR2 and LGI1.

600 mg/day) can be considered as treatment of first choice if the symptoms are severe.

Isaacs Syndrome and Morvan Syndrome

These conditions are much rarer than the cramp-fasciculation syndrome. Symptoms and signs of both disorders include muscle stiffness, generalized myokymia (muscle twitching and undulation) (**Video 18.1**), and autonomic symptoms such as hyperhidrosis, sialorrhoea, and orthostatic hypotension. Paraesthesia and neuropathic pain can also occur. EMG shows spontaneous motor unit activities including fasciculation potentials and myokymic and neuromyotonic discharges. Often, anti-CASPR2 and anti-LGI1 antibodies, both part of the voltage-gated potassium channel (VGKC) complex, can be found. Especially in these patients, neoplasms, notably thymoma, may co-exist, and some of these patients also have myasthenia gravis with anti-AChR antibodies.

Isaacs syndrome is diagnosed if confined to peripheral nerves. In Morvan syndrome, there are also signs of central nervous system involvement, notably insomnia, hallucinations, and agitation. Morvan syndrome shares these features with limbic encephalitis, which is also associated with anti-LGI1 and CASPR2 antibodies but lacks in general features of peripheral nerve hyperexcitability (Fig. 18.1).

The clinical course of Isaacs and Morvan syndromes is usually slowly progressive, with fluctuations. Therapy with plasma exchange, intravenous immunoglobulins, and/or high-dose corticosteroids and rituximab may ameliorate the symptoms.

Suggested Reading

De Wel B, Claeys KG. Neuromuscular hyperexcitability syndromes. *Curr Opin Neurol* 2021;34(5):714–720. doi: 10.1097/WCO.0000000000000963. PMID: 34914668.

Sawlani K, Katirji B. Peripheral nerve hyperexcitability syndromes. *Continuum (Minneap Minn)* 2017;23(5, Peripheral Nerve and Motor Neuron Disorders):1437–1450. doi: 10.1212/CON.0000000000000520. PMID: 28968370.

Idiopathic Brachial Plexus Neuropathy, Neuralgic Amyotrophy (NA)

Clinical History

A 33-year-old man was referred because of winging of the right scapula. History taking disclosed that seven months prior to referral he had experienced excruciating pain in the neck, irradiating to the right arm and thumb. The pain, which was particularly severe in the right scapular region, kept him initially awake and lasted for approximately six weeks. A week after the pain had started, he noticed having difficulty raising his right arm and hand. The latter is no longer present but at referral he still had a right-sided winged scapula and sensory disturbances of the radial part of the right medial forearm and of part of his thumb. Family history was negative for neuromuscular diseases.

Examination

He was athletically built, and on neurological examination a scapula alata on the right was observed (Fig. 19.1). Slight atrophy of the right infraspinatus and rhomboid muscle was observed. There was moderate weakness of the right serratus anterior and rhomboid muscle and hypaesthesia of the radial part of the right forearm and the thumb. Right biceps reflex was absent. Otherwise, there were no abnormalities.

Diagnostic Considerations

The acute onset of severe, nonradicular pain followed by paresis of arm muscles, innervated by more than one nerve, is characteristic of a diagnosis of idiopathic neurologic amyotrophy (NA).

Ancillary Investigations

EMG showed polyphasic, long-duration motor unit action potentials in the infraspinatus and serratus anterior muscles.

General Remarks

NA, also known as idiopathic brachial plexus neuropathy or Parsonage–Turner syndrome, is a monophasic acute-onset upper brachial plexopathy. It is characterized by severe pain that is usually worse at night. In Table 19.1 other characteristics are described. When a patient presents with a typical history and classic clinical symptoms of the disorder, any further investigation (e.g., EMG, MRI) does not contribute to the diagnosis.

NA often manifests with winging of the scapula due to involvement of the long thoracic nerve, usually unilateral, but bilateral involvement is found in 20–30%. This classic phenotype is observed in about 70% of patients. NA can also manifest with involvement of other peripheral nerves, such as the median nerve (resembling anterior interosseous nerve syndrome) and radial nerve (resembling posterior interosseous nerve syndrome), or the lower brachial plexus with sympathetic nervous system involvement (resembling complex regional pain syndrome), lumbosacral involvement (resembling radiculopathy), and phrenic nerve involvement. The lumbosacral variant of neuralgic amyotrophy (lumbosacral radiculoplexus neuropathy) typically occurs in patients with mild type 2 diabetes mellitus, but it can also occur in non-diabetics. All NA patients with phrenic nerve involvement (manifesting with exertional dyspnoea, orthopnoea, sleep disturbance, excessive daytime fatigue in both unilateral and bilateral cases) have brachial plexus involvement.

NA is not a rare disease given a one-year incidence rate for the classic phenotype of 1 per 1,000. NA can occur at all ages, with a median onset age of around 40 years for the idiopathic form. It may occur in neonates and elderly people as well. Paediatric NA is similar to adult-onset NA. Painless episodes are more frequent in children and long-term recovery seems to be better. Men are affected twice as frequently as women. Recurrences may occur in 25% in 5–10 years after the first attack.

NA is considered an organ-specific, immune-mediated disorder. The exact cause of NA is not clear. Immunological, mechanical, and genetic factors have been implicated.

More than half of the patients report an antecedent event, infection being the most frequent event, followed by exercise and surgery. About 10% of NA patients have a concomitant hepatitis E virus (HEV) infection in the acute phase. These patients appear to have a distinctive clinical phenotype. They are older, have bilateral and more extensive involvement of the brachial plexus, and are more likely to have phrenic nerve and

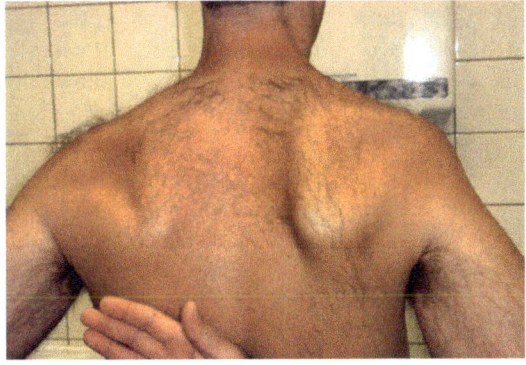

Figure 19.1 Atrophy of rhomboid muscle and winging of the right scapula due to serratus anterior and rhomboid muscle weakness.

Table 19.1 Clinical features of neuralgic amyotrophy

Pain	In ~90% pain precedes weakness, in only a minority attacks are painless	Stuttering onset in a proportion of patients	Duration: average 40 days (1–60), males have a longer duration than females	Localization: mostly shoulder or cervical spine/neck into arm, sometimes scapular/dorsal region to chest wall and/or arm, and rarely lower plexus distribution or chest wall region
Motor involvement	In one-third first signs of weakness < 24 h	In ~40% after 1–7 days	In a minority after 1–2 weeks	Muscle atrophy occurs in the majority of patients, 2–5 weeks after onset of attack
Site of motor involvement	Plexus brachialis – unilateral in ~70%, bilateral in 20–30%	Upper and/or middle plexus including long thoracic nerve in half of the patients; lower plexus is rare	Predominantly interior inter-osseous nerve is rare	In a proportion of patients, the lumbosacral plexus is affected; rarely the phrenic nerve, recurrent laryngeal nerve, or other nerves, e.g., intercostal nerves
Sensory involvement	~70%, mainly hypaesthesia			
Recovery	In ~60% between first and sixth month, in ~20% 6–12 months, in ~20% < 1 month or > 1 year	Chronic pain in about half of NA and ~60% of hereditary neuralgic amyotrophy (HNA) patients; mild persistent paresis in NA (~70%), moderate to severe paresis in a small proportion. In HNA more frequently persistent moderate or severe weakness		One-third of NA and HNA patients reported a 90–99% recovery; most HNA patients and a proportion of NA patients, respectively, report < 50% recovery

lumbosacral plexus involvement compared with NA cases without HEV infection.

Management and Prognosis

Managing the acute pain is a priority. However, the pain is mostly therapy-resistant. In a large cohort study, the best option proved to be a combination of a long-acting opioid with an NSAID, which was found to relieve pain in 60% of patients.

There are no sufficient data to support efficacy of corticosteroids or intravenous immunoglobulins (IVIg). One exception is patients with hereditary neuralgic amyotrophy (HNA) (see below) with proven, recurrent postprocedural attacks in whom preventive steroids (with or without IVIg) prevented surgery- or labour-induced attacks.

Most patients have substantial recovery of strength in their weak muscles over the course of 6–18 months, except for recovery from distal upper limb and phrenic nerve involvement, which can take up to 3–4 years. Approximately 60% of NA patients still suffer pain on follow-up after 6 to more than 24 months, and more than 80% have impaired shoulder movements. Regular physical therapy, mostly consisting of strength training, is ineffective or may worsen symptoms in half of NA patients. A non-blinded randomized controlled trial showed that a multidisciplinary rehabilitation programme focused on motor relearning to improve scapular dyskinesia, combined with self-management strategies for reducing pain and fatigue, had more beneficial effects on shoulder, arm, and hand functional capability than usual care in patients with NA.

When there is a (near-)complete paralysis without recovery after 6 months, surgical neurolysis is indicated within 6–12 months to allow reinnervation. With this treatment, improvement was seen in 90% of the patients.

In case of diaphragm dysfunction due to phrenic neuropathy noninvasive ventilation is indicated when the patient shows signs of night-time hypoventilation or orthopnoea.

Hereditary Neuralgic Amyotrophy (HNA)

Ten percent of NA patients have a positive family history of the disorder compatible with the hereditary variant of NA (HNA). The symptomatology of their attacks is similar, albeit onset is at a younger age (average 20 years) as compared with NA, there are more recurrences (75%), and there is more involvement beyond the plexus brachialis. HNA is genetically heterogeneous; about half of the families show variations in the septin-9 (*SEPT9*) gene.

As in NA, a fair proportion of HNA patients suffer from chronic pain or have residual weakness, and only a few patients report a full recovery (see Table 19.1).

Suggested Reading

IJspeert J, Janssen RMJ, van Alfen N. Neuralgic amyotrophy. *Curr Opin Neurol* 2021;34(5):605–612. doi: 10.1097/WCO.0000000000000968. PMID: 34054111.

Janssen RMJ, Lustenhouwer R, Cup EHC, et al. Effectiveness of an outpatient rehabilitation programme in patients with neuralgic amyotrophy and scapular dyskinesia: a randomised controlled trial. *J Neurol Neurosurg Psychiatry* 2023;94(6):474–481. doi: 10.1136/jnnp-2022-330296. Epub 2023 Jan 25. PMID: 36697215.

Klein CJ, Barbara DW, Sprung J, Dyck PJ, Weingarten TN. Surgical and postpartum hereditary brachial plexus attacks and prophylactic immunotherapy. *Muscle Nerve* 2013;47(1):23–27. doi: 10.1002/mus.23462. Epub 2012 Oct 5. PMID: 23042485; PMCID: PMC3528817.

van Eijk JJJ, Dalton HR, Ripellino P, et al. Clinical phenotype and outcome of hepatitis E virus-associated neuralgic amyotrophy. *Neurology* 2017;89(9):909–917. doi: 10.1212/WNL.0000000000004297. Epub 2017 Aug 2. PMID: 28768846.

Case 20 Diabetic Neuropathy

Clinical History

A 76-year-old man was referred with a diagnosis of 'motor neuron disease' or 'polyneuropathy'. For about eight months he had noticed progressive muscle weakness in his right leg associated with pain, initially more intense than at referral, and a numb feeling around the right knee. Two years previously his left hand had become weak and wasted, associated with loss of sensation of the ring finger, the little finger, and the ulnar part of the palm of his hand. He had lost weight (5 kg) unintentionally over the past six months. He had always been very active, but was now no longer able to walk his dog or do some gardening. He was recently diagnosed with diabetes mellitus (DM) for which oral antidiabetics were prescribed. Family history was unremarkable.

Examination

Atrophy of the m. interosseous I and the hypothenar on the left, and of the right thigh was noted. There was slight weakness (grade 4+ out of MRC 5) of the left-sided mm. interossei and severe paresis of the right-sided iliopsoas and quadriceps femoris muscle (MRC grade 2) and slight (MRC grade 4+) weakness of the hamstrings. Arm reflexes were normal, knee jerks and Achilles tendon jerks were absent. Hypoaesthesia and hypoalgaesia of the fourth and fifth fingers on the left, lateral thigh, lateral and anterior lower leg, and lateral side of the right foot were noted. Vibration sense and joint position test were reduced in the right leg.

Diagnostic Considerations

Motor neuron disease was unlikely given the sensory abnormalities. The presence of pain, numbness, and muscle weakness in the right leg suggested a lumbosacral plexopathy, and the findings in the left arm were consistent with an ulnaropathy. Areflexia in the legs was consistent with a polyneuropathy.

Given the history of diabetes mellitus, a diagnosis of neurological complications of diabetes mellitus was considered.

Ancillary Investigations

Serum glucose was elevated (16.4 mmol/L), HbA1c 108 mmol/mol (normal < 53).

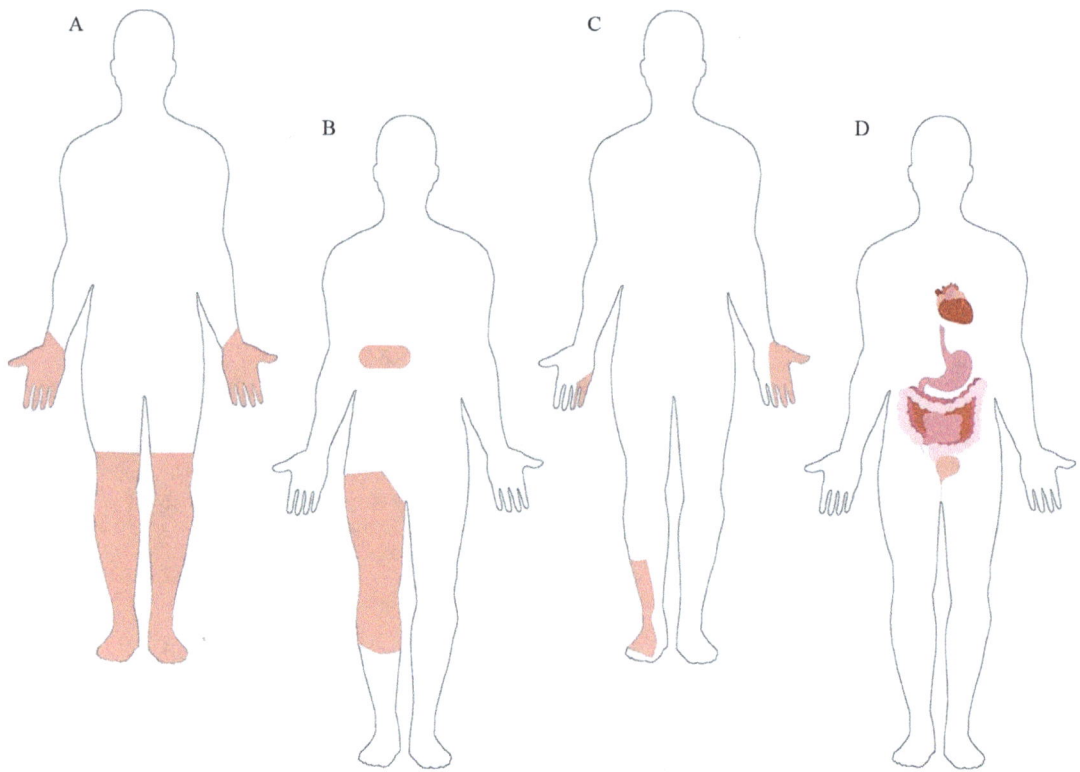

Figure 20.1 (A–D) Patterns of nerve injury in diabetic neuropathy. Several different patterns of neuropathy can present in individuals with diabetes. The following patterns are shown in the figure: diabetic sensorimotor polyneuropathy, small-fibre-predominant (most common) or treatment-induced neuropathy (A); radiculopathy (B); mononeuropathy (C); autonomic neuropathy (the most commonly affected organs are shown) including treatment-induced neuropathy (D). Small-fibre neuropathy has the same pattern as diabetic sensorimotor polyneuropathy but neurological examination and electrodiagnostic studies are different. Diabetic radiculoplexopathy or radiculopathy can respond to immunotherapy and usually improves with time, unlike other types of nerve injury in individuals with diabetes. Treatment-induced neuropathy is under-recognized, is caused by overaggressive glycaemic control, and can present in multiple forms. From Peltier A, et al., *BMJ* 2014; 348:g1799, with permission.

EMG findings were consistent with a left-sided ulnaropathy, a lumbosacral plexopathy on the right, and sensorimotor axonal polyneuropathy.

Follow-Up

We discussed the diagnosis with the patient and informed him about the often spontaneous albeit not always complete recovery of the plexopathy over a couple of months. We recommended that he should see his GP for better diabetes regulation.

General Remarks

Diabetic neuropathy is the most common neuropathy in developed countries and may affect about half of the patients with diabetes. By far, distal symmetric sensorimotor polyneuropathy (DSPN) is the most common presentation manifesting with sensory symptoms and pain, which may worsen during periods of rest and at night (Fig. 20.1) . Diabetic polyneuropathy is initially often asymptomatic. Autonomic involvement, in particular sexual disturbances, a neurogenic bladder, and gastrointestinal complaints, can be found in patients with a longer duration of diabetes. Patients with diabetic polyneuropathy are at risk of developing foot complications (ulceration, gangrene, or amputation), increasing with age and diabetes duration, regardless of its type. Foot ulceration is a preventable condition by identifying and treating the risk factors and careful foot care.

History taking and clinical examination suffice for the diagnosis of polyneuropathy. Blood glucose and HbA1c are the first tests to be done in a patient with painful polyneuropathy. In patients with typical signs and symptoms, an EMG is usually of no added value, since electrodiagnostic testing rarely changes the management of these

Table 20.1 Classification of diabetic neuropathy

Generalized neuropathy
- Diabetic distal symmetric sensorimotor polyneuropathy with/without autonomic neuropathy
- Acute painful sensory neuropathy variants
    o Insulin neuropathy (can occur if serum glucose drops too quickly)
    o Acute painful neuropathy associated with severe weight loss

Focal and multifocal neuropathy
- Cranial neuropathy
    o Abducens nerve most frequently involved, especially in elderly patients
    o Oculomotor nerve, in half of the cases associated with retro-orbital pain and often with responsive pupils
    o Other cranial neuropathies include facial nerve and (very rarely) phrenic nerve, recurrent laryngeal nerve
- Focal neuropathy of the limbs
    o Carpal tunnel syndrome (median nerve), ulnaropathy, peroneal/fibular neuropathy
- Thoracolumbal radiculoneuropathy
- Lumbosacral radiculoplexoneuropathy
- Cervical radiculoplexoneuropathy

patients. Additional blood tests, however, need to be done to exclude other treatable causes of polyneuropathy.

Risk factors for polyneuropathy in patients with diabetes include duration of diabetes, obesity, hypertension, dyslipidaemia (features of metabolic syndrome), and a history of smoking.

Less frequent manifestations of diabetic neuropathy include (multi)focal neuropathies of the limbs, trunk, or cranial nerves (see Table 20.1). Lumbosacral and cervical plexopathies usually present with excruciating pain, exacerbating at night, followed by muscle weakness and wasting. Initially, there is asymmetric involvement, but often the contralateral side becomes affected as well. History commonly discloses unintentional weight loss. These manifestations can occur in both diabetes types 1 and 2 and in particular in elderly men. The illness is usually monophasic. Recovery of multifocal neuropathies takes several months and is not always complete. EMG can also show generalized polyneuropathy or signs of other focal neuropathies. MRI may be performed in cases of diagnostic doubt to exclude structural changes implicating the lumbar plexus.

Various subtypes of diabetic neuropathy can be found in individual patients as is also the case in the reported patient. However, the pathophysiology is different. In DSPN there is an assumed metabolic aetiology as a result of hyperglycaemia and focal neuropathy usually also has a vascular component.

Management

Treatment consists of optimal glycaemic control and risk factor management and adequate pain treatment.

There are some indications that in type 2 DM an active life style, a diet low in carbohydrates and fat, and weight reduction may be beneficial.

About 10% of patients who undergo rapid glycaemic control by intensive insulin treatment will experience a treatment-induced neuropathy manifesting with severe burning and lancinating pain in a distal symmetric pattern with pain and/or autonomic dysfunction within eight weeks of significant glycaemic control.

Clinical guidelines on pain relief recommend the following:

- Drug of first choice: serotonin and noradrenalin reuptake inhibitors, SNRI (duloxetine and venlafaxine)
- Drug of second choice: tricyclic antidepressant (amitriptyline, nortriptyline) or an antiepileptic drug (gabapentin, pregabalin)
- Drug of third choice: carbamazepine or topical 0.075% capsaicin
- One should start with low dosages and titrate according to the effect and adverse events. Opioids are not recommended because of the adverse events and risk of tolerance.

Suggested Reading

Feldman EL, Callaghan BC, Pop-Busui R, et al. Diabetic neuropathy. *Nat Rev Dis Primers* 2019;5(1):41. doi: 10.1038/s41572-019-0092-1. PMID: 31197153.

Izenberg A, Perkins BA, Bril V. Diabetic neuropathies. *Semin Neurol* 2015;35(4):424–430. doi: 10.1055/s-0035-1558972. Epub 2015 Oct 6. PMID: 26502765.

Ng PS, Dyck PJ, Laughlin RS, et al. Lumbosacral radiculoplexus neuropathy: incidence and the association with diabetes mellitus. *Neurology* 2019;92(11):e1188–e1194. doi: 10.1212/WNL.0000000000007020. Epub 2019 Feb 13. PMID: 30760636; PMCID: PMC6511105.

Case 21 — Alcoholic Polyneuropathy

Clinical History

A 66-year-old man with slowly progressive tingling and a dull feeling in his feet for two years visited our outpatient clinic. He noticed some imbalance when walking after rising from a chair or from bed. He had no complaints about his hands, and he did not notice weakness. He loved to play golf with his friends several times a week. He was known to have a steatotic liver and hypertension. He did not smoke, but he admitted that he had been drinking six glasses of beer or wine a day for many years. He used anti-hypertensive drugs and vitamin B complex.

Examination

He was obese, had a red-coloured face, and rather warm and red feet. There was some hyperhidrosis. Neurological examination revealed a symmetric glove-and-stocking diminished sense of touch and pain in the hands and distally from 15 cm below the knees. Vibration sense was reduced at the ankles and absent at the halluces. Position sense was normal. There was minor weakness of his anterior tibial and extensor hallucis muscles. Achilles tendon reflexes were absent. The knee–heel test showed minor ataxia. Romberg sign was just positive.

Diagnostic Considerations

A chronic length-dependent polyneuropathy can be due to many causes. In particular, potentially treatable causes should be ruled out: diabetes, vitamin deficiencies (B1, B6, B12, folic acid) or intoxications (alcohol, vitamin B6, chemotherapy, certain other drugs), paraproteinaemia, kidney and thyroid dysfunction. We considered alcohol overuse as the cause of a slowly progressive axonal polyneuropathy.

Ancillary Investigations

Glucose, kidney, and thyroid functions were normal. Liver enzymes, especially gamma glutamyl transpeptidase (gamma-GT), were elevated. No monoclonal protein. Vitamin B1 and B6 levels were within normal limits (especially pyridoxine was not increased, which is important because a vitamin B6 intoxication can cause a polyneuropathy). EMG examination showed a predominantly sensory axonal polyneuropathy (compatible with a polyneuropathy due to overuse of alcohol).

Follow-Up

We strongly advised the patient to stop or reduce alcohol intake. When we examined the patient a year later, he said he had reduced the use of alcohol. His complaints had not worsened. On neurological examination, the abnormalities were unchanged.

General Remarks

A chronic alcoholic polyneuropathy is characterized by a predominantly distal symmetric sensory neuropathy, sometimes associated with hyperesthaesia and pain. Weakness may occur. Achilles tendon reflexes are reduced or absent. There often are associated features such as thin and tender muscles, and autonomic features such as hyperhidrosis, especially in severe cases. EMG typically reveals features of a length-dependent symmetric sensory more than motor axonal neuropathy.

The pathogenic mechanisms for the development of polyneuropathy in chronic alcohol users are unclear, and it is unknown whether it is caused by the direct toxic effects of ethanol or by another, currently unidentified factor. Why some people develop signs and symptoms of a polyneuropathy relatively rapidly is also unknown. It is not known how much alcohol consumption leads to symptoms of an alcoholic neuropathy. Patients taking over 100 grams of alcohol (about 10 glasses) per day over a period of several years and especially those who skip proper meals are at risk. Although the most important risk factor for alcohol-related peripheral neuropathy seems to be the total lifetime dose of ethanol, other risk factors have also been identified, including genetic variables and male sex. The development of an alcoholic polyneuropathy is also associated with nutritional deficiency. Vitamin (thiamine) deficiency plays a role. It seems likely that other metabolic factors ('metabolic syndrome') play an additional role. It is important to always check for other, potentially treatable causes of polyneuropathy. Therefore, laboratory investigation should check for a range of risk factors of chronic axonal polyneuropathy.

Alcoholism associated with a severe thiamine deficiency can also cause an acute polyneuropathy. This syndrome, also called beriberi, usually starts with impairment of sensory functions (touch, pain, and temperature), which is followed by weakness and autonomic disturbances, which may mimic Guillain–Barré syndrome. Signs and symptoms of Wernicke encephalopathy may also be present in these patients.

Management and Prognosis

There is currently sparse data to support a particular management strategy in chronic alcohol-related peripheral neuropathy, but the limited data available appear to support the use of vitamin supplementation, particularly of B vitamins including thiamine. It is recommended to start treatment with thiamine supplementation (50 mg orally, one to three times daily; in severe cases start with 100 mg thiamine SC/IM) and vitamin B complex, in combination with the advice to stop drinking alcohol or reduce alcohol consumption, and switch to a healthy diet when indicated. Symptoms and signs may remain stable or partially disappear over months. If the neuropathy clearly worsens, consider continued alcohol overconsumption. Clinical examination is important, but biomarkers, that is, gamma-GT or carbohydrate-deficient transferrin (CDT), can be very helpful. Other metabolic risk factors for polyneuropathy such as diabetes mellitus and vitamin B6 (pyridoxine) intoxication should be excluded.

Suggested Reading

Hamel J, Logigian EL. Acute nutritional axonal neuropathy. *Muscle Nerve* 2018;57(1):33–39. doi: 10.1002/mus.25702. Epub 2017 Jun 19. PMID: 28556429.

Hanewinckel R, van Oijen M, Ikram MA, van Doorn PA. The epidemiology and risk factors of chronic polyneuropathy. *Eur J Epidemiol* 2016;31(1):5–20. doi: 10.1007/s10654-015-0094-6. Epub 2015 Dec 23. PMID: 26700499; PMCID: PMC4756033.

Julian T, Glascow N, Syeed R, Zis P. Alcohol-related peripheral neuropathy: a systematic review and meta-analysis. *J Neurol* 2019;266(12):2907–2919. doi: 10.1007/s00415-018-9123-1. Epub 2018 Nov 22. PMID: 30467601; PMCID: PMC6851213.

Chronic Idiopathic Axonal Polyneuropathy (CIAP)

Clinical History

A 60-year-old man reported slowly progressive symptoms over a period of five years. He experienced tingling in his toes that gradually spread halfway up the lower legs. He also developed a stiff feeling in his lower legs and nightly cramps in both calves, but no pain. For one year, he complained of numb fingertips with some loss of dexterity. He had no symptoms of autonomic dysfunction, was not known to have diabetes, ate a healthy, balanced diet, drank one glass of alcohol a day, and had not been treated with neurotoxic medication. His family history indicated no other relatives with similar complaints.

Examination

There were no foot deformities (pes cavus, hammer toes) or calf atrophy. Normal walking was nearly unremarkable, but standing on one leg was difficult. He had weakness of his toe extensors (MRC grade 4), but could walk well on his heels. Vibration sense was absent at the toes and diminished at the ankles. Position sense of the toes was decreased. Pain and tactile sense were abnormal at his fingertips and below the knees. The Achilles tendon reflexes were absent; the other reflexes were normal.

Diagnostic Considerations

Based upon the symptoms and neurological examination, a clinical diagnosis of chronic polyneuropathy was made. There was no obvious cause for the polyneuropathy. A long disease history, the length-dependent abnormalities (distal, symmetric complaints), the absence of prominent pain, and the absence of asymmetry were compatible with a possible metabolic cause of the polyneuropathy (such as diabetes, alcohol overuse, or a vitamin deficiency), or a polyneuropathy related to a monoclonal IgG or IgM paraprotein. Considered unlikely were a paraneoplastic neuropathy (develops more rapidly) and immune-mediated neuropathy such as chronic inflammatory demyelinating polyneuropathy (CIDP) or vasculitis (which often also gives proximal or asymmetric weakness, respectively). The absence of affected family members in combination with the absence of foot deformities and atrophy of the lower legs made a hereditary neuropathy less likely. Before the diagnosis of chronic idiopathic axonal polyneuropathy (CIAP) can be made, additional laboratory investigations are required and need to be normal.

Ancillary Investigations

Laboratory analysis tests, including glucose, Hb1Ac, ESR, hemoglobin, leucocytes, RBCs, platelets, gamma-GT, ALAT, creatinine, vitamins B1, B6, and B12, folic acid, and TSH, were all normal. Immunofixation revealed no M-protein (paraprotein).

EMG showed absent sural nerve action potentials and a minor decrease of the median and ulnar sensory nerve action potentials (SNAPs). Compound muscle action potentials (CMAPs) of motor nerves were within normal limits. Nerve conduction velocities were normal. These findings indicate a mild (predominantly sensory) axonal polyneuropathy.

Follow-Up

Based on history taking, neurological examination, and laboratory findings including EMG examination, the diagnosis of CIAP was made. The patient subsequently experienced slow progression of these symptoms over years. Later, he used a cane when walking on uneven surfaces or when he needed to walk longer distances.

General Remarks

Chronic Polyneuropathy

Chronic polyneuropathy (progression > 2 months, usually in many months to years) is a frequently occurring disorder. Its prevalence increases with age, ranging from about 2% in patients aged 50–60 years to over 12% in patients over the age of 80 (Fig. 22.1).

Polyneuropathy is a clinical diagnosis. The Erasmus Polyneuropathy Symptom Score (E-PSS) is a simple, validated six-item tool that takes the presence and frequency of six different symptoms into account and may be helpful in screening individuals for the presence of chronic polyneuropathy. These six items are numb feet and tingling feet, walking on cotton wool and allodynia of the feet, tingling feelings in both hands, and balance problems. Numb feet and tingling feet are the most frequently reported symptoms by patients with chronic polyneuropathy and have the highest sensitivity compared with normal controls. Walking on cotton wool and allodynia have the highest specificity. The other informative questions concern the presence of tingling feelings in both hands and balance problems. Nerve

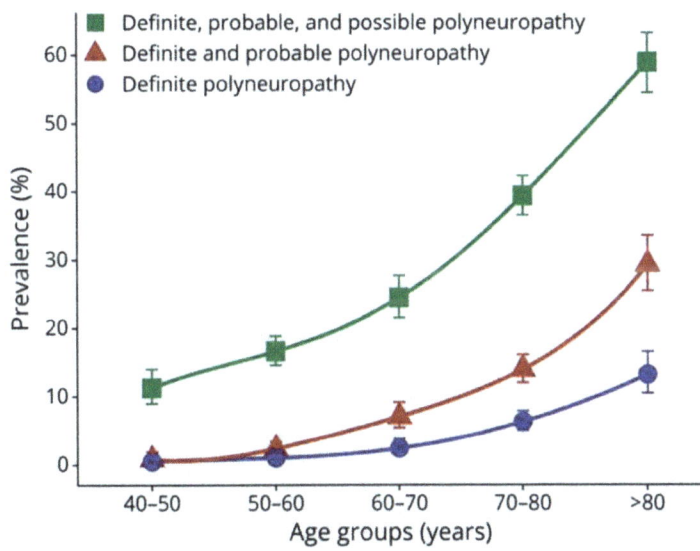

Figure 22.1 Prevalence of chronic polyneuropathy clearly increases with age. Level of diagnostic certainty (definite, probable, and possible) for polyneuropathy is based upon a screening procedure used in a population-based study. From Taams et al., *Neurology* 2022;99:e2234–e2240, with permission.

Table 22.1 Chronic axonal polyneuropathy: diagnoses to be considered.

Disease[a]	Appropriate tests (suggestions)[b]
Diabetes mellitus	Glucose and glycosylated haemoglobin (HbA1c)
Renal insufficiency[c]	Creatinine, urea
Alcohol abuse	γ-glutamyl transferase (gamma-GT), alanine aminotransferase (ALAT)
Hypothyroidism	TSH
Vitamin B1 deficiency	Thiamine
Vitamin B6 deficiency[d]	Pyridoxine
Vitamin B6 intoxication[e]	Pyridoxine
Vitamin B12 deficiency[f]	Cyanocobalamin (B12), methylmalonic acid (increased)
Monoclonal gammopathy	Serum (and urine) M-protein immunofixation, free light chains
Systemic disease[g]	ESR, ANA, SS-A, SS-B
Malignancy[h]	Anti-neuronal antibodies

[a] Table indicates prevalent diseases (not exhaustive) related to polyneuropathy
[b] Additional tests should be ordered related to possible other causes
[c] Neuropathy is not an early sign, motor signs predominate.
[d] Ataxic signs usually predominate.
[e] When used for a long period (months) in high dosages as a vitamin supplement.
[f] Pyramidal signs can also be present; consider also use of nitrous oxide gas
[g] For example, Sjögren disease, vasculitis (the latter often painful and asymmetric).
[h] Rapid progression, sensory and ataxic, may precede tumour signs.

conduction studies can confirm the diagnosis, and – importantly – are used to make the distinction between an axonal and a demyelinating polyneuropathy, which have different causes. Patients with a chronic polyneuropathy most frequently have an axonal polyneuropathy.

If a patient is diagnosed with a chronic polyneuropathy, additional laboratory investigations need to be done (Table 22.1). The first step is to exclude the most frequent risk factors: diabetes, vitamin B12 deficiency, exposure to toxic agents (medication or use of, e.g., nitric oxide gas, or overuse of alcohol). Recent studies have found that in about 10% of patients with a chronic axonal polyneuropathy, more than one risk factor (such as diabetes, alcohol overuse, or vitamin deficiency) for polyneuropathy can be identified when conducting standard laboratory investigations. Because some of these factors can be modified, this indicates that it is worth the effort to test also for additional risk factors (such as a vitamin deficiency) if a single risk factor for polyneuropathy is already known to be present.

Chronic Idiopathic Axonal Polyneuropathy (CIAP)

If a patient has a slowly progressive axonal polyneuropathy and no cause is found (which is the case in about 30% of patients who visit a neurological outpatient clinic for their polyneuropathy, and in about 40–50% of patients in the general population), the diagnosis of sCIAP can be made. Characteristics of CIAP are shown in Table 22.2

In a population-based study it was found that about half of the individuals diagnosed with a chronic axonal polyneuropathy were unaware of having this disease (Fig. 22.2). CIAP runs a slowly progressive course over many years. Patients may need ankle-foot orthosis or a cane to walk. Few patients eventually need a wheelchair. CIAP is usually less painful than diabetic polyneuropathy, and there is generally no need for medication to reduce neuropathic pain.

The cause of CIAP is currently still unknown. Recent findings indicate that a metabolic syndrome contributes to the occurrence of polyneuropathy. It is not known, however, whether treatment of hypertension or hypercholesterolaemia is useful.

Low Ankle Reflexes at Older Age ('Normal Ageing')

As mentioned above, polyneuropathy is a clinical diagnosis. In this respect, it is important to realize that decreased ankle reflexes and reduced vibration sense at the hallux (great toe) are not always

Table 22.2 Main features of chronic idiopathic axonal polyneuropathy (CIAP)

- Onset > 50 years
- Site of onset in toes, soles of feet, can start somewhat asymmetric
- Sensory or sensory and motor, not purely motor
- Progression in years
- Ankle dorsal flexor weakness in 2/3 of patients
- Weakness of hand muscles in 1/6 of patients
- CK elevation (rarely > 2 × ULN) in < 5% of patients
- Walking aids[a] needed by ¼ of patients
- Autonomic signs[b] or severe pain absent/not predominant

[a] Walking aids: cane, adjusted shoes, ankle-foot orthosis, wheeled walker (rarely needed in patients < 65 years of age)

[b] If early autonomic signs are evident, consider again diabetes, monoclonal protein, and hereditary TTR amyloidosis.

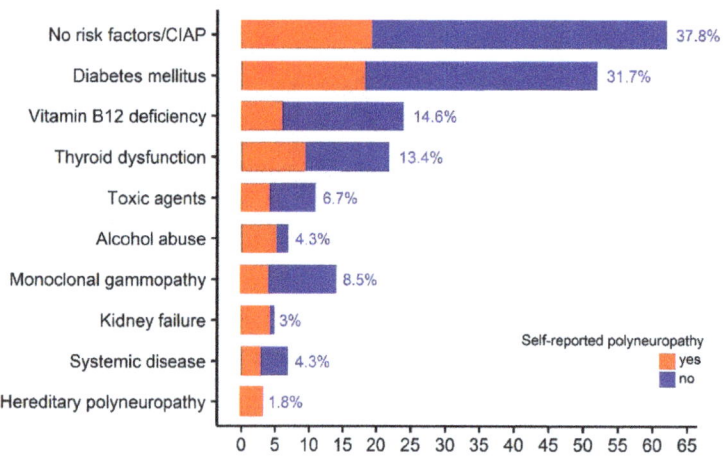

Figure 22.2 Risk factors of polyneuropathy in the general population. Percentages (%) indicate individuals with a certain risk factor as percentage of the total group of patients with polyneuropathy. In this case, nearly 38% had CIAP. High percentage of 'no self-reported polyneuropathy' indicates that many individuals diagnosed with polyneuropathy did not know that their signs and symptoms were due to this disease. From Taams et al., *Neurology* 2022;99:e2234–e2240), with permission.

signs of polyneuropathy, as this can also occur in normal ageing in persons over 70 years of age.

Suggested Reading

Hanewinckel R, van Oijen M, Ikram MA, van Doorn PA. The epidemiology and risk factors of chronic polyneuropathy. *Eur J Epidemiol* 2016 Jan;31(1):5–20. doi: 10.1007/s10654-015-0094-6. Epub 2015 Dec 23. PMID: 26700499; PMCID: PMC4756033.

Hanewinckel R, van Oijen M, Taams NE, et al. Diagnostic value of symptoms in chronic polyneuropathy: the Erasmus Polyneuropathy Symptom Score. *J Peripher Nerv Syst* 2019;24(3):235–241. doi: 10.1111/jns.12328. Epub 2019 Jul 9. PMID: 31172622.

Taams NE, Drenthen J, Hanewinckel R, Ikram MA, van Doorn PA. Prevalence and risk factor profiles for chronic axonal polyneuropathy in the general population. *Neurology* 2022:10.1212/WNL.0000000000201168. doi: 10.1212/WNL.0000000000201168. Epub ahead of print. PMID: 36008153.

Visser NA, Notermans NC, Linssen RS, van den Berg LH, Vrancken AF. Incidence of polyneuropathy in Utrecht, the Netherlands. *Neurology* 2015;84(3):259–264. doi: 10.1212/WNL.0000000000001160. Epub 2014 Dec 12. PMID: 25503982.

Vrancken AF, Franssen H, Wokke JH, Teunissen LL, Notermans NC. Chronic idiopathic axonal polyneuropathy and successful aging of the peripheral nervous system in elderly people. *Arch Neurol* 2002;59(4):533–340. doi: 10.1001/archneur.59.4.533. PMID: 11939887.

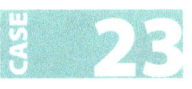

Critical Illness Polyneuropathy and Myopathy (CIPM)

Clinical History

A 64-year-old man with hypertension had acute-onset dysarthria and left-sided ataxia. A haematoma in the left cerebellar hemisphere was diagnosed. When he developed severe headaches and vertical gaze paresis, the neurosurgeon was consulted and a decision to evacuate the haematoma was made. After surgery, he acquired pneumonia, necessitating artificial ventilation. Further complications included metabolic alkalosis, sepsis, and haemodynamic instability. One week after surgery, he developed a tetraparesis.

Examination

He opened his eyes quickly when spoken to. Compression of the nail bed caused facial grimacing. His eye movements were normal. His limbs were paralytic with areflexia. After a few days, his best motor response was protrusion of the tongue on demand and blinking the eyes. Weaning from the ventilator could not be achieved. He had not been treated with neuromuscular blocking agents and was given small doses of sedative drugs.

Diagnostic Considerations

There was severe, symmetric weakness of arms and legs, with preserved facial and ocular motor function, areflexia, and normal consciousness. Because of the early areflexia, Guillain–Barré syndrome was a possible explanation, but critical illness polyneuropathy and myopathy (CIPM) was considered much more likely in view of the setting of severe illness on the intensive care unit (ICU). Other diagnostic possibilities were myasthenia gravis or locked-in syndrome.

Ancillary Investigations

Nine days after surgery, a brain MRI scan showed a hypodensity within the left cerebellar hemisphere, but no other abnormalities. Serum CK activity and serum electrolyte concentrations were normal. Two weeks following surgery, needle EMG showed spontaneous muscle fibre activity in both anterior tibial muscles, but not in proximal leg muscles. Nerve conduction studies showed normal distal latencies and normal motor and sensory conduction velocities, with decreased amplitudes of the compound muscle action potentials and sensory nerve action potentials. A diagnosis of CIP or CIPM was made.

Table 23.1 Main features of critical illness polyneuropathy (CIP) and critical illness myopathy (CIM)

- Symmetric, proximal more than distal limb weakness
- Weakness of diaphragm hampering weaning from mechanical ventilation
- No weakness of facial and ocular muscles
- CK is normal in CIP and can be mildly elevated in CIM
- CIP and CIM often occur together
- CIP is an axonal, predominantly motor polyneuropathy
- Recovery rate is higher in CIM than in CIP

Follow-Up

Complications were treated successfully. He received whole-body rehabilitation consisting of interruption of sedation and physical and occupational therapy. Weaning from the ventilator remained difficult and was successful only after eight weeks. He had developed severe skeletal muscle atrophy, distal more than proximal, and was transferred to a rehabilitation clinic. Six months later, he was able to walk with a walker.

General Remarks

Critical Illness Polyneuropathy (CIP) and Critical Illness Myopathy (CIM) (Table 23.1)

With the current longer survival of severely ill patients in the ICU, CIP and CIM are increasingly recognized as frequent complications of sepsis and multi-organ failure. Patients hospitalized in the ICU for more than one week are at risk. This risk can be diminished by avoiding hyperglycaemia and early parenteral feeding. CIP or CIM should be suspected if patients at awakening have flaccid, symmetric, proximal more than distal limb weakness, or cannot be weaned from the ventilator, if confounding effects of drugs have been ruled out. Facial and ocular muscles are typically spared, distinguishing CIP and CIM from, for example, severe Guillain–Barré syndrome and myasthenia gravis. CIM and CIP often occur together (critical illness polyneuromyopathy, CIPM). CIP is an axonal, motor more than sensory polyneuropathy and establishing abnormalities of sensation can be difficult in ill patients in an ICU setting. Thus, the distinction between CIM and CIP may require electrophysiological testing, showing reduced amplitudes of sensory nerve action potentials (SNAPs) in CIP. One might argue, however, that making this distinction does not influence the therapeutic approach. Neuromuscular electrical stimulation and various pharmacological interventions have been shown to be ineffective, and the efficacy of early rehabilitation is uncertain to date. CIP and CIM are both associated with an increased duration of hospital stay, increased in-hospital and one-year mortality, and reduced physical quality of life after five years. One year after discharge, 50–75% of patients with CIM or CIP have persisting muscle weakness. The prognosis of CIM is better in this regard.

Intensive Care Unit (ICU)-Acquired Weakness

The terms 'CIP' and 'CIM' are often used interchangeably with the term 'ICU-acquired weakness'. The latter, however, also includes severe generalized muscle atrophy due to disuse and a catabolic state, which will usually become manifest after one to two weeks in the ICU. Electrophysiological findings are normal in contrast to CIP and CIM. Prognosis is better than in CIP and CIM. Full recovery is to be expected once the patient becomes more active.

Difficulties with Weaning in Patients with a Hitherto Unknown Neuromuscular Disorder

In patients who cannot be weaned from the ventilator, CIP and CIM should also be differentiated from weakness of respiratory muscles due to a neuromuscular disorder that was present but not manifest or not recognized before admission to the ICU. Acute, severe bulbar weakness and diaphragmatic weakness may be triggered by stress factors such as surgery and critical illness in patients with myasthenia gravis, who had no or only minor and unrecognized symptoms until then. In some myopathies (e.g., myotonic dystrophy type 1 or Pompe disease), patients may be unaware of having a muscle disease, while there is a disproportional, gradually increasing weakness of the diaphragm. If these patients need mechanical ventilation for an unrelated condition, acute further deterioration of respiration function ('acute-on-chronic') may easily result from lying flat, aspiration, oxygen therapy, or the use of neuromuscular blocking agents. It is paramount not to erroneously consider these disorders as CIP or CIM. Myasthenic respiratory weakness will generally respond quickly to intravenous immunoglobulins or plasma exchange. In most cases, patients with a myopathy will eventually be weaned from the ventilator and start noninvasive ventilation. If appropriate, causal treatment will be initiated, for example in Pompe disease.

Suggested Reading

Kress JP, Hall JB. ICU-acquired weakness and recovery from critical illness. *N Engl J Med* 2014;370(17):1626–1635. doi: 10.1056/NEJMra1209390. PMID: 24758618.

Vanhorebeek I, Latronico N, Van den Berghe G. ICU-acquired weakness. *Intensive Care Med* 2020;46(4):637–653. doi: 10.1007/s00134-020-05944-4. Epub 2020 Feb 19. PMID: 32076765; PMCID: PMC7224132.

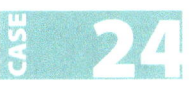

Drug-Induced Polyneuropathies: Amiodarone Polyneuropathy

Clinical History

A 76-year-old man complained about progressive dull feelings and weakness of the distal lower limbs that gradually progressed over a couple of months to the proximal legs and the hands. In addition, there was minor myalgia in the proximal muscles. He had had a myocardial infarction with cardiac arrhythmia three years earlier. He was treated with amiodarone afterwards. He did not have visual complaints and was otherwise healthy. He did not drink alcohol or use other drugs. He had not been treated with cytostatic drugs.

Examination

The patient had problems with rising from a chair and walking. We found diffuse weakness of muscles of both arms and legs, distally more pronounced (MRC grade 4) than proximally. He had distal stocking-and-glove sensory disturbances and areflexia. Tremor and gait ataxia were absent, and visual acuity was normal. Additionally, he had a somewhat blue-greyish discolouration of his face and hands, which suggested treatment with amiodarone.

Diagnostic Considerations

A length-dependent sensory-motor polyneuropathy was diagnosed. Although a relationship with amiodarone was considered because of the facial blue-greyish discolouration, additional investigations of other risk factors for polyneuropathy were done.

Ancillary Investigations

Routine blood investigation was normal (especially no paraprotein was found, and there was no vitamin B1, B6, or B12 deficiency). CSF revealed a slightly elevated protein (0.7 g/L) without pleiocytosis. EMG showed signs of a demyelinating polyneuropathy, which did not fulfil the EAN/PNS criteria for chronic inflammatory demyelinating polyneuropathy.

Follow-Up

The diagnosis of amiodarone-related polyneuropathy was made. Amiodarone was stopped. The neuropathy gradually improved after about one year. When he was seen four years later, he was in good condition and symptoms and signs of neuropathy were almost absent. The blue-greyish discolouration of his face had virtually disappeared.

General Remarks

Polyneuropathies can be caused by a variety of drugs and toxic substances (Table 24.1). It is important to consider toxic aetiologies when searching for the cause of a polyneuropathy, in particular because some of these risk factors are among the treatable forms of peripheral nerve dysfunction.

A large number of drugs can cause neuropathy. Some of these are not very frequently used. Especially if the full side effect profile is not well known, one should check whether a drug can be

Table 24.1 Examples of toxins and drugs that can cause a polyneuropathy

Axonal

Acrylamide, alcohol, arsenic, bortezomib, colchicine, dapsone, dioxin, disulfiram, ethambutol, IFN-a, isoniazid, lead, lithium, metronidazole, nitrofurantoin, nitrous oxide (inhalation) organophosphates, phenytoin, platinum analogs, pyridoxine, paclitaxel, vinca alkaloids

Demyelinating

Amiodarone, chloroquine, tacrolimus, perhexiline, procainamide, zimelidine

associated with polyneuropathy. It is remarkable that chronic use of high-dosage vitamin B6 (pyridoxine), likely > 100–200 mg per day or more, which is about 50–125 times the daily intake from food, can cause a mainly sensory ataxic neuropathy. The precise mechanism is not well understood, but it is suggested that the inactive form of pyridoxine competitively inhibits the active vitamin B6 form (pyridoxal-5 ×-phosphate), causing the symptoms of vitamin B6 deficiency.

In particular, cytostatic drugs are well known for their relation with polyneuropathy (Table 24.2). Several chemotherapy drug classes cause neuropathy with high incidence in a dose-dependent fashion. To prevent this often serious complication (chemotherapy-induced peripheral neuropathy, CIPN), it may be required to reduce the dose or even to switch to alternative medication, if possible. Toxic neuropathies most frequently give rise to pure sensory or sensorimotor symptoms. Pain can be a prominent

Table 24.2 Cytostatic drugs that may cause polyneuropathy[a]

Drug	Symptoms and signs	Reversible?
Proteasome inhibitors, e.g., bortezomib	Sensory, painful	Gradually, with dose reduction or when stopped
Taxanes, e.g., paclitaxel	Paresthesias, dysesthesias, pain, (weakness), ataxia	Partially (may persist for years)
Vincristine	Sensorimotor, autonomic, ataxia	Yes (in general)
Platinum-based, e.g., cisplatin	Sensory axonopathy, ataxia, neuronopathy), Lhermitte sign	May worsen after discontinuation ('coasting' effect)

[a] Neuropathy due to cytostatic drugs is usually dose-related.

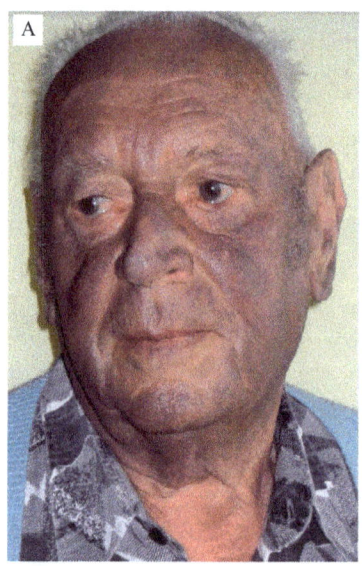
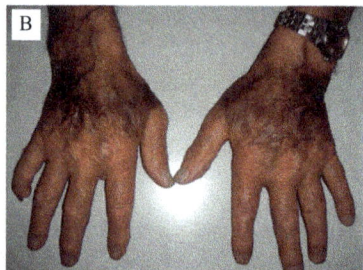

Figure 24.1 Blue-grey discolouration of the face and the hands due to amiodarone. Exposure to sunlight causes more blueish discolouration. From Stähli BE, Schwab S, *QJM* 2011;104:723–724, with permission.

feature. Most toxic polyneuropathies are axonal or predominantly axonal. Some, however, can be (predominantly) demyelinating and may mimic CIDP. Amiodarone is one of these. The overt proximal weakness that can also occur in amiodarone neuropathy may mimic CIDP. A blue discolouration of the skin – especially after sun exposure – is a well-known side effect of amiodarone (Fig. 24.1). It is explained by accumulation of lipofuscin, or deposits of electron-dense granules. Symptoms can develop anywhere from a few months to years of amiodarone therapy. Optic neuropathy occurs in 1–2% of patients who are treated with amiodarone. Peripheral neuropathy is less prevalent. As with most toxic neuropathies, it has been shown that the risk of developing an amiodarone-related neuropathy is dependent on the dose and duration of treatment. Stopping amiodarone can result in virtual disappearance of the neuropathy. When informing a patient, it should be kept in mind that progression of symptoms and signs of neuropathy may continue for three to six months after cessation of the causative agent. This is the so-called coasting effect.

Suggested Reading

Orr CF, Ahlskog JE. Frequency, characteristics, and risk factors for amiodarone neurotoxicity. *Arch Neurol* 2009;66(7):865–869. doi: 10.1001/archneurol.2009.96. PMID: 19597088.

Peters J, Staff NP. Update on toxic neuropathies. *Curr Treat Options Neurol* 2022;24(5):203–216. doi: 10.1007/s11940-022-00716-5. Epub 2022 Apr 6. PMID: 36186669; PMCID: PMC9518699.

Smyth D, Kramarz C, Carr AS, Rossor AM, Lunn MP. Toxic neuropathies: a practical approach. *Pract Neurol* 2023;23(2):120–130. doi: 10.1136/pn-2022-003444. Epub 2023 Jan 25. PMID: 36697225.

Stähli BE, Schwab S. Amiodarone-induced skin hyperpigmentation. *QJM* 2011;104(8):723–724. doi: 10.1093/qjmed/hcq131. Epub 2010 Jul 30. PMID: 20675394.

Vassallo P, Trohman RG. Prescribing amiodarone: an evidence-based review of clinical indications. *JAMA* 2007;298(11):1312–1322. doi: 10.1001/jama.298.11.1312. PMID: 17878423.

CASE 25 Lyme Radiculopathy

Clinical History

A previously healthy 13-year-old boy was referred because of fatigue and progressive weakness in the legs for one month. His right leg seemed more affected than the left one. He also had difficulty getting up from his bed and needed support of the arms. For one week, strength in the arms also decreased. When looking in the mirror, he had the impression that there was thinning of the upper arms and legs. He had lower back pain as well as nonradiating pain in the knee cavities, especially at night. He also had significant weight loss, from 40 to 35 kg. There had been no previous illness, skin changes, or insect bites.

Examination

There was axial weakness and asymmetric muscle weakness of both arms and legs. Shoulder abduction was MRC grade 4 on both sides, and there was winging of the left scapula (Fig 25.1A). Hip abductors and flexors were weak, MRC grade 4 on the right and grade 3 on the left side. Trendelenburg sign was positive when standing on the left leg (Fig. 25.1B). He needed to roll to his side in order to get up from a lying position due to weakness of the abdominal wall muscles. By contrast, there was no bulbar weakness or weakness of neck flexors and extensors. He could not rise from a kneeling position or stand up from a chair without support of the arms. There was also weakness of the right ankle dorsiflexion and extension preventing him from standing on his heel and on tiptoes. Tendon reflexes of the arms and knee jerks were hypoactive. Both Achilles tendon reflexes were absent. Sensory examination was normal. There were no abnormalities of the skin or the joints. A few days after the initial examination, his back pain

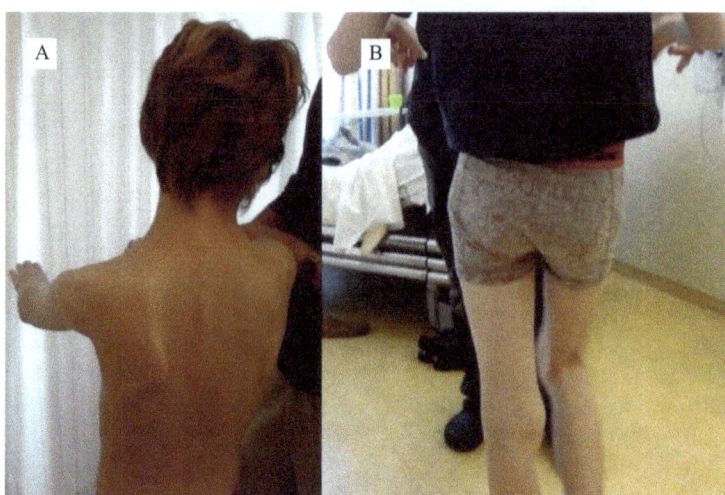

Figure 25.1 (A,B) Asymmetric scapular winging (A) and positive Trendelenburg sign due to hip abductor weakness on the left (B).

worsened. Elevation of the legs (straight leg raise test) was now positive with fixation in the hips and causing pain in the knee cavities. There were no skin abnormalities.

Diagnostic Considerations

The pattern of a pure motor disorder with acquired axial and limb muscle weakness, fatigue, and weight loss initially directed thoughts towards a myositis, although this is generally more symmetric and does not show distinct distal involvement. The absence of skin changes makes dermatomyositis highly unlikely in children, but other forms of myositis occur also in children. In case of acquired weakness, pain, and reduced or absent tendon reflexes at any age, acute inflammatory demyelinating polyneuropathy, or polyradiculitis should be considered. However, the absence of sensory abnormalities several weeks after onset is exceptional, as pure motor forms of Guillain–Barré syndrome are extremely rare in children. The positive Lasègue sign that became clear after admission pointed towards nerve root involvement.

Ancillary Investigations

CK was normal. Nerve conduction studies were normal, but needle EMG of the left anterior tibial, vastus lateralis, and deltoid muscle showed polyphasic motor unit action potentials of low amplitude (< 1 mV). Muscle MRI including T1 and fat-suppressed T2 sequences was then performed, but no areas of

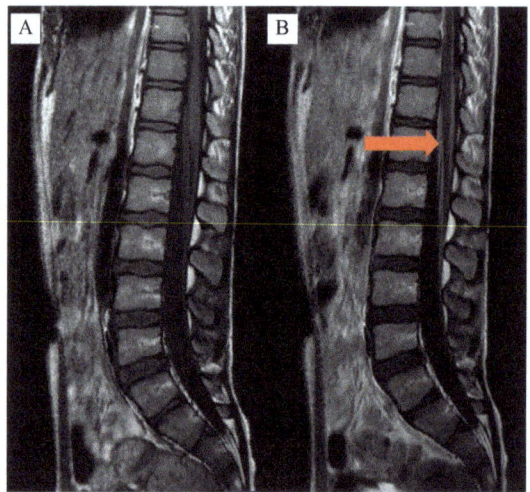

Figure 25.2 (A,B) T1-weighted MRI of the lumbar spine (A) showing gadolinium enhancement of the nerve roots (B).

intramuscular high T2 signal could be found in any affected muscle. MR imaging of the spinal cord showed gadolinium enhancement of the meninges, conus medullaris, and spinal nerve roots (Fig. 25.2). A lumbar puncture was performed, yielding a pleiocytosis (230 cells/3 μL) with predominantly polymorphic cells, increased protein level of 1.66 g/L (ref 0.15 to 0.45), and oligoclonal bands compatible with intrathecal IgG synthesis. This polymorphic cell reaction ruled out Guillain–Barré syndrome and made polyradiculitis due to a malignancy less likely. Finally, IgG and IgM antibodies to *Borrelia* were detected in serum, and intrathecal antibody production was found in CSF, which confirmed a diagnosis of neuroborreliosis with meningoradiculitis.

Follow-Up

Ceftriaxone 2 g IV daily was given for two weeks. The pain resolved within a few days and muscle strength and function recovered completely within five months. No recurrence of infection was observed one year after treatment.

General Remarks

Lyme disease is caused by various *Borrelia burgdorferi* genotypes, transmitted by species of the *Ixodes* ticks, depending on geographical location. Incidence is highest in endemic areas within the 30°–60° latitudes of the northern hemisphere and in springtime. Classification can be done according to time and distribution of symptoms. Acute localized disease is hallmarked by erythema migrans (EM) or rarely a *Borrelia* lymphocytoma. Disseminated disease includes, among others, multiple EM, neuroborreliosis, carditis, arthritis, uveitis, panophthalmitis, hepatitis, myositis, and orchitis. Chronic Lyme disease involves a skin condition known as acrodermatitis chronic atrophicans, chronic neuroborreliosis, or chronic arthritis.

The described patient did not report a tick bite or EM, but this is not exceptional. In adult patients with neuroborreliosis, a tick bite is noted in 39% and EM in 25%. Neuromuscular manifestations of neuroborreliosis include unilateral or bilateral facial nerve palsy, single or multiple radiculitis, mononeuritis multiplex, plexitis, and rarely myositis. Radiculitis is typically painful and radiating in contrast to the patient described here in whom a positive Lasègue sign could only be elicited during the first week after admission. In children, the most common presentation is facial nerve palsy (Table 25.1). A unilateral facial nerve palsy is more prevalent in children than in adults. Radiculitis or meningoradiculitis (Bannwarth syndrome) by contrast is very rare in children (3%).

Lyme disease is diagnosed in blood by demonstrating antibodies to *B. burgdorferi* using enzyme-linked immunoassay or Western blot. Antibodies are generally detectable between two and six weeks after onset of symptoms. The test can thus be false-negative in the acute setting and repeat testing should be considered. Neuroborreliosis is hallmarked by lymphocytic mononuclear cell pleiocytosis in CSF in more than 95% of the cases. The diagnosis is confirmed by intrathecal antibody production (IgM and/or IgG) or the demonstration of *Borrelia* DNA in CSF by PCR, which is recommended if there is strong clinical suspicion of neuroborreliosis. Diagnostic sensitivity of specific ELISAs to demonstrate antibody production in CSF is much higher than that of a PCR to test for DNA, but PCR may be useful during early stages of neuroborreliosis, as antibody production can be lagging behind.

The recommended treatment is with intravenous antibiotics. Ceftriaxone is most often used; penicillin and cefotaxime are alternatives. However, oral doxycycline may be equally effective according to an open label study in adults. Doxycycline, however, is not recommended in children below eight years and in pregnant or breastfeeding women because of negative effects on bone development and teeth. A complete recovery as in the presented case is more common in children (83%) than in adults (40%).

Suggested Reading

Dutta A, Hunter JV, Vallejo JG. Bannwarth syndrome: a rare manifestation of pediatric Lyme neuroborreliosis. *Pediatr Infect Dis J* 2021;40(11): e442–e444. doi: 10.1097/INF.0000000000003245. PMID: 34636801.

Garcia-Monco JC, Benach JL. Lyme neuroborreliosis: clinical outcomes, controversy, pathogenesis, and polymicrobial infections. *Ann Neurol* 2019;85(1):21–31. doi: 10.1002/ana.25389. PMID: 30536421; PMCID: PMC7025284.

Kortela E, Kanerva MJ, Puustinen J, et al. Oral doxycycline compared to intravenous ceftriaxone in the treatment of Lyme neuroborreliosis: a multicenter, equivalence, randomized, open-label

Table 25.1 Main features of Lyme neuroborreliosis in children

- Preceded by tick bite or erythema migrans in a minority of patients
- Unilateral or bilateral facial nerve palsy more frequent in children than in adults
- Polyradiculitis, meningoradiculitis, and meningitis rare in children
- Diagnosis by demonstration of antibodies to *Borrelia burgdorferi*, PCR, pleiocytosis
- Treatment with IV ceftriaxone or oral doxycycline, or IV penicillin or IV cefotaxime according to prevailing guideline

trial. *Clin Infect Dis* 2021;72(8):1323–1331. doi: 10.1093/cid/ciaa217. PMID: 32133487.

Nordberg CL, Bodilsen J, Knudtzen FC, et al.; DASGIB study group.Lyme neuroborreliosis in adults: a nationwide prospective cohort study. *Ticks Tick Borne Dis* 2020;11(4):101411. doi: 10.1016/j.ttbdis.2020.101411. Epub 2020 Feb 24. PMID: 32178995.

van Samkar A, Bruinsma RA, Vermeeren YM, et al. Clinical characteristics of Lyme neuroborreliosis in Dutch children and adults. *Eur J Pediatr* 2023;182 (3):1183–1189. doi: 10.1007/s00431-022-04749-5. Epub 2023 Jan 6. PMID: 36607413.

CASE 26 Leprosy

Clinical History

A 14-year-old girl born in Brazil who moved to Europe at a young age presented with weakness and a dull feeling in her right hand. The symptoms had been progressive over a period of one year. Initially, she had diminished sensation of her right index finger. This gradually progressed to affect the whole of her right hand, which eventually became numb. She was right-handed and could no longer use a pen for writing. Otherwise, her history was unremarkable.

Examination

She had a claw hand with atrophy of the intrinsic muscles of the right hand (Fig. 26.1). There was a paresis (MRC grade 2–4) of all hand muscles innervated by the median, ulnar, and radial nerves. She had sensory disturbances of all modalities except for the position sense. The biceps, brachioradial, and triceps reflexes were diminished in the right arm. We noticed some discolouration of the distal part of her right arm, compatible with depigmentation. There were no abnormalities of the left arm and legs. On palpation, the ulnar, median, and radial nerves of the right forearm appeared to be enlarged.

Diagnostic Considerations

The initial differential diagnosis included a middle or lower brachial plexus lesion, a cervical syrinx, hereditary neuropathy with liability to pressure palsy (HNPP), multifocal chronic inflammatory demyelinating polyneuropathy (multifocal CIDP, also called multifocal acquired demyelinating sensory and motor (MADSAM) neuropathy or Lewis–Sumner syndrome), and leprosy. Leprosy was suggested by the combination of the enlarged nerves with hypopigmented skin lesions and diffuse motor and sensory disturbances of one hand.

Ancillary Investigations

The referring neurologist had already performed routine blood examination and an MRI of the cervical spine and brachial plexus. None of the tests revealed abnormalities. Ultrasound imaging demonstrated enlarged nerves in both arms. Because leprosy was considered, she was referred to a dermatologist. A skin biopsy of the depigmented lesion showed perivascular and peri-adnexal infiltrates with granuloma formation, compatible

Figure 26.1 Claw hand of a patient with lepromatous neuropathy. Claw hand with some atrophy of the intrinsic muscles. Damage to the tip of the index finger and nail beds is due to wounds following loss of sensation.

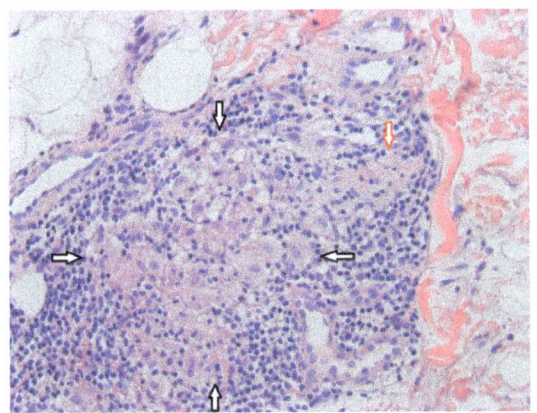

Figure 26.2 Skin biopsy of depigmented lesion. White arrows indicate the perivascular and peri-adnexal infiltrate and granuloma formation, and the red arrow identifies a dermal nerve.

with leprosy, of the borderline-tuberculoid type (Fig. 26.2).

Follow-Up

Once the patient had been diagnosed with leprosy of the borderline-tuberculoid type, treatment with dapsone, rifampicin, clofazimine, and prednisolone was started. After several months of treatment, she burned her hand when using a hairdryer even though sensation had improved. The muscles of her right hand were trained by a hand therapist, and there was some increase in muscle function over a period of one year.

General Remarks

Every year, about 200,000 new leprosy cases are diagnosed worldwide. In Europe and North America, the incidence is low. When taking the medical history, information about migration must be included, as more than 80% of all registered leprosy cases are from India, Brazil, Surinam, Myanmar, Indonesia, Madagascar, and Nepal. Leprosy is caused by a chronic granulomatous immune response to infection of the skin and nerves with *Mycobacterium leprae*, which resides in macrophages and Schwann cells. The infection is transmitted via droplets from the nose and mouth during close and frequent contact with untreated cases. As the replication of *M. leprae* is slow, the incubation period can range from a few years to over 30 years (mean 2–7 years). *M. leprae* can penetrate nerves presumably by binding to laminin, and very often causes signs of neuropathy. As the optimal replication temperature of *M. leprae* is low, it will probably preferentially affect the more superficial parts of nerves. Subsequently, enlarged nerves are more vulnerable to compression. In combination with inflammation and the formation of granulomata, this could easily produce symptoms and signs of mononeuropathy, multiple mononeuropathy (most frequent), or polyneuropathy. The peripheral nerves that are usually affected are – in order of frequency – the posterior tibial, ulnar, median, and peroneal/fibular nerves.

Leprosy is a clinical diagnosis requiring the presence of at least one of the following: a hypopigmented or erythematous skin lesion with a local hypaesthesic area through involvement of dermal nerves, thickened peripheral nerve (clinical or high-resolution nerve sonography) with loss of sensation and/or weakness of the muscles supplied by that nerve, or the identification of acid-fast bacilli (*M. leprae*) in a biopsy from a depigmented lesion or sural nerve.

The primary goal of leprosy multidrug treatment with dapsone, rifampicin, minocycline, and other drugs is to stop the active infection with *M. leprae* to avoid progressive inflammation with formation of granulomata and to stop further progression of the neuropathy, skin lesions, and erosion of hand digits and feet. The ultimate goal is also to improve sensory and muscle function. Occupational and physical therapy may also be helpful. Education is important to prevent further damage due to (burn) wounds.

Suggested Reading

Giesel LM, Hökerberg YHM, Pitta IJR, et al. Clinical prediction rules for the diagnosis of neuritis in leprosy. *BMC Infect Dis* 2021;21(1):858. doi: 10.1186/s12879-021-06545-2. PMID: 34425777; PMCID: PMC8381570.

Tomaselli PJ, Dos Santos DF, Dos Santos ACJ, et al. Primary neural leprosy: clinical, neurophysiological and pathological presentation and progression. *Brain* 2022;145(4):1499–1506. doi: 10.1093/brain/awab396. PMID: 34664630.

World Health Organization. *Towards Zero Leprosy: Global Leprosy (Hansen's Disease) Strategy 2021–2030*. (who.int). Jan 27, 2023. ISBN: 978 92 9022 850 9

Case 27: Charcot–Marie–Tooth Disease (CMT) Type 1A/Hereditary Neuropathy with Liability for Pressure Palsies (HNPP)

Clinical History

A 24-year-old woman had difficulty with walking since early childhood. At age 18 months she was able to walk without support. She often stumbled and could not keep up with her peers in gym class. However, she still had been able to walk 5 km during a four-day walking event. Management included physiotherapy, and she had orthopaedic shoes. She underwent surgery at age eight years (tendon repositions of both feet). Family history was not available because she was adopted. Previous history includes bilateral congenital hip dysplasia and congenital hypothyroidism.

Examination

She had claw hands (Fig. 27.1) and pes cavus. Atrophy and weakness of arms and legs were distal more than proximal. Proximal weakness of arms and legs was MRC grade 4 and distal grade 3–4. She was not able to walk on heels due to anterior tibial muscle weakness, but could stand on tiptoes, which indicates normal strength of the calf muscles. All tendon reflexes were absent. There were severe sensory disturbances: pinprick was decreased at the forearms and lower legs, vibration sense was absent below the knees, and joint position sense was impaired at the ankles.

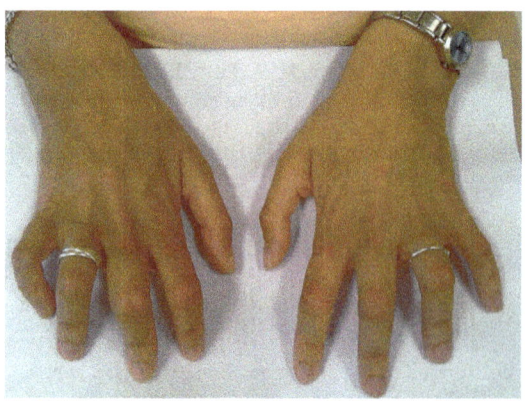

Figure 27.1 Claw hands in a patient with Charcot–Marie–Tooth disease (CMT) type 1A (CMT1A).

Diagnostic Considerations

The clinical picture is that of an early-childhood-onset, slowly progressive motor-sensory polyneuropathy associated with hand and foot deformities. There was no information about the inheritance pattern, but the clinical picture was compatible with Charcot–Marie–Tooth disease (CMT). For further subclassification, nerve conduction studies and DNA analysis (multiplex ligation-dependent probe amplification (MLPA)) were done, first aimed at the *PMP-22* gene, since a duplication is found in close to 50% of all CMT cases.

Ancillary Investigations

Electrodiagnostic studies showed markedly decreased nerve conduction velocities compatible with a demyelinating polyneuropathy. Motor conduction velocity of the n. ulnaris was slow (12 m/sec; normal value > 38 m/sec); the compound muscle action potential (CMAP) amplitude was 1.1 mV (moderately reduced). The sensory nerve action potential (SNAP) amplitude of the ulnar nerve was 2.6 µV (considerably reduced) and the sensory nerve conduction velocity was slow (13 m/s; demyelinating range). A *PMP-22* duplication was found, which led to a diagnosis of CMT type 1A (CMT1A).

Follow-Up

Over a period of 15 years there was progression of muscle weakness. The patient had to use a wheelchair for outdoors transportation and was no longer able to cycle. She was referred to a geneticist for genetic counselling.

General Remarks

Charcot–Marie–Tooth (CMT) disease (hereditary motor and sensory neuropathies; HSMN) is one of the most common inherited neuromuscular disorders.

Dominant and recessive demyelinating forms are classified as CMT1 and type 4 (CMT4), respectively; dominant and recessive axonal forms are classified as CMT type 2 (CMT2) and autosomal recessive CMT2 (AR-CMT2), respectively. Other hereditary neuropathies include hereditary neuropathy with liability to pressure palsies (HNPP), X-linked dominant CMT, distal spinal muscular atrophy (or hereditary motor neuropathy), and hereditary sensory (and autonomic) neuropathies (HS(A)N) (Table 27.1).

CMT1 disease (demyelinating) and CMT2 disease (axonal) can be distinguished using upper limb motor nerve conduction velocities (MNCVs), measured at the median or ulnar nerves. CMT1 is defined by MNCVs < 38 m/s (usually around 25 m/sec) and CMT2 by MNCVs > 38 m/s (usually > 45 m/sec). There is also an intermediate type, with median or ulnar nerve MNCVs between the demyelinating and axonal range (between 25 and 45 m/s). However, there is

Table 27.1 Classification of most frequent types of CMT (> 100 genes), HMN (> 30 genes), HSAN, and HNPP

Name/inheritance	Gene	Features	Comments
CMT1A/AD	PMP-22	Distal weakness and atrophy; legs > arms; pes cavus, claw hands; distal sensory disturbances	Congenital hypomyelinating neuropathy (severe phenotype), AD or AR may also occur
CMT1B/AD	MPZ	Distal weakness and atrophy; legs > arms; pes cavus, claw hands; distal sensory disturbances	Axonal phenotype with pupillary changes and hearing loss may also occur, as does a congenital hypomyelinating neuropathy (severe phenotype), AD or AR
CMT2/AD/rarely AR (see **Case 28**)	MFN2	Distal weakness and atrophy; legs > arms; pes cavus, claw hands; distal sensory signs; sometimes pyramidal signs	Severely affected patients have optic atrophy.
CMT2/dHMN/AR	SORD	Distal motor axonal neuropathy	Most frequent AR CMT2/dHMN; ~70% of cases sporadic. Mean age of onset late adolescence. Sensory symptoms in 50% of cases. Accumulation of sorbitol in blood and tissue. Potentially treatable.
X-CMT/X-linked dominant CMT	GJB1	Distal weakness and atrophy; legs > arms; pes cavus, claw hands; distal sensory signs; CNS white matter lesions may occur	Females mildly affected; demyelinating EMG Males: more severely affected; axonal EMG
CMT4C/AR	SH3TC2	Distal weakness and atrophy; legs > arms; pes cavus, claw hands; distal sensory signs result in sensory ataxia in 70%; scoliosis in 75%; deafness in 70%	Deafness and unresponsive pupils in severely affected patients
CMT4E/AD or AR	EGR2	Neonatal hypotonia, arthrogryposis, generalized weakness	
HS(A)N1/AD (see **Case 29**)	SPTLC1	Age at onset 2nd–3rd decade (average 25 years); pansensory loss; acromutilation; autonomic dysfunction usually not prominent. SPTLC1 is also associated with juvenile ALS and HSP	Most common type of HSAN. Weakness late in course.
HMN(dSMA)/AD	HSPB1, HSPB8, GARS1, BSCL2, SETX, DCTN1	Distal muscle weakness; legs > arms (except GARS1)	Extensor plantar responses in BSCL2, SETX; upper limb predominance in GARS1; vocal cord involvement in DCTN1

Table 27.1 (cont.)

Name/inheritance	Gene	Features	Comments
Distal SMA with diaphragmatic involvement/AR	IGHMBP2	Onset < 2 years; generalized muscle weakness, respiratory insufficiency	Later onset associated with milder neuropathy (AR-CMT2)
HNPP/AD	PMP-22	Episodes of nerve dysfunction with asymmetric motor and/or sensory features; recovery over days to months	Weakness may be permanent; in some patients, phenotype evolves in CMT2

AD = autosomal dominant; AR = autosomal recessive; ALS = amyotrophic lateral sclerosis; CMT1 = Charcot–Marie–Tooth disease, demyelinating phenotype; CMT2 = Charcot–Marie–Tooth disease, axonal phenotype; dHMN = distal hereditary motor neuropathy; HNPP = hereditary neuropathy with liability to pressure palsies; HS(A)N = hereditary sensory (autonomic) neuropathy; HSP = hereditary spastic paraplegia.

an ongoing debate whether the intermediate type is a separate entity, since within a single family individuals can have predominantly demyelinating neuropathy, whereas other family members may have an axonal neuropathy, for example, in X-linked dominant CMT. In X-linked CMT, females usually have an axonal and males a demyelinating phenotype.

In the past, the Dejerine–Sottas syndrome phenotype manifesting in infancy or early childhood and very slow nerve conduction velocities (< 12 m/sec) was considered to be autosomal recessively inherited. However, this phenotype can also be caused by dominant de novo mutations in peripheral myelin protein 22 (*PMP22*), myelin protein zero (*MPZ*), or early growth response 2 (*EGR2*, autosomal dominant or recessive). Our patient was first diagnosed with Dejerine–Sottas because of the very slow conduction velocity.

Clinical features can help the clinician to decide whether a neuropathy is likely to be genetic (Table 27.2). It is important not to rule out an inherited neuropathy in the absence of a positive family history. These apparently sporadic patients are frequently encountered in clinical practice and usually have a pathogenic variant in one of the common autosomal dominantly inherited genes, including *de novo* dominant mutations jn some cases. Pathogenic variants in autosomal recessively inherited genes are less common. A carefully taken family history may help the clinician to further refine the diagnosis. Sometimes, one is not aware of the occurrence of the disease in the family, albeit a 'funny walk' is acknowledged.

Table 27.2 Clinical features of a hereditary neuropathy

- Positive family history (can be absent due to clinical variability or a *de novo* mutation)
- Usually early presentation (infancy–adolescence), but in CMT2 onset may be as late as the seventh decade
- Slow disease progression; autosomal recessive inheritance associated with worse prognosis as compared with autosomal dominant inheritance
- Foot and hand deformities are frequently present

It may be helpful to examine asymptomatic family members for foot deformities and/or areflexia.

Since the identification of the 1.4 Mb duplication of chromosome 17 containing the peripheral myelin protein 22 (*PMP22*) gene as the cause of CMT1A – making *PMP22* the first causative gene for CMT to be identified – there have been rapid advances in understanding the molecular basis for many forms of CMT, and more than 100 causative genes have now been identified. There is a considerable overlap between genes causative of a demyelinating or axonal CMT and between axonal CMT and HMN. Over 80% to 90% of the genetic abnormalities are due to copy number variation in *PMP22* (formerly called duplication or deletion) and single nucleotide variant in *GJB1*, *MPZ*, and *MFN2* genes. It is important to realize that only in one-third of the cases negative for a *PMP22* duplication/deletion a molecular genetic diagnosis can be established, more so in demyelinating as compared with axonal CMT. Next-generation sequencing is the preferred technique for establishing the genetic diagnosis in CMT, including copy number variations.

The lack of a family history does not exclude CMT1A, as about 10% of the CMT1A cases are sporadic. In European populations, CMT1A accounts for ~70% of all CMT1 cases. Point mutations in the *PMP22* gene are associated with a wider spectrum of phenotypes including classic CMT1A and more severe CMT1.

CMT1A patients usually present with a 'classic CMT phenotype' that is length-dependent, the upper limbs becoming affected later than the lower limbs. The onset is in the first two decades, and the clinical picture is characterized by walking difficulty and foot deformity (e.g., pes cavus) associated with distal atrophy and weakness, sensory loss, and hyporeflexia (Fig. 27.2, **Video 27.1**).

CMT1A can also present either at birth or in the first years of life. Symptoms include not only congenital foot deformities, but also delayed motor milestones and more proximal muscle weakness. Tendon reflexes are usually decreased, but not necessarily absent.

There is a marked clinical variability, about 10% of cases being asymptomatic or paucisymptomatic. At the other end of the spectrum, patients (also ~10%) lose ambulation, as was also noticed during follow-up in our patient. Atrophy of hand muscles can also vary (Fig. 27.3). If severe, clawing of the fingers can occur. Respiratory insufficiency due to involvement of the diaphragm is very rare.

The disease course in CMT1A is slowly progressive, rather reflecting a process of normal ageing than ongoing active disease, on top of early dysmyelination causing the clinical picture of weakness and wasting.

Treatment in CMT is still based on symptomatic pharmacological treatment, surgery for skeletal deformities, and rehabilitation therapy. There is yet no disease-modifying therapy for any type of CMT. Strength or endurance training improves functionality and activities of daily life of affected patients.

Pain is a frequent complaint in CMT. Mostly this is biomechanical in nature, but neuropathic pain due to small nerve fibre involvement also occurs. The former requires treatment with analgesic drugs and the latter should be treated with tricyclic antidepressants, SSRI drugs, anticonvulsants (pregabalin, gabapentin, carbamazepine, etc.), or local capsaicin. Fatigue and cramps are also frequent complaints for which there is no clear efficacious treatment.

In general, the patients are referred to the rehabilitation physician for regular follow-up and aids (e.g., orthopaedic shoes, orthoses, cane, or crutches). Education of the patient about the implications of genetic testing, course of the disease, to remain active, and to avoid drugs that may worsen neuropathy is strongly recommended. Surgical interventions are carried out if the foot deformities increase and cannot be corrected by orthopaedic shoes.

Hereditary neuropathy with liability to pressure palsies (HNPP) is an autosomal dominantly inherited disorder; 85% of cases have a copy

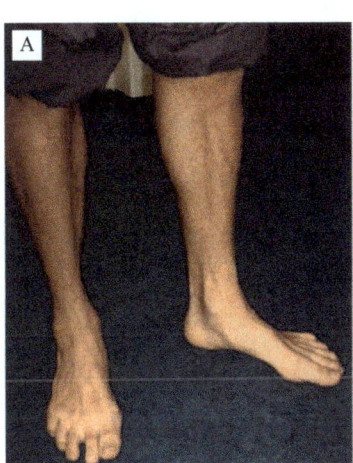
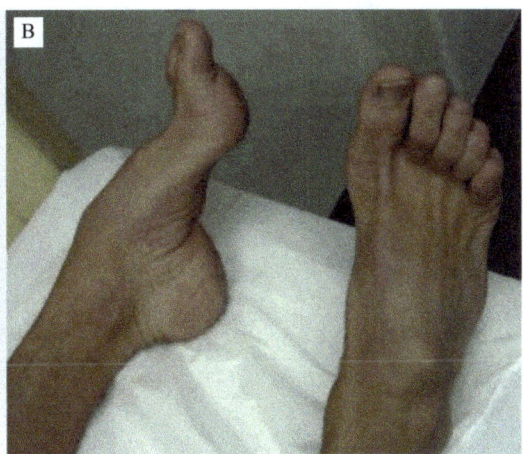

Figure 27.2 (A,B) Muscle atrophy of the lower legs (A), and pes cavus (B) in a patient with CMT1A.

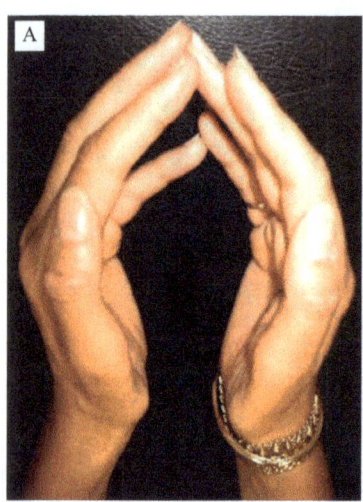 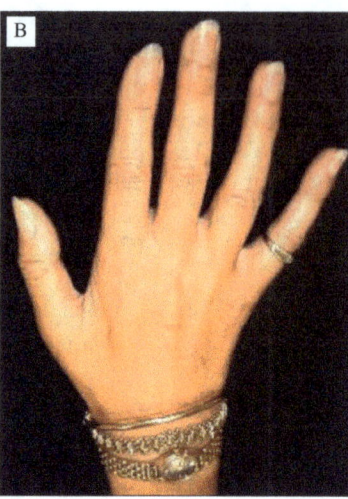

Figure 27.3 (A,B) Thenar atrophy (A) and first interosseal dorsal muscle atrophy (B) in a patient with CMT1A.

number variation (deletion) identical to the region where, in CMT1A, duplication can be found. In the remaining cases with HNPP, point mutations in the *PMP22* gene are causative. More than one-third of the cases have no positive family history. There is reduced penetrance signifying that clinical severity is markedly variable within families. This notion may partly explain the 'negative' family history in many cases. However, 20% of patients affected with HNPP and a *PMP22* deletion have a *de novo* mutation.

Age at onset is usually in the second and third decade. Onset in childhood is rare. Pressure palsies are the hallmark of the disease. Mild trauma or compression is the cause in 40% of patients; other causes are repeated local exercise or stretching. The ulnar and peroneal/fibular nerves are most frequently involved, but virtually every nerve can be affected, even the brachial plexus. The absence of pain discriminates the condition from idiopathic and hereditary neuralgic amyotrophy (NA), albeit that about 5% of these patients report no pain before the NA attack. Usually, the symptoms and signs are mild and transient with full recovery over a period of a few days to months. In due course and with repeated minor nerve injuries, there may be persistent, often asymmetric weakness, especially in the hand. This may cause claw fingers and foot drop. In some advanced cases, the phenotype is close to the classic form of CMT.

Suggested Reading

Bird TD. Charcot-Marie-Tooth hereditary neuropathy overview. 1998 Sep 28 [updated 2023 Feb 23]. In Adam MP, Mirzaa GM, Pagon RA, et al., editors. *GeneReviews®* [Internet]. Seattle, WA: University of Washington; 1993–2023. PMID: 20301532.

Corrado B, Ciardi G, Bargigli C. Rehabilitation management of the Charcot-Marie-Tooth syndrome: a systematic review of the literature. *Medicine (Baltimore)* 2016;95(17):e3278. doi: 10.1097/MD.0000000000003278. PMID: 27124017; PMCID: PMC4998680.

Klein CJ. Charcot-Marie-Tooth disease and other hereditary neuropathies. *Continuum (Minneap Minn)* 2020;26(5):1224–1256. doi: 10.1212/CON.0000000000000927. Erratum in: Continuum (Minneap Minn). 2021 Feb 1;27(1):289. PMID: 33003000.

Kramarz C, Rossor AM. Neurological update: hereditary neuropathies. *J Neurol* 2022;269(9):5187–5191. doi: 10.1007/s00415-022-11164-1. Epub 2022 May 21. PMID: 35596796; PMCID: PMC9363318.

Nagappa M, Sharma S, Taly AB. Charcot-Marie-Tooth disease. 2022 Aug 22. In *StatPearls* [Internet]. Treasure Island, FL: StatPearls Publishing; 2023 Jan–. PMID: 32965834.

Zambon AA, Pini V, Bosco L, et al. Early onset hereditary neuronopathies: an update on non-5q motor neuron diseases. *Brain* 2023;146(3):806–822. doi: 10.1093/brain/awac452. PMID: 36445400; PMCID: PMC9976982.

Charcot–Marie–Tooth Disease (CMT) Type 2A and Type 2B

Clinical History

A 40-year-old man was referred because he wished to be informed about the genetic nature of his disorder. He was diagnosed with Charcot–Marie–Tooth (CMT) disease. At 14 months of age, he started walking, but awkwardly due to a bilateral drop foot for which braces were prescribed. On first examination at age 2 years and 8 months, there was marked atrophy, hypotonia, and areflexia of the lower legs, and slight wasting of the thenar and hypothenar. At that time, nerve conduction studies showed normal motor conduction velocities of arm nerves. No motor unit action potentials could be recorded in the lower leg muscles on concentric needle examination.

Weakness and atrophy were progressive, leading to wheelchair dependency at the age of 11. He had decreased vision for years and had complaints about the quality of his voice. He had no other symptoms, in particular no breathlessness.

The family history disclosed that his father, who died at age 63 years, probably due to respiratory insufficiency, had been evaluated at the age of 35 with an identical clinical picture. He started to walk at 14 months of age, but his gait had always been clumsy. Progression was relentless and he became wheelchair bound by the age of 14. Examination was similar to that described in his son, consisting of bilateral opticopathy with marked decreased visual acuity of 2/60 and severe wasting, weakness, and contractures of all four limbs. In addition, he had severe sensory disturbances and generalized areflexia.

The index patient's older brother was affected with an identical clinical picture of polyneuropathy and opticopathy. In addition, he was found to have bilateral vocal cord paralysis. From the age of 42 years he had received nocturnal noninvasive ventilatory support. At 43, he died unexpectedly, probably due to pneumonia.

Examination

On examination, the patient, who was wheelchair bound, had a high-pitched and hoarse voice, decreased movement of the vocal cords, marked atrophy and weakness of the arms and legs, distal more than proximal, with contractures of the major joints and the finger flexors, scapulae alatae, pectus excavatum, marked lumbar hyperlordosis, and a scoliosis (Fig. 28.1).

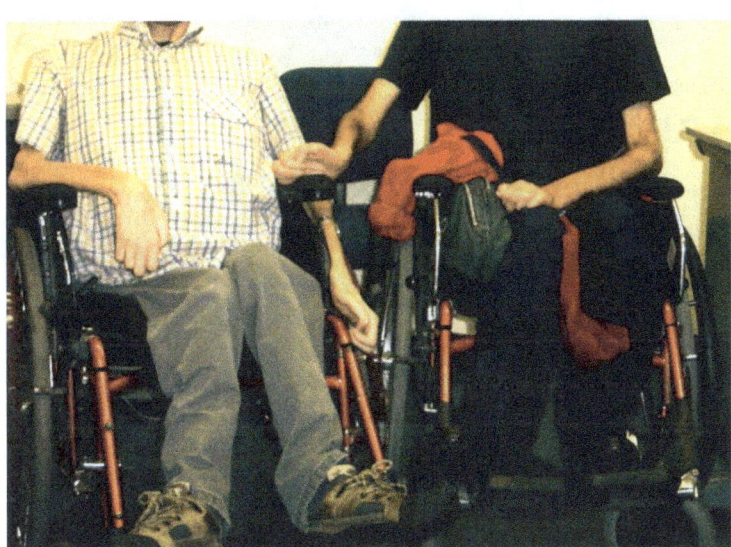

Figure 28.1 The described two brothers with CMT2A caused by an MFN2 mutation. From Züchner et al., Axonal neuropathy with optic atrophy is caused by mutations in mitofusin 2. *Ann Neurol* 2006;59:276–281, with permission.

He had marked distal sensory disturbances, with absent position sense of toes and fingers, and generalized areflexia.

Ophthalmological examination revealed a visual acuity of 4/20. There was mild anisocoria, the left pupil being slightly larger. The pupillary reactions were slow and symmetric. There was no ophthalmoparesis or ptosis. Ophthalmoscopic examination revealed very pale optic discs with a small cup. The macula, peripheral retina, and blood vessels were normal.

Diagnostic Considerations

The combination of autosomal dominantly inherited motor and sensory symptoms and signs is consistent with a hereditary polyneuropathy. Nerve conduction velocities had been examined at age 2 years and 8 months and were normal, which is more compatible with an axonal than a demyelinating neuropathy. The presence of an optic neuropathy narrows down the differential diagnosis to CMT2A caused by variants in mitofusin 2 (*MFN2*) or pyridoxal kinase (*PDXK*).

Ancillary Investigations

Additional investigation with electrophysiology showed an abnormal visual evoked potential (VEP). The pattern VEP was flat, and with a flash VEP, very weak responses were elicited. The electroretinogram was normal. It was concluded that there was a severe optic atrophy that had been stable for at least 13 years.

Vital capacity was decreased (62% of expected). EMG showed severe axonal sensorimotor polyneuropathy with absent CMAPs and SNAPs of the distal nerves of arms and legs.

DNA analysis revealed a missense mutation (c.1090C>T, p.R364W) in the mitofusin 2 (*MFN2*) gene on chromosome 1p36.2.

Follow-Up

There was progression over a 10-year follow-up period. He had difficulty sitting in an upright position in his wheelchair. He also complained about morning headache and shortness of breath while talking and therefore he was referred to the department of home mechanical ventilation. A severely restricted lung function was found, but there was no nocturnal hypoventilation. He died unexpectedly a few months after his last follow-up visit at age 52 years.

General Remarks

Axonal CMT (CMT2) represents approximately one-third of the total CMT, and may be associated with unusual clinical features, such as delayed motor development, ankle contracture, kyphoscoliosis, pyramidal features, vocal cord paralysis, hearing loss, optic atrophy, and abnormal pupillary reaction.

CMT2A is caused by mutations in the mitofusin 2 gene (*MFN2*). Among autosomal dominantly inherited CMT2, CMT2A is the most frequent form, accounting for approximately 10–40% of axonal CMT cases and 4–7% of all CMTs with a genetic diagnosis (*SORD* is probably the most frequent form of autosomal recessively inherited CMT2). There is clinical heterogeneity: there are mild cases, but mostly there is severe involvement from early childhood onwards, leading to wheelchair dependency. Axonal CMT with optic atrophy caused by *MFN2* mutations, as found in the case report, is often referred to as HMSN type VI or CMTVI.

A peculiar CMT2 subtype is CMT2B caused by variants in the RAS-associated protein gene (*Rab7*) and mainly manifesting with sensory abnormalities and ulceromutilating features (Fig. 28.2). Most patients have pes cavus and some also have distal muscle weakness in the legs. There is an overlap with hereditary sensory and autonomic neuropathies

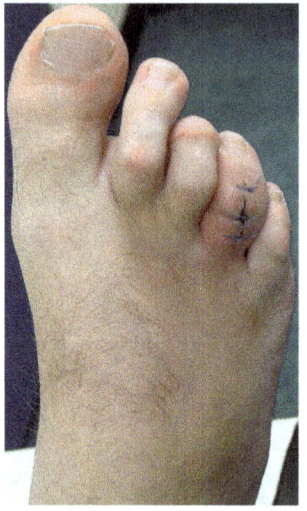

Figure 28.2 Patient with CMT2B (*RAB7*) in whom the distal part of his third digit of the right foot was amputated because of poorly healing ulcers and osteomyelitis. He recently underwent surgery for another ulcer.

(HSAN). Rarely, *RAB7* variants can also cause the classic CMT2 phenotype with motor predominance.

Suggested Reading

Abati E, Manini A, Velardo D, et al. Clinical and genetic features of a cohort of patients with MFN2-related neuropathy. *Sci Rep* 2022;12(1):6181. doi: 10.1038/s41598-022-10220-0. PMID: 35418194; PMCID: PMC9008012.

Cortese A, Zhu Y, Rebelo AP et al. Biallelic mutations in SORD cause a common and potentially treatable hereditary neuropathy with implications for diabetes. Nat Genet. 2020 May;52 (5):473-481. doi: 10.1038/s41588-020-0615–4. Epub 2020 May 4.

Case 29: Hereditary Sensory and Autonomic Neuropathy (HSAN) Type 4

Clinical History

Within a period of a few days, a 34-year-old woman developed progressive weakness of the right leg without pain. Having suffered spontaneous bone fractures as a child, she had been diagnosed with insensitivity to pain syndrome. She had never been able to perspire; this meant warm weather was not well tolerated and it resulted in an increase in body temperature. The tip of the right thumb had been amputated following a skin ulcer ('panaritium').

Her 36-year-old sister also had had several spontaneous bone fractures without pain. She had similar but less severe complaints. The parents are full cousins.

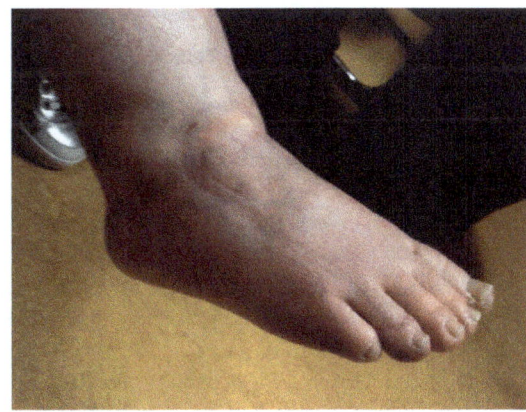

Figure 29.1 HSAN 4 (*NTRK1*): Charcot deformity of the foot.

Examination

The patient was of short stature. Sharp–dull discrimination was diminished in the arms, more pronounced distally. Passive movements of the legs caused some back pain. Muscle strength and pain sense in the right leg were diminished. Below the knees, sharp–dull discrimination was absent and warm–cold sensation impaired. Vibration sense was normal. She had Charcot deformities and neuropathic arthropathy of the right knee and ankle (Fig. 29.1).

Neurological examination of the sister showed normal pain sensation in the arms with decreased pain sense below the knees.

Diagnostic Considerations

Both sisters had neuropathy with congenital insensitivity to pain, decreased cold and warm sensation, anhidrosis, and skin ulcers. Proprioception, muscle strength, and reflexes were normal. Early onset with fractures and consanguinity of the healthy parents was compatible with autosomal recessive hereditary sensory and autonomic neuropathy. Due to sensory disturbances, microtrauma and the resulting inflammatory response passed unnoticed.

Ancillary Investigations

The MRI of the lumbosacral spine showed collapse of the first and second lumbar vertebrae compatible with Charcot arthropathy of the spine (CSA), also known as spinal neuroarthropathy. In addition, the MRI of the cervical spine showed neurogenic arthropathy at the level C4–C7 (Fig. 29.2). Needle EMG and motor nerve conduction velocities were normal. SNAPs were reduced in arm nerves and could not be elicited in lower limb nerves, suggesting dying back axonal degeneration. Short stimuli of 30 mA caused pain. DNA analysis revealed homozygous pathological variants in the neurotrophic receptor tyrosine kinase (NTRK) 1 gene, confirming a diagnosis of hereditary sensory and autonomic neuropathy (HSAN) type 4.

Follow-Up

After decompression and fixation of the spine, she complained of stiffness when walking, altered sensation and decreased strength in both hands, and tingling in the fingertips that progressed over periods of weeks. A cervical MRI showed severe degeneration of cervical vertebrae leading to spinal stenosis and myelopathy. She had no pyramidal signs. Following C3–C6 cervical laminectomy and spondylodesis, her neurological condition improved.

General Remarks

The hereditary sensory and autonomic neuropathies (HSANs) are a group of heterogeneous disorders characterized by slowly progressive loss of the unmyelinated and small myelinated peripheral nerves, leading to loss of pain and temperature sensation and dysautonomia (Table 29.1). Touch and vibration are relatively preserved in most cases. Several autosomal dominant and autosomal recessive types are distinguished based on the gene involved. Nerve conduction studies show reduced sensory nerve action potentials, and sometimes reduced compound muscle action potentials. The diagnosis is made by means of next-generation sequencing gene panel analysis.

In autosomal recessively inherited subtypes, the clinical features are apparent from birth and include hypotonia, feeding difficulties, increased secretions, vomiting, inappropriate temperature control, or apnoea. In autosomal dominantly inherited subtypes, onset is in the second to fourth decade.

In some subtypes there is predominant dysautonomia, notably type 3 (familial dysautonomia, Riley–Day syndrome, *IKBKAP/ELP1*). In other subtypes, symptoms and signs are primarily related to loss of pain and temperature sensation (congenital insensitivity to pain (CIP), hereditary sensory neuropathy (HSN)). Dysautonomic crises manifest as

Table 29.1 Main features of hereditary sensory and autonomic neuropathies (HSANs)

- AR types: *WNK1, IKBKAP/ELP1, FAM134B, KIF1A, SCN9A, NTRK1, NGFβ, DST, PRDM12*. Clinical features present at birth.
- AD types: *SPTLC1, SPTLC2, ATL1, DNMT1, ATL3, SCN11A*. Onset in second to fourth decade.
- Insensitivity to pain can lead to unnoticed burns and ulceration, osteomyelitis, amputation, and Charcot arthropathy.
- Dysautonomia includes anhidrosis complicated by hyperpyrexia and dystrophic hair and nails, hyperhidrosis, bladder dysfunction, sexual dysfunction, postural hypotension, gastrointestinal dysmotility, alacrima, pruritus.
- Slow progression with reduced life expectancy in case of severe dysautonomia.
- Multidisciplinary management to minimize orthopaedic complications and symptoms of dysautonomia is paramount.

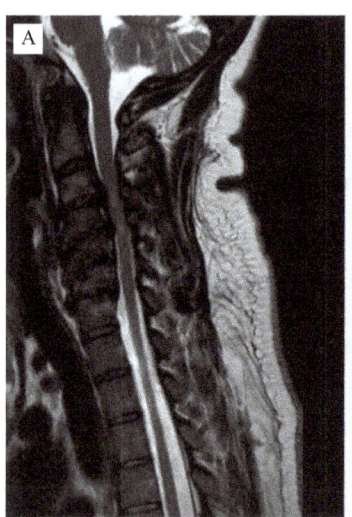 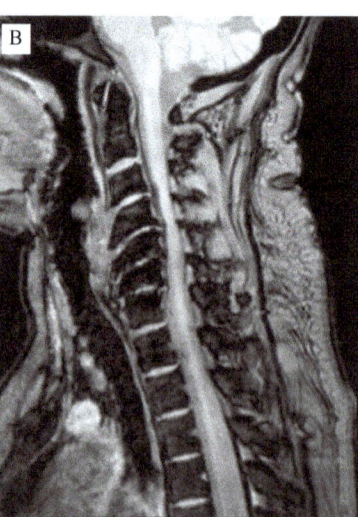

Figure 29.2(A,B) HSAN 4 (*NTRK1*): T2-weighted MRI scan shows loss of height of the 4th to 6th cervical vertebrae and abnormal bone formation causing cervical stenosis and myelopathy (A). T2-weighted fast field echo showing abnormal bone formation around the 4th to 6th cervical vertebrae (B).

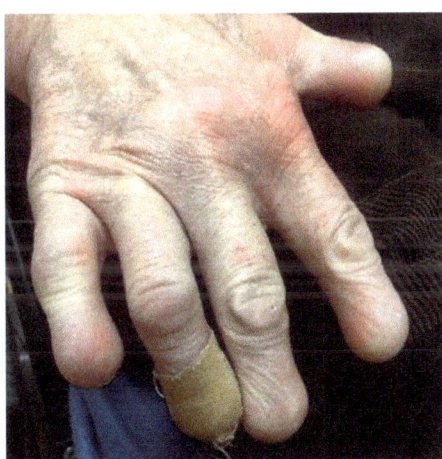

Figure 29.3 HSAN 2B (*FAM134B*). 65-year-old man showing amputations and distal contractures. Earlier, he had been diagnosed with hereditary spastic paraplegia because of hyperreflexia.

Table 29.2 Charcot arthropathy

Causes

- Myelopathy
- Syringomyelia
- Spina bifida
- Trauma
- Tabes dorsalis
- Neuropathies:
  - Diabetes mellitus
  - Leprosy
  - Hereditary sensory and autonomic neuropathy
  - Charcot–Marie–Tooth disease (rare)

Symptoms and signs

- Erythema, oedema, elevated temperature of the affected joint
- Pain (can be absent in HSAN)
- Thickening of the joint
- Deformity of the joint
- Loss of function
- Crepitation at palpation

nausea, vomiting, hypertension, tachycardia, hyperhidrosis, among others. Insensitivity to pain and temperature, together with autonomic dysregulation, can eventually lead to serious complications such as mutilating amputations (Fig. 29.3), osteomyelitis, fatal sepsis, and Charcot deformities. Charcot arthropathy may affect all axial and peripheral joints with the knee, foot, and spine being predominantly affected (Table 29.2). Sensitivity to visceral pain is preserved. Several subtypes are characterized by distinctive features such as burning or lancinating pain, intellectual disability and distal weakness (type 1A, *SPTLC1*), chronic cough (type IB), absent lingual fungiform papillae (type 3, *IKBKAP/ELP1*), or hyperreflexia and spasticity (e.g., type 2B, *FAM134B*, Fig. 29.3). In severe dysautonomia, life expectancy is reduced.

Treatment should be provided in a multidisciplinary setting. Podiatrists, dermatologists, physical and occupational therapists, prosthetists, and orthopaedic surgeons can provide foot and limb care, which is paramount in minimizing complications. Other disciplines include dentists (in case of tongue ulcerations), ophthalmologists (in case of alacrima), and gastroenterologists (in case of vomiting and reflux). Prevention of overheating in case of anhidrosis is recommended. Management of orthostatic hypotension comprises several supportive measures. Carbidopa reduces the severity of nausea, vomiting attacks, and blood pressure variability. Hypertension in autonomic crises can be treated with α_2-adrenergic agonists such as clonidine and intranasal dexmedetomidine. Neuropathic pain and restless legs syndrome are treated with pregabalin or gabapentin. *HSAN1* missense mutations reduce the affinity of the encoded enzyme SPT for L-serine, leading to the formation of neurotoxic sphingolipids. In adults with HSAN1A, a randomized, placebo-controlled trial showed that high-dose oral L-serine during one year is safe and effective as measured by the Charcot–Marie–Tooth Neuropathy Score, but the primary endpoint was not met (Fridman et al., 2019).

Suggested Reading

Farrugia PR, Bednar D, Oitment C. Charcot arthropathy of the spine. *J Am Acad Orthop Surg* 2022;30(21): e1358–e1365. doi: 10.5435/JAAOS-D-22-00212. Epub 2022 Aug 25. PMID: 36007201.

Fridman V, Suriyanarayanan S, Novak P, et al. Randomized trial of L-serine in patients with hereditary sensory and autonomic neuropathy type 1. *Neurology* 2019;92(4):e359–e370. doi: 10.1212/WNL.0000000000006811. Epub 2019 Jan 9. PMID: 30626650; PMCID: PMC6345118.

González-Duarte A, Cotrina-Vidal M, Kaufmann H, Norcliffe-Kaufmann L. Familial dysautonomia. *Clin Auton Res* 2023;33(3):269–280. doi: 10.1007/s10286-023-00941-1. Epub 2023 May 19. PMID: 37204536.

Schwartzlow C, Kazamel M. Hereditary sensory and autonomic neuropathies: adding more to the classification. *Curr Neurol Neurosci Rep* 2019;19 (8):52. doi: 10.1007/s11910-019-0974-3. PMID: 31222456.

Sethi PK, Sethi NK. Charcot joint. *Ann Neurol* 2022;91 (3):436–437. doi: 10.1002/ana.26310. Epub 2022 Feb 10. PMID: 35084055

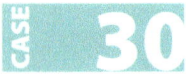

Hereditary Transthyretin (TTR) Amyloidosis

Clinical History

A 70-year-old man noticed a feeling of walking on cotton wool for the past two years. Numbness had progressed from the toes to the knees, and for half a year there was tingling and numbness in the fingertips. These complaints were symmetric and there was no pain. Walking had become insecure. For one year he had no erections, whereas sexual function had previously been normal. There were no other signs of autonomic dysfunction. In the past two years there was also shortness of breath on exertion. A diagnosis of cardiomyopathy had been made recently.

The family history revealed vitreous opacities in the father and several siblings. A brother also had sensory disturbances in his feet and a thickened heart muscle. His four daughters did not have any complaints.

Examination

There was atrophy of the extensor digitorum brevis muscles and symmetric weakness of all foot and toe dorsal flexors (MRC grade 4) and plantar flexors (MRC 4+). Sensation was impaired for touch and pain at the fingers and distally from the knees. Vibration was absent distal from the ankles. Tendon reflexes in the arms and the knee tendon reflexes were low, and the Achilles tendon reflexes were absent. Walking was insecure and walking on heels and tiptoes was not possible.

Diagnostic Considerations

The family history suggests autosomal dominant hereditary disease, but the rate of progression is faster than what is usual in Charcot–Marie–Tooth disease. Vasculitis neuropathy is unlikely because there is no pain and because symptoms and signs were not multifocal. In chronic inflammatory demyelinating polyneuropathy (CIDP), there often is generalized areflexia after two years, and autonomic dysfunction is usually not prominent. The combination of a sensorimotor polyneuropathy with autonomic dysfunction, cardiomyopathy, and vitreous opacities is strongly suggestive of familial TTR-amyloidosis, which can be confirmed by sequencing of the *TTR* gene.

Ancillary Investigations

Nerve conduction studies showed a symmetric axonal sensorimotor polyneuropathy. Standard laboratory investigations for causes of axonal polyneuropathy were normal. There was no paraprotein and free kappa/lambda light chain ratio was also normal. Analysis of the *TTR* gene showed the pathogenic c.148G>A (p.Val50Met) variant.

Follow-Up

At the time of the diagnosis, the patient did not qualify for treatment with tafamidis or liver transplantation because the polyneuropathy was already too severe. He started treatment with diflunisal and was also treated with drugs for imminent congestive heart failure. He also started using ankle-foot orthoses because of the foot drop. The sensory complaints deteriorated, causing difficulties with activities of daily living. Two years later, the diflunisal was discontinued because he started participation in the APOLLO trial (patisiran vs. placebo). He continued to get worse: he could no longer work at his computer because of the sensory disturbances. He became wheelchair dependent because of progressive weakness in the legs. Five years after onset of the first complaints, there was weakness of proximal muscles in arms and legs

(MRC grade 4), distal arm muscles grade 4, and distal leg muscles grade 0. Eating was difficult because he became nauseous even after a light meal. There were cardiac conduction disturbances, but before a pacemaker was implanted, he died, aged 74 years.

General Remarks

Amyloidosis

Amyloid is a misfolded protein which is deposited extracellularly as insoluble amyloid fibrils. In systemic amyloidosis, there is progressive loss of function in multiple organs, notably heart, kidney, lung, liver, spleen. Polyneuropathy and myopathy can occur in any form of amyloidosis and may cause progressive sensorimotor and autonomic polyneuropathy and progressive proximal weakness, sometimes as a presenting feature. Amyloid can be demonstrated by means of the Congo-red stain in unpolarized or crossed-polarized light in a biopsy, preferably of an involved organ (Fig. 30.1). Abdominal subcutaneous fat aspiration is the most used technique to diagnose amyloidosis at a surrogate site. The reported sensitivity is 72–93% in specialized centres.

Many small proteins are susceptible to forming amyloid under certain circumstances, and the many amyloid disorders, acquired and hereditary, are classified according to these amyloid precursor proteins. In light chain amyloidosis (AL), which is the most frequent type of amyloidosis, amyloid is formed by high serum levels of either lambda or kappa immunoglobulin-free light chains, demonstrable in chronic plasma cell dyscrasias. The second most frequent form of amyloidosis, AA, is caused by amyloid formed by serum amyloid A protein (SAA). This is an acute phase reactant, which can be present in high levels in chronic autoimmune or infectious inflammation.

The third most frequent form of amyloidosis is TTR amyloidosis (ATTR), encompassing a non-familial variant and an autosomal dominantly inherited variant. The precursor protein is transthyretin (TTR), a transport protein. In the non-familial variant (ATTRw), normal ('wild type') TTR may form amyloid with ageing, especially in men, causing cardiomyopathy and carpal tunnel syndrome. The hereditary form (ATTRv), also called hATTR, arises from a point mutation in the *TTR* gene, resulting in an amino acid substitution. More than 150 amyloidogenic mutations have been identified.

Neuropathic Hereditary Transthyretin Amyloidosis

The most frequent clinical manifestation of hereditary ATTR amyloidosis is an adult-onset, severe, symmetric distal sensorimotor polyneuropathy (neuropathic hereditary transthyretin amyloidosis, or hereditary transthyretin amyloidosis-polyneuropathy (ATTRv-PN), formerly called transthyretin familial amyloid polyneuropathy (TTR-FAP)), see Table 30.1. There can be predominantly small fibre involvement, resulting in autonomic symptoms and burning neuropathic pain, sometimes as presenting symptoms. Even if there is no positive family history, TTR-FAP should be suspected in case of rapid progression, autonomic dysfunction, concomitant cardiac abnormalities, vitreous opacities, bilateral carpal tunnel syndrome, weight loss, or renal impairment. Misdiagnoses, delaying appropriate treatment, are

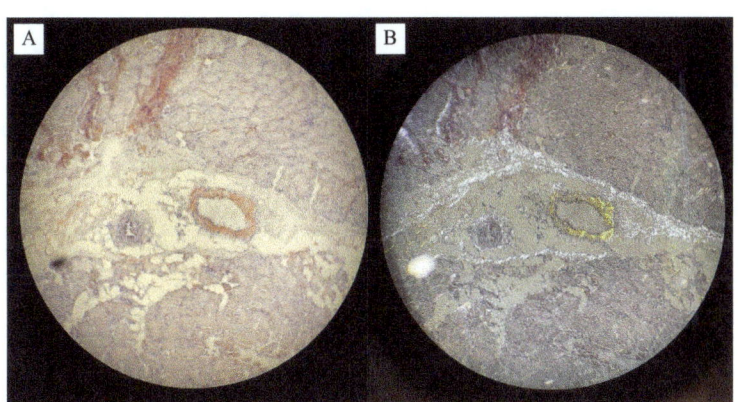

Figure 30.1(A,B) Amyloid deposition in a vessel wall (centre) in a frozen muscle biopsy section. Amyloid appears salmon-pink on a Congo-red stain with unpolarized light (A) and yellow-green by birefringence in cross-polarized light imaging (B). This 67-year-old woman presented with subacute weakness of pelvic girdle muscles, CK 302, as a first manifestation of light chain (AL) amyloidosis. Courtesy Professor Eleonora Aronica and Dr. Wim van Hecke.

Table 30.1 Main clinical features of neuropathic hereditary TTR amyloidosis

- Early or late adult-onset distal symmetric sensorimotor polyneuropathy
- Small fibre involvement with burning pain and dysautonomia. Erectile dysfunction may precede sensory symptoms.
- Time to needing a walking aid 3–6 years.
- Cardiac arrhythmias, conduction abnormalities, restrictive cardiomyopathy (80%)
- Bilateral carpal tunnel syndrome

CIDP, lumbar radiculopathies, paraproteinemic neuropathy, and light chain amyloidosis.

Several modes of treatment for TTR-FAP are now known to be effective. Diflunisal (a non-steroidal anti-inflammatory drug) and tafamidis stabilize the TTR tetramer, preventing its dissociation into amyloidogenic monomers. These drugs have been shown to delay disease progression. Inotersen, an antisense oligonucleotide drug (ASO), and patisiran, a small interfering RNA (siRNA), can strongly decrease levels of TTR (which is dispensable) and both drugs were shown in recent phase 3 randomized controlled trials to be effective in preventing disease progression. These treatments may, however, be limited by serious side effects. A liver transplant can be an option in early-onset ATTR-Val30Met patients. Other therapeutic approaches such as CRISPR-Cas9–based in vivo gene editing are currently under investigation. Without treatment, median survival in TTR-FAP is 10 years.

Suggested Reading

Aimo A, Castiglione V, Rapezzi C, et al. RNA-targeting and gene editing therapies for transthyretin amyloidosis. *Nat Rev Cardiol* 2022;19(10):655–667. doi: 10.1038/s41569-022-00683-z. Epub 2022 Mar 23. PMID: 35322226.

Carroll A, Dyck PJ, de Carvalho M, et al. Novel approaches to diagnosis and management of hereditary transthyretin amyloidosis. *J Neurol Neurosurg Psychiatry* 2022;93(6):668–678. doi: 10.1136/jnnp-2021-327909. Epub 2022 Mar 7. PMID: 35256455; PMCID: PMC9148983.

Gillmore JD, Gane E, Taubel J, et al. CRISPR-Cas9 in vivo gene editing for transthyretin amyloidosis. *N Engl J Med* 2021;385(6):493–502. doi: 10.1056/NEJMoa2107454. Epub 2021 Jun 26. PMID: 34215024.

Kaku M, Berk JL. Neuropathy associated with systemic amyloidosis. *Semin Neurol* 2019;39(5):578–588. doi: 10.1055/s-0039-1688994. Epub 2019 Oct 22. PMID: 31639841.

Magrinelli F, Fabrizi GM, Santoro L, et al. Pharmacological treatment for familial amyloid polyneuropathy. *Cochrane Database Syst Rev* 2020;4(4):CD012395. doi: 10.1002/14651858.CD012395.pub2. PMID: 32311072; PMCID: PMC7170468.

Plante-Bordeneuve V. Transthyretin familial amyloid polyneuropathy: an update. *J Neurol* 2018;265(4):976–983. doi: 10.1007/s00415-017-8708-4. Epub 2017 Dec 16. PMID: 29249054.

Wisniowski B, Wechalekar A. Confirming the diagnosis of amyloidosis. *Acta Haematol* 2020;143(4):312–321. doi: 10.1159/000508022. Epub 2020 Jun 16. PMID: 32544917.

Disorders of the Neuromuscular Junction

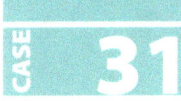

Myasthenia Gravis with Acetylcholine Receptor Antibodies (AChR MG)

Clinical History

A 70-year-old woman was referred by her GP because of progressive nasal speech and difficulties with chewing and swallowing, shortly after abdominal surgery because of a borderline malignant cystoadenofibroma of the uterus. Weeks later, she also noticed drooping of both eyelids and a tendency for her head to drop at the end of a day. In retrospect, mild nasal speech had been present for some months prior to surgery.

Examination

An asymmetric ptosis increased after looking upward for 20 seconds, with the eyelid covering the pupil. She had no diplopia. There was mild bulbar dysarthria and mild weakness of neck extensor muscles. Atrophy and fasciculation of the tongue were absent. There was no limb weakness.

Diagnostic Considerations

Both the clinical history and the neurological examination provided evidence of fluctuating oculobulbar muscle weakness. The clinical diagnosis of generalized (i.e., not exclusively ocular) myasthenia gravis can be confirmed in most patients by the finding of an increased level of serum anti-acetylcholine receptor (anti-AChR) or anti-muscle-specific kinase (anti-MuSK) autoantibodies.

Ancillary Investigations

Vital capacity was normal. The level of serum AChR autoantibodies was increased and autoantibodies to striated muscle proteins were detectable. CT scan of the chest showed signs of a thymoma measuring 1.4 inch × 1.1 inch.

Follow-Up

Pyridostigmine had no effect and the bulbar weakness worsened over days. She improved quickly on intravenous immunoglobulins (IVIg) and high-dose oral prednisolone (1 mg/kg/day). Azathioprine was not well tolerated. Thymoma surgery was successful. In subsequent years, she had several periods of increased bulbar weakness when under physical or emotional stress. These were successfully treated with an increase in prednisolone dose or with IVIg. Seven years after presentation, she had surgery for a colon carcinoma. During the ensuing years, myasthenia gravis remained stable on low-dose prednisolone.

General Remarks

Of all acquired disorders of the neuromuscular junction, myasthenia gravis (MG) caused by autoantibodies directed to the skeletal muscle nicotine AChR at the post-synaptic membrane is the most common. About 85% of patients with generalized weakness have these antibodies. In half of the remaining 15% of patients, antibodies targeting other molecules at the postsynaptic neuromuscular junction can be demonstrated (MuSK, 6%) and low-density lipoprotein receptor-related protein 4 (LRP4, 2%). Antibody testing is becoming more sensitive with improved immunoassay techniques.

The clinical hallmark of AChR MG is weakness of striated muscles, which is aggravated by activity of these muscles and improves with rest (Table 31.1). Fluctuating, asymmetric external ophthalmoplegia is the most frequent presentation (Fig. 31.1), and

Table 31.1 Main features of AChR-myasthenia gravis

- Fatigable weakness of extra-ocular muscles (diplopia) and asymmetric, fatigable ptosis (**Video 31.1**).
- Fatigable weakness of muscles involved in swallowing, chewing, speech (bulbar weakness), holding up the head, may extend to weakness of limb girdle muscles.
- Treatment with pyridostigmine, prednisone, conventional non-steroidal immunosuppressants, C5 complement inhibitors, neonatal Fc receptor inhibitors.
- Thymectomy has been shown to be effective in adult patients with disease duration < 5 years.
- Myasthenic crisis: rapidly evolving bulbar weakness and respiratory insufficiency. Good effect of IVIg and plasma exchange.
- Patients with early onset (< 50 years) are commonly women.
- Patients with very late onset (> 65 years) are commonly men. They may present with severe disease and respond well to timely and appropriate treatment.

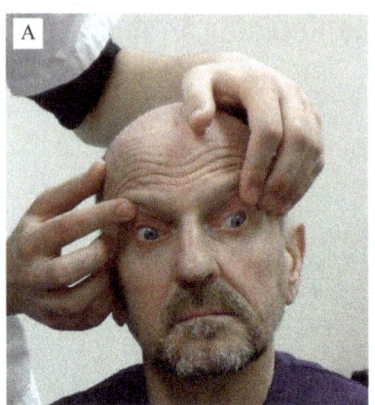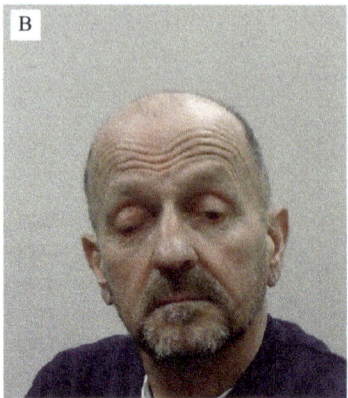

Figure 31.1 (A,B) External ophthalmoplegia (A) and severe disabling ptosis (B) in myasthenia gravis.

generalized weakness usually develops within two years. The disease remains confined to extraocular weakness (ptosis, diplopia) in 15% of patients. In early-onset myasthenia gravis (< 50 years), patients are most frequently female. Spontaneous long-lasting remission occurs occasionally in this group. Isolated myasthenic bulbar weakness in younger women is relatively frequently caused by anti-MuSK. Several drugs may induce or worsen myasthenia gravis via diverse mechanisms (see **Case 33**).

Diagnosis

Provocation tests often support the diagnosis if the clinical history points to myasthenia gravis (Fig. 31.2, **Video 31.1**). An increased level of serum antibody to muscle AChR confirms the diagnosis. Antibody testing has high sensitivity and specificity in generalized AChR MG, but not in isolated ocular myasthenia. In this group, approximately 50% are seronegative. Useful electrophysiological tests include repetitive 3 Hz nerve stimulation of the ulnar, accessory, and facial nerves, showing a decremental response of the compound muscle action potential (CMAP) in a symptomatic muscle (Fig. 31.3). Single-fibre EMG of the orbicularis oculi muscles is particularly sensitive for a diagnosis of ocular myasthenia gravis and also reaches high specificity in combination with a positive ice pack test in these patients. The neostigmine test can be performed at the bedside but may be difficult to interpret. Autoantibodies to striated muscle proteins (titin, ryanodine receptors) are associated with more severe disease, with oropharyngeal weakness, myasthenic crises, and with thymoma.

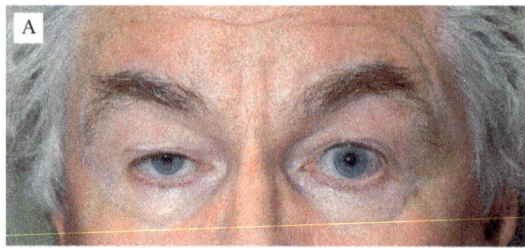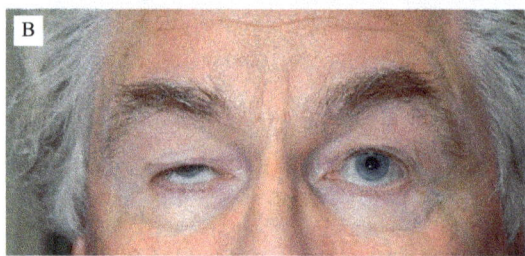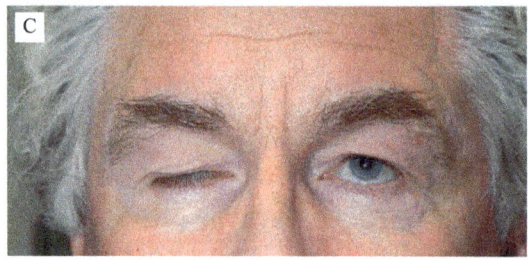

Figure 31.2 (A–C) A 62-year-old man with AChR-positive ocular myasthenia gravis. Right-sided slight ptosis at rest (A), worsening to almost complete ptosis (B,C) and slight left-sided ptosis when looking upwards for 30 seconds (C).

Treatment and Prognosis

The treatment of first choice is a cholinesterase inhibitor (pyridostigmine) in sufficiently high and frequent doses. Most patients need 6 × 60 mg/day.

Case 31 AChR Myasthenia Gravis

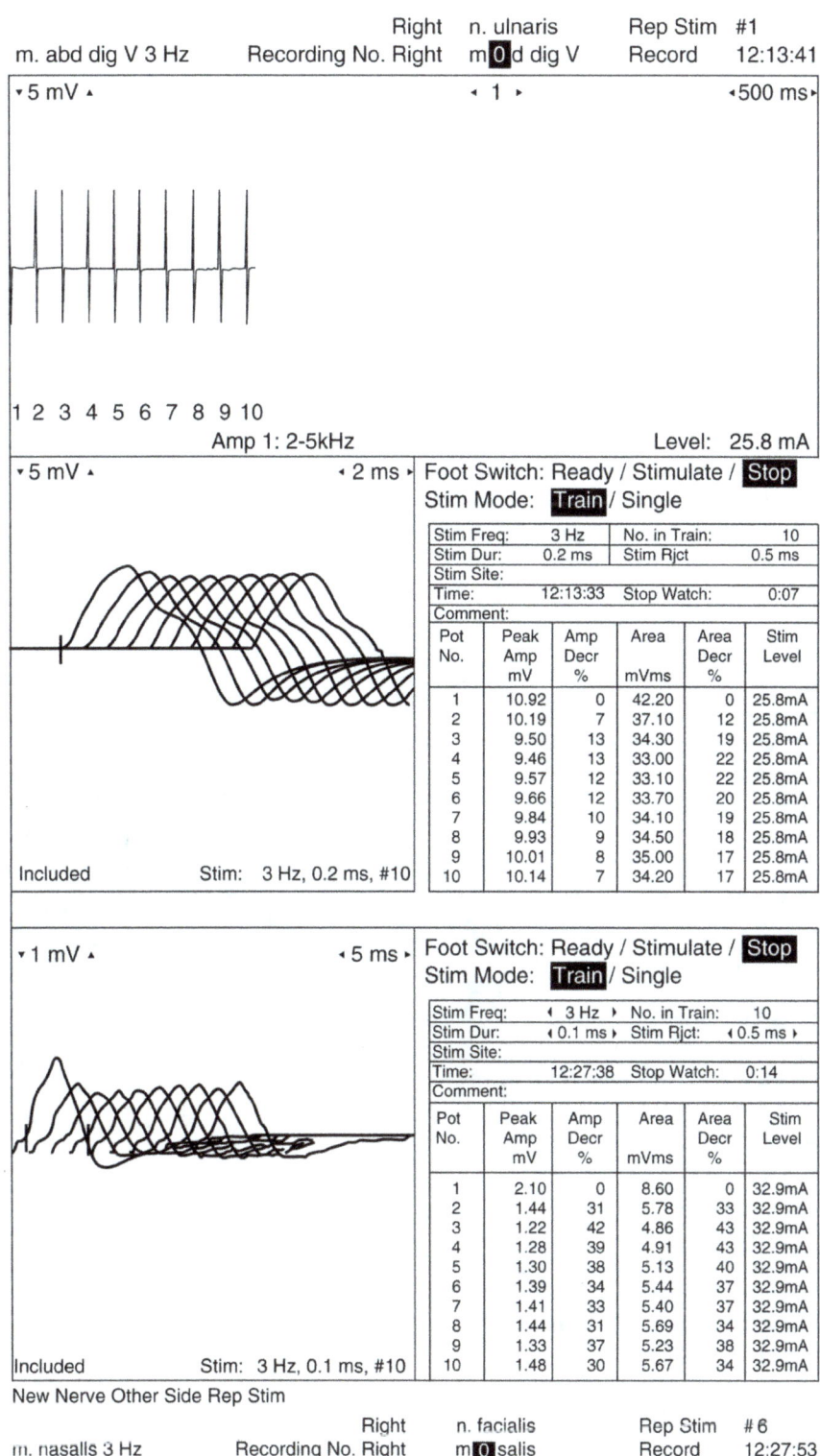

Figure 31.3 Decrement of the CMAP during 3 Hz stimulation in a patient with myasthenia gravis. The CMAP decrease is most prominent with the fourth or fifth stimulus and becomes less pronounced thereafter. Upper and middle panels: Stimulus of the ulnar nerve at the wrist with recording from the abductor digiti minimi muscle shows a decrement of up to 13%. Lower panel: stimulation of a facial nerve branch at the cheek with recording from the nasal muscle shows a decrement of up to 42%.

Some need a controlled-release formulation before the night. Pyridostigmine is usually well tolerated. Diarrhoea can be treated with atropine sulphate 0.125–0.250 mg per dose of pyridostigmine or with loperamide, but can be avoided by starting with a lower dose. Cramps and fasciculation may also occur. Thymomas should always be surgically removed because of the risk of infiltrative growth. In the absence of a thymoma, thymectomy is recommended in adult patients <65 years of age with AChR-positive generalized MG as soon as possible within 5 years of disease duration. Thymectomy may be considered in younger patients, and in ocular AChR-positive myasthenia and seronegative myasthenia but has no proven efficacy in these groups.

If the effect of pyridostigmine is not satisfactory, the benefits of prednisolone (1–1.5 mg/kg daily, max 80 mg, 30 mg in ocular MG) together with azathioprine (or methotrexate) as prednisolone-sparing agent should be weighed against the adverse effects with long-term use. Many patients with bulbar weakness will need corticosteroid treatment. Transient worsening may occur at the end of the first week or in the second week of treatment. High-dose prednisolone is administered for four to six weeks. After this period, the dosage can be tapered gradually and slowly to a maintenance therapy of 15–25 mg on alternate days, for example. Once stabilization has been achieved and the patient has improved, further tapering can be tried. Some patients are kept on azathioprine for years. It is not clear whether antibody levels can be used as biomarkers for disease activity in individual patients, and their use to guide treatment strategies is currently not recommended.

Beside azathioprine and methotrexate, other non-steroidal immunosuppressants such as mycophenolate mofetil, cyclosporine, tacrolimus, and rituximab can be used as steroid-sparing drugs, or as monotherapy if prednisolone is contraindicated, but their use is in general not supported by clinical evidence. With treatment, most patients will be able to return to work and be socially active. However, 10–30% of AChR-positive generalized MG patients prove treatment resistant. Some patients with severe and prednisone-resistant bulbar or respiratory weakness require chronic treatment with IVIg or chronic plasma exchange.

Newly developed drugs include humanized monoclonal antibodies against the C5 complement molecule (e.g., eculizumab, ravulizumab). These drugs block complement activation and the formation of the membrane attack complex and so aim at reducing the disruption of AChR clusters and the destruction of the postsynaptic membrane. These drugs have shown efficacy and safety and are recommended in adult refractory AChR-positive generalized MG. Another therapeutic approach is blocking of the neonatal Fc receptor (FcRn), thus inhibiting IgG recycling and lowering IgG antibodies (e.g., efgartigimod). Efgartigimod also has shown to be efficacious and well tolerated as add-on treatment of adult AChR-positive patients with generalized myasthenia gravis. These three new drugs are administered intravenously, with varying intervals. The use of new drugs is limited by their very high costs. Phase 2 and phase 3 clinical trials with other new drugs are underway, and practice guidelines are bound to be adjusted in the coming years.

As anti-AChR antibodies cause increased AChR internalization and depletion, pyridostigmine may become less effective with time. New endplates will develop on the muscle nearby (Fig. 31.4), but this

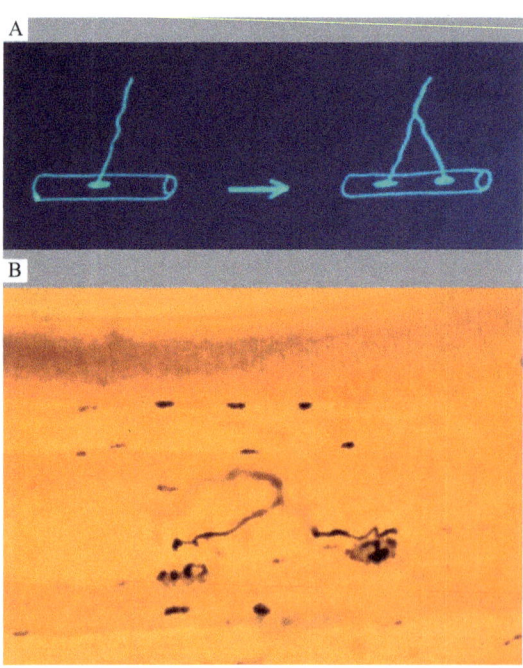

Figure 31.4 (A,B) Normally, one muscle fibre has a single endplate area. Anti-AChR antibodies induce the destruction of endplates through activation of complement. As a repair mechanism, new endplates are formed nearby destructed ones (A). The lower muscle fibre has two endplates with one newly induced by a preterminal nerve sprout. Nuclei and endplates stained dark on a silver-cholinesterase stain (B).

regenerative process may fail in elderly or severely affected patients. Patients who have myasthenia gravis for a long period of time may, therefore, develop residual atrophy of muscles. This argues for initiating drugs with proven efficacy early in the disease course.

In principle, the treatment of 'triple-negative' MG, ocular MG, and MG in children is the same as in generalized AChR-positive adults. However, FDA and EMA approvals of new drugs hold only for AChr-positive generalized disease in adults.

Myasthenic Crisis

Myasthenic crisis (rapid deterioration of dysarthria, swallowing, dropped head, dyspnoea in supine position) occurs in 20% of patients, more often in the elderly, and may be the first manifestation of the disease. Respiratory failure can evolve in hours, and these patients therefore should be monitored very closely (vital capacity, single breath counting) to ensure timely intubation. Functional tests are more useful indicators of imminent respiratory failure than blood gas analysis, because levels of carbon dioxide rise only late in the process of rapidly weakening respiratory muscles. Patients with myasthenia gravis should be carefully instructed to immediately contact their doctor in case of rapidly increasing bulbar symptoms or difficulty lying flat. Patients in a crisis respond well in days–weeks to treatment with IVIg or plasma exchange and an increase of corticosteroid dose.

Suggested Reading

Doughty CT, Guidon AC. Diagnostic testing for ocular myasthenia gravis: stronger together. *Neurology* 2020;95 (13):563–564. doi: 10.1212/WNL.0000000000010616. Epub 2020 Aug 11. PMID: 32788244.

Gilhus NE. Myasthenia gravis can have consequences for pregnancy and the developing child. *Front Neurol* 2020;11:554. doi: 10.3389/fneur.2020.00554. PMID: 32595594; PMCID: PMC7304249.

Gilhus NE, Tzartos S, Evoli A, et al. Myasthenia gravis. *Nat Rev Dis Primers* 2019;5(1):30. doi: 10.1038/s41572-019-0079-y. PMID: 31048702.

Menon D, Bril V. Pharmacotherapy of generalized myasthenia gravis with special emphasis on newer biologicals. Drugs 2022;82(8):865–887. doi: 10.1007/s40265-022-01726-y. Epub 2022 May 31. PMID: 35639288; PMCID: PMC9152838.

Narayanaswami P, Sanders DB, Wolfe G, et al. International consensus guidance for management of myasthenia gravis: 2020 Update. *Neurology* 2021;96 (3):114–122. doi: 10.1212/WNL.0000000000011124. Epub 2020 Nov 3. PMID: 33144515; PMCID: PMC7884987.

Vanoli F, Mantegazza R. Current drug treatment of myasthenia gravis. *Curr Opin Neurol* 2023;36(5):410–415. doi: 10.1097/WCO.0000000000001196. Epub 2023 Aug 30. PMID: 37678337.

Verschuuren JJ, Palace J, Murai H, et al. Advances and ongoing research in the treatment of autoimmune neuromuscular junction disorders. *Lancet Neurol* 2022;21(2):189–202. doi: 10.1016/S1474-4422(21)00463-4. Erratum in: *Lancet Neurol* 2022 Mar;21(3):e3. PMID: 35065041.

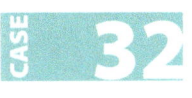

Myasthenia Gravis with Muscle-Specific Kinase Antibodies (MuSK MG)

Clinical History

Over a period of months, a 45-year-old woman noticed that she had difficulty raising her arms. She also reported double vision in the evening that, in retrospect, had been present for some years. Three years later, it became difficult to keep her head up without support, to chew, and to swallow, which sometimes worsened over a period of weeks.

Examination

There was asymmetric diplopia after 15 seconds of looking sideways, mild dysarthria, and MRC grade

4 weakness of neck extensor and flexor muscles, and shoulder abduction.

Diagnostic Considerations

The diplopia and bulbar symptoms and signs that vary in intensity were suggestive of myasthenia gravis. Most patients (85%) with myasthenia gravis have anti-acetylcholine receptor (AChR) antibodies. Bulbar signs and axial weakness are common in muscle-specific kinase myasthenia gravis (MuSK MG), and transient diplopia and ptosis are also often present early in the disease. Electrophysiological testing to confirm a postsynaptic transmission disorder should be performed if the serology is negative, but it should be kept in mind that the interpretation of a negative test result is difficult if the patient has started pyridostigmine.

Ancillary Investigations

Forced vital capacity was normal. EMG showed a pathological (20%) decrement on 3 Hz stimulation of the nasalis and trapezius muscles that confirmed a defect of neuromuscular transmission in these muscles. Autoantibodies to AChR were not detected, but autoantibodies to MuSK were present.

Follow-Up

During subsequent years, weakness progressed, and she was treated with various combinations of pyridostigmine, prednisolone, azathioprine, intravenous immunoglobulins (IVIg), and mycophenolate mofetil. Fifteen years after disease onset, the myasthenic symptoms are reasonably well controlled, but at the cost of continuous medication with prednisolone 15 mg and azathioprine 100 mg daily, and she had to cope with prednisolone-related hypertension, diabetes mellitus, and gastric complaints.

General Remarks

About 15% of patients with generalized MG do not have detectable anti-AChR antibodies with current standard methods. Among the AChR-negative MG patients, a varying proportion have MuSK MG, according to an ethnic–geographical gradient, with higher prevalence in people of Mediterranean or African origin. MuSK MG occurs predominantly in young women. MuSK is a transmembrane protein that is responsible for the development and maintenance of clustering of AChR at the neuromuscular junction.

As in AChR MG, ocular symptoms (diplopia and ptosis) are frequent first manifestations, but in MuSK MG these features are less conspicuous and may go unnoticed. Compared with AChR MG, in MuSK MG there is prominent and early involvement of bulbar, axial, and respiratory muscles (Table 32.1). Bulbar weakness

Table 32.1 Main clinical features of MuSK myasthenia gravis

- Much rarer than AChR MG
- Predominant in young women (third decade)
- Ocular manifestations usually present at onset, but often symmetric, and less striking than in AChR MG
- Prominent fatigable bulbar weakness
- Respiratory weakness may be presenting sign. Myasthenic crisis is treated as in AChR MG
- Muscle atrophy (e.g., tongue), fixed weakness and myopathic abnormalities may appear with time

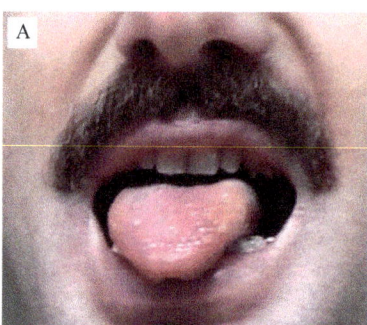

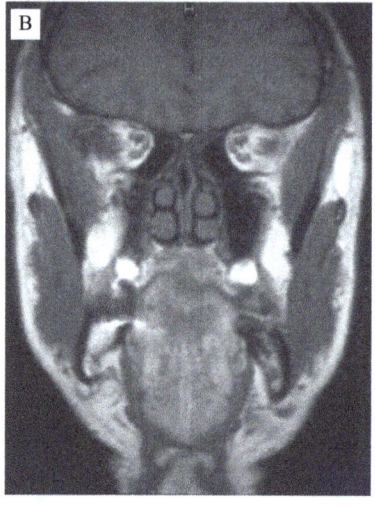

Figure 32.1 (A,B) Atrophy of the tongue in a man with MuSK myasthenia gravis. Note also the vertical position of the nasolabial folds (A). T1-weighted MRI shows the replacement of the tongue muscle (dark-grey) by fat (white-grey) (B). Courtesy Professor Jan Verschuuren.

manifests with dysarthria (often with nasal voice), dysphonia, and dysphagia (mainly for fluids). Respiratory crises occur in one-third of patients and may be the presenting feature. With long-standing disease, facial and tongue atrophy may develop (Fig. 32.1).

Treatment

Compared to AChR MG, MuSK MG is more difficult to treat. Symptoms and signs tend to be more severe and the response to pyridostigmine is poorer, with many patients reporting muscle twitching and cramping. A high proportion of MuSK MG patients require combined therapy with prednisone and non-steroidal immunosuppressants to achieve satisfactory symptom control. Recent studies suggest that rituximab, which depletes B cells, has a favourable result in MuSK MG. This drug is now advocated not only in refractory MuSK MG, but also in early stages of the disease. The optimum infusion dose and scheme have yet to be established. The complement pathway does not play a role in MuSK MG, since the autoantibodies are mainly of the IgG4 subclass, which do not activate complement. Eculizumab and other complement inhibitors are not recommended in MuSK-MG.

Thymoma usually does not occur in MuSK MG. Thymus hyperplasia is also very rare, and thymectomy is not recommended.

As in AChR MG, several points of attention should be taken into account with respect to pregnancy and delivery; see Chapter 8 in Part I.

Suggested Reading

Brauner S, Eriksson-Dufva A, Hietala MA, et al. Comparison between rituximab treatment for new-onset generalized myasthenia gravis and refractory generalized myasthenia gravis. *JAMA Neurol* 2020;77:974–981. doi: 10.1001/jamaneurol.2020.0851.

Gilhus NE. Myasthenia gravis can have consequences for pregnancy and the developing child. *Front Neurol* 2020 Jun 12;11:554. doi: 10.3389/fneur.2020.00554. PMID: 32595594; PMCID: PMC7304249.

Cao M, Koneczny I, Vincent A. Myasthenia gravis with antibodies against muscle specific kinase: an update on clinical features, pathophysiology and treatment. *Front Mol Neurosci* 2020;13:159. doi: 10.3389/fnmol.2020.00159

Narayanaswami P, Sanders DB, Wolfe G, et al. International consensus guidance for management of myasthenia gravis: 2020 update. *Neurology* 2021;96:114–122. doi:10.1212/WNL.0000000000011124

Verschuuren JJ, Palace J, Murai H, et al. Advances and ongoing research in the treatment of autoimmune neuromuscular junction disorders. *Lancet Neurol* 2022;21(2):189–202. doi: 10.1016/S1474-4422(21)00463-4. Erratum in: Lancet Neurol. 2022 Mar;21(3):e3. PMID: 35065041.

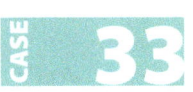

Drug-Induced Myasthenia Gravis: Immune Checkpoint Inhibitor (ICI)-Related

Clinical History

A 73-year-old man was referred by his oncologist because of dyspnoea occurring for one and a half weeks, and high CK levels (1341 U/L). For four years he was treated for a melanoma with pulmonary and cerebral metastases. Treatment included nivolumab that had been started three months previously. The dyspnoea was worse on exertion and when lying down. He also experienced some difficulties speaking clearly, and choking had occurred a few times during the past week. He had no diplopia. The complaints did not fluctuate. There was some recent myalgia, but he had not noticed any muscle weakness.

Examination

He spoke in short sentences and there was mild dysarthria. There were no other neurological abnormalities. Ptosis, diplopia, or weakness of neck or arm muscles could not be provoked.

Diagnostic Considerations

The dyspnoea was contributed to weakness of the diaphragm because of orthopnoea. This was considered to be caused by myositis based on the combination of myalgia and high CK level, although diaphragmatic weakness and dysphagia are not common signs of myositis in the absence of severe proximal limb weakness. Rapidly progressive diaphragmatic weakness can be more readily explained by myasthenia. Although the clinical features were not typical, myasthenia gravis was also considered based on the mild dysarthria and dysphagia. The combined features of myasthenia and myositis can occur as a complication of immune checkpoint inhibitors such as nivolumab. Myocarditis co-exists frequently.

Ancillary Investigations

Forced vital capacity was 46% of expected in sitting position and 39% supine. Arterial pCO2 was 47 mmHg (6.3 kPa), troponin-1 was 191 ng/L (normal < 18). The level of anti-acetylcholine receptor (AChR) antibodies was 0.6 nmol/L (normal < 0.4). Anti-muscle-specific kinase (MuSK) antibodies were not detected. There was a standstill of the diaphragm on ultrasound examination. The ECG showed atrial flutter and fibrillation. Cardiac ultrasound and MRI were negative for signs of myocarditis. Whole-body MRI showed oedema in anterior and posterior proximal leg muscles. Repetitive stimulation of the ulnar and accessory nerves was normal. Single-fibre EMG and muscle biopsy were not performed.

Follow-Up

Treatment with nivolumab was discontinued. Intravenous immunoglobulins (IVIg) and high-dose corticosteroids were initiated immediately. Sotalol and rivaroxaban were added because of the atrial flutter. Within two weeks, myalgia had disappeared and CK values had normalized. After two months, the dyspnoea had improved, although lying flat remained unpleasant, daytime CO_2 retention had disappeared, vital capacity had increased significantly, and the diaphragm showed a steady improvement of movement when studied with ultrasound imaging. Troponin levels remained elevated, and the cardiac arrhythmia persisted. Overall, the patient felt fine. Four months later, he was re-admitted because of intracranial bleeding from a brain metastasis and he subsequently died.

General Remarks

Immune checkpoint inhibitors (ICIs) are a new class of effective anti-cancer drugs. These monoclonal antibodies act by blocking a protein on T cells (CTLA-4, PD-1) or the ligand present on various normal and cancer cells (PD-L1), which inhibit T cells. By blocking the inhibition of T cells, the anti-tumor response of T cells is enhanced. Immune-related adverse events by ICIs (also called immune-related adverse effects, irAEs) involve mainly the gut, skin, endocrine glands, liver, and lung. Neuromuscular irAEs affect 1-2% of patients and are more frequent than irAEs involving the central nervous system. Neurological complications should be recognized promptly, because they can be life-threatening and react favourably to therapeutic interventions.

Neuromuscular irAEs comprise various forms of poly(radiculo)neuropathy including Guillain–Barré syndrome and cranial neuropathy, myasthenia, and inflammatory myopathy. Onset is commonly within a few weeks after initiation of treatment, but may also follow after several months. It is unclear yet whether these complications are dose related.

In one-quarter of patients, ICI-related myasthenia gravis is accompanied by myositis, and less frequently by myocarditis. An in-hospital mortality rate of 60% has been reported in the myasthenia gravis–myositis-myocarditis overlap syndrome.

In patients with the clinical features of generalized myasthenia, anti-AChR autoantibodies are positive in two-thirds of patients, and repetitive nerve stimulation shows a pathological decrement in almost half the patients. Available data from case reports and retrospective studies indicate that ICI-related myasthenia is more severe and more rapidly progressive than classic myasthenia gravis and has a higher risk of myasthenic crisis and fatal outcome. Diaphragm involvement seems to be more severe in combination with myositis, and mortality in combined myasthenia and myositis is higher as compared with myasthenia alone. ICI-induced myasthenia-myositis-myocarditis is more severe when ICIs are combined (e.g., nivolumab and ipilimumab) than with ICI monotherapy.

Management of neuromuscular complications involves withholding ICI treatment unless symptoms are very mild, and quickly starting adequate treatment (IVIg, high-dose corticosteroids). Retrospective data suggest that after resolution of mildly or moderately severe ICI-related myasthenia, ICI treatment can be re-administrated, under continuation of myasthenia treatment, without increased risk of recurrence of myasthenia symptoms.

Other Drugs That Can Induce or Worsen Myasthenia Gravis

Many drugs have been reported to worsen or induce myasthenia gravis, with varying levels of evidence. The presumed mechanisms vary. It is recommended to weigh the needs against the risks in individual patients. Table 33.1 lists drugs to avoid or to prescribe with caution and close monitoring.

Table 33.1 Drugs to avoid or to use with caution in patients with myasthenia gravis (non-exhaustive)

D-penicillamine. Avoid use
Chloroquine and hydroxychloroquine. Avoid use
Interferon-alpha. Avoid use
Antibiotics: aminoglycoside, macrolide, polypeptide, tetracycline, chinolone antibiotics, penicillin, ritonavir
Beta blockers
Botulinum toxin. Avoid use
Corticosteroids. May worsen MG in the first 2 weeks
Magnesium. Avoid high-dose intravenous use
Immune checkpoint inhibitors
Quinidine, procainamide, piperazine
Depolarizing muscle relaxants (succinylcholine) Avoid use. Non-depolarizing muscle relaxants (vecuronium, pancuronium). Use in lower dose, see Chapter 8 in Part I
Live-attenuated vaccines are contraindicated in patients who use immunosuppressive treatment

Suggested Reading

Astaras C, de Micheli R, Moura B, Hundsberger T, Hottinger AF. Neurological adverse events associated with immune checkpoint inhibitors: diagnosis and management. *Curr Neurol Neurosci Rep* 2018;18(1):3. doi: 10.1007/s11910-018-0810-1. PMID: 29392441.

Huang YT, Chen YP, Lin WC, Su WC, Sun YT. Immune checkpoint inhibitor-induced myasthenia gravis. *Front Neurol* 2020;11:634. doi: 10.3389/fneur.2020.00634. PMID: 32765397; PMCID: PMC7378376.

Narayanaswami P, Sanders DB, Wolfe G, et al. International consensus guidance for management of myasthenia gravis: 2020 Update. *Neurology* 2021;96 (3):114–122. doi: 10.1212/WNL.0000000000011124. Epub 2020 Nov 3. PMID: 33144515; PMCID: PMC7884987.

Rossi S, Gelsomino F, Rinaldi R, et al. Peripheral nervous system adverse events associated with immune checkpoint inhibitors. *J Neurol* 2023;270(6):2975–2986. doi: 10.1007/s00415-023-11625-1. Epub 2023 Feb 17. PMID: 36800019; PMCID: PMC10188572.

Safa H, Johnson DH, Trinh VA, et al. Immune checkpoint inhibitor related myasthenia gravis: single center experience and systematic review of the literature. *J Immunother Cancer* 2019;7(1):319. doi: 10.1186/s40425-019-0774-y. PMID: 31753014; PMCID: PMC6868691.

Schneider BJ, Naidoo J, Santomasso BD et al. Management of Immune-Related Adverse Events in Patients Treated With Immune Checkpoint Inhibitor Therapy: ASCO Guideline Update. *J Clin Oncol.* 2021 Dec 20;39(36):4073–4126. doi: 10.1200/JCO.21.01440. Epub 2021 Nov 1. Erratum in: J Clin Oncol. 2022 Jan 20;40(3):315. PMID: 34724392.

Lambert–Eaton Myasthenic Syndrome (LEMS)

Clinical History

A 33-year-old-woman who was diagnosed with chronic fatigue syndrome several years ago noticed a 'heavy feeling' and progressive weakness of the upper legs over a period of four months. Climbing stairs became very difficult, and eventually she could no longer walk independently. She did not complain about weakness in her arms. There were no sensory complaints. During the past months, her voice had changed. Especially if she was tired, she would speak 'like a drunk'. There were no complaints about double vision, drooping eyelids, or swallowing. There were no clear symptoms of autonomic dysfunction. She did not drink alcohol but had smoked at least a pack of cigarettes per day for over 10 years.

Examination
The patient was in a wheelchair, could barely stand, and could walk only with help. She had a bulbar dysarthria. There was symmetric ptosis that increased after looking upward, but there was no diplopia. She had mild weakness of the neck flexor muscles. Overt skeletal muscle atrophy and fasciculations were absent. She had a symmetric paresis of the arms, proximal (MRC grade 4) more than distal. The proximal muscles of the legs were severely paretic (MRC grade 2), distal weakness MRC grade 4. There were no sensory disturbances. The tendon reflexes were reduced. Interestingly, repetitive movements against force clearly improved muscle force of the arms and legs, and the biceps tendon reflexes increased after bending the upper arm against resistance.

Diagnostic Considerations
The patient presented with severe limb girdle weakness that had been progressive over months. This pattern of weakness is compatible with myositis or thyroid dysfunction, among others. However, because during neuromuscular examination some muscle groups showed improvement in muscle force after repetitive movements, a neuromuscular transmission disorder was also considered. Myasthenia gravis would be most likely based on the prevalence of disease, and because some patients with this disease may present with limb girdle weakness. However, because of her many years of smoking heavily, and because muscle strength and tendon reflexes increased after repetitive movements or exercise, a presynaptic disease (i.e., Lambert–Eaton myasthenic syndrome (LEMS)) was suspected. Therefore, she was tested for the presence of antibodies against acetylcholine receptors (AChR) and voltage-gated calcium channels (VGCC). We also considered repetitive nerve stimulation (RNS) and a single-fibre EMG in case of negative serology for VGCC (or AchR) antibodies, especially to test for the presence of a presynaptic neuromuscular transmission defect.

Ancillary Investigations
Anti-AChR antibodies were negative, but anti-VGCC antibodies were demonstrated. Compound muscle action potentials (CMAPs) had low amplitudes. RNS with 20 Hz revealed a clear increase in CMAPs, showing a presynaptic failure of neuromuscular transmission compatible with LEMS.

Follow-Up
After it became evident that the patient had LEMS following heavy smoking for many years, a thoracic CT showed that she likely had lung cancer. Further investigations revealed that she had small-cell lung cancer (SCLC), after which treatment with cytostatics was started. We also started pyridostigmine treatment (40 mg tid). Unfortunately, increase of pyridostigmine did not result in further improvement of muscle weakness. Treatment with 3,4-diaminopyridine (3,4-DAP) was then started, which resulted in improved muscle strength. Treatment of SCLC may also have a therapeutic effect on symptoms of LEMS.

General Remarks
LEMS is a rare autoimmune disease that is characterized by proximal muscle weakness, autonomic features, and low or absent reflexes (Table 34.1). Men are more frequently affected than women. In addition, patients may have mild and usually transient ptosis. Proximal leg muscle weakness is usually the first symptom (in 80%). Weakness of the arms is present or develops quickly. Weakness spreads proximally to distally, and caudally to cranially, including eventually the oculobulbar region. The speed of progression is much more pronounced in SCLC–LEMS than in non-tumour (NT)-LEMS (Fig. 34.1). In patients with LEMS, nerve conduction studies typically show low CMAPs at rest (due to impaired release of acetylcholine), with facilitation after brief exercise. RNS at 3 Hz shows a distinct pattern, with a decrement of more than 10% at rest, and a post-exercise facilitation (amplitude increment) of at least 60% after 10 seconds of exercise or after fast stimulation at 20–50 Hz.

Half of the patients with LEMS have SCLC. In these cases, LEMS is a paraneoplastic neuromuscular junction disorder. Rarely, other types of tumour have been described. The remaining half have a primary autoimmune disease. The disease is caused by pathogenic (cross-reactive) autoantibodies directed against presynaptic (P/Q-type) VGCCs, also present on the surface of SCLC cells. These antibodies play a role in decreasing the release of acetylcholine, which is triggered by Ca^{2+} influx. More than 85–90% of patients with LEMS have antibodies

Case 34 Lambert–Eaton Myasthenic Syndrome

Table 34.1 Comparison between Lambert–Eaton myasthenic syndrome (LEMS) and myasthenia gravis

	LEMS	**Myasthenia gravis**
Prevalence	Very rare	Rare
Clinical	Onset: often proximal muscle weakness Autonomic symptoms Reduced or absent tendon reflexes	Onset: often oculobulbar weakness No autonomic dysfunction Normal tendon reflexes
Electrophysiology	Low CMAP at rest Low-frequency (3 Hz) RNS: CMAP decrement High-frequency (20–50 Hz) RNS or aftermaximum voluntary contraction: CMAP increment	Normal CMAP at rest Low-frequency (3 Hz) RNS: CMAP decrement High-frequency (20–50 Hz) RNS: CMAP decrement
Serology	Anti-VGCC antibodies (> 90%)	Anti-AChR antibodies (85%), anti-MuSK (6%)
Tumour association	SCLC	Thymoma

AChR = acetylcholine receptor; CMAP = compound muscle action potential; MuSk = muscle-specific kinase; RNS = repetitive nerve stimulation; SCLC = small-cell lung cancer; VGCC = voltage-gated calcium channel.

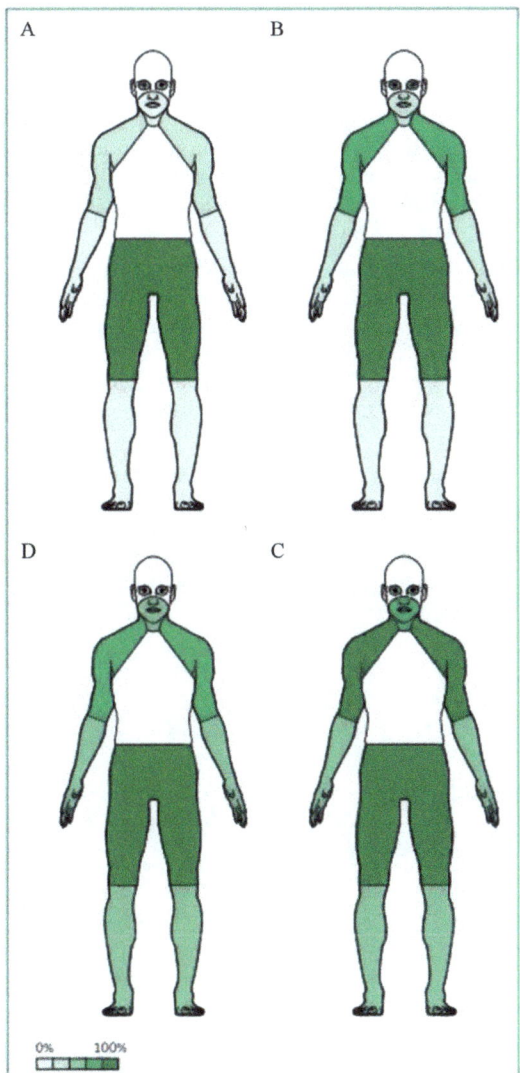

Figure 34.1 (A–D) Spreading of symptoms in patients with NT–LEMS and SCLC–LEMS. Frequency of symptoms at 3 months (A) and 12 months (B), respectively, in patients with NT–LEMS, and frequency of symptoms at 3 months (C) and 12 months (D), respectively, in patients with SCLC–LEMS. The percentages describe the approximate proportion of patients who have a particular symptom within the given time frame. From Titulaer et al., *Lancet Neurol* 2011;10:1098–1107, with permission.

directed against these presynaptic VGCCs. The presence of these VGCC antibodies do not distinguish between primary autoimmune and paraneoplastic LEMS. However, antibodies against Sry-like high-mobility group box protein 1 (SOX1) are likely specific for paraneoplastic disease.

Screening for SCLC is mandatory in all patients presenting with LEMS. In almost all cases, symptoms of LEMS occur before SCLC is diagnosed, and in approximately two-thirds of patients with LEMS, SCLC is in an early stage when diagnosed. The mean age of disease onset in SCLC-related LEMS is around 60 years, whereas in NT–LEMS there are two peaks, one at the age of around 35 years and a second peak around the age of 60 years. Independent predictors for SCLC in LEMS are age at onset (> 50 years), smoking, weight loss, Karnofsky score < 60, bulbar involvement, impotence, and the presence of SOX1 serum antibodies. Using the Dutch–English LEMS Tumour Association Prediction (DELTA-P) score, the chance whether a LEMS patient has SCLC can be determined. In LEMS patients in whom initially no SCLC is shown, cancer screening (thoracic CT, FGD-PET) should continue every three to six months for at least two years from symptom onset. In patients with LEMS finally shown to have SCLC, this was found in 92% within three months, and in 96% within a year.

Treatment and Prognosis

For SCLC–LEMS, tumour therapy is essential. Symptoms of LEMS in patients with SCLC may stabilize or improve after SCLC surgery. Patients with NT–LEMS require treatment for several months or – more likely – years, after which they can be completely asymptomatic even after tapering the medication. For all patients with LEMS, symptomatic therapy is with 3,4-DAP, a potassium channel blocker that increases acetylcholine release. Treatment with pyridostigmine is usually much less effective in comparison with patients with myasthenia gravis. Immunosuppression and immunomodulation with corticosteroids, azathioprine, intravenous immunoglobulin, and possibly also with other medication including rituximab can be helpful to treat symptoms of LEMS.

Suggested Reading

Huijbers MG, Marx A, Plomp JJ, et al. Advances in the understanding of disease mechanisms of autoimmune neuromuscular junction disorders. *Lancet Neurol* 2022;21(2):163–175. doi: 10.1016/S1474-4422(21)00357-4. PMID: 35065039.

Kesner VG, Oh SJ, Dimachkie MM, Barohn RJ. Lambert-Eaton myasthenic syndrome. *Neurol Clin* 2018;36(2):379–394. doi: 10.1016/j.ncl.2018.01.008. PMID: 29655456; PMCID: PMC6690495.

Titulaer MJ, Lang B, Verschuuren JJ. Lambert-Eaton myasthenic syndrome: from clinical characteristics to therapeutic strategies. *Lancet Neurol* 2011;10(12):1098–1107. doi: 10.1016/S1474-4422(11)70245-9. PMID: 22094130.

Titulaer MJ, Maddison P, Sont JK, et al. Clinical Dutch-English Lambert-Eaton myasthenic syndrome (LEMS) tumor association prediction score accurately predicts small-cell lung cancer in the LEMS. *J Clin Oncol* 2011;29(7):902–908. doi: 10.1200/JCO.2010.32.0440. Epub 2011 Jan 18. PMID: 21245427.

Verschuuren JJ, Palace J, Murai H, et al. Advances and ongoing research in the treatment of autoimmune neuromuscular junction disorders. *Lancet Neurol* 2022;21(2):189–202. doi: 10.1016/S1474-4422(21)00463-4. Erratum in: Lancet Neurol. 2022 Mar;21(3):e3. PMID: 35065041.

CASE 35 Congenital Myasthenic Syndromes (CMS): Dok7

Clinical History

A 7-year-old girl visited the outpatient clinic because of difficulty walking. She had never managed to run properly, and experienced frequent falls ever since she began walking independently at the age of 18 months. Jumping was not possible, and when stepping up or down, she needed support below her arms. There was no fluctuation of symptoms during the day, but she had suffered from periods that could last several weeks in which using the stairs was completely impossible. She was unable to blow up a balloon and her speech was slow and poorly articulated. There were no complaints about chewing or swallowing. She had a healthy non-identical twin sister and the family history was unremarkable.

Examination

There was symmetric ptosis with normal eye movements. Elevation of the eyebrows was barely possible and the eyelashes remained visible upon eye closure. Proximal and symmetric muscle weakness of the legs led to a waddling gait with an endorotation of the right leg (**Video 35.1**). She was barely able to increase her speed and unable to jump. Stair climbing could only be done step by step and by pulling herself up using the handrail. Although she was able to perform 10 squats with significant difficulty, there was no clear fatigability. Prolonged walking also did not increase weakness.

Diagnostic Considerations

Generalized weakness originating in early infancy with involvement of facial muscles and a stable course over time is compatible with a congenital myopathy. This was also the clinical diagnosis upon referral. There was also a history of worsening of symptoms that could last several weeks and resolve spontaneously. Fluctuating weakness is the hallmark of disorders of neuromuscular transmission, although typically, fatigability is more prominent in the history and can be provoked during clinical examination by repeated or sustained muscular efforts.

Ancillary Investigations

The previous diagnosis of a congenital myopathy had been based on the phenotype and a biopsy taken from the right vastus lateralis muscle, which showed increased variability in fibre size, as a nonspecific finding (Fig. 35.1), as well as an abnormal needle EMG with low-amplitude motor unit action potentials. Serum CK was normal, which is not uncommon in milder phenotypes, but somewhat remarkable in view of the severe weakness. In an attempt to classify the myopathy, muscle imaging was performed. Ultrasound showed a normal echogenicity throughout, even in clearly affected muscles like those of the upper

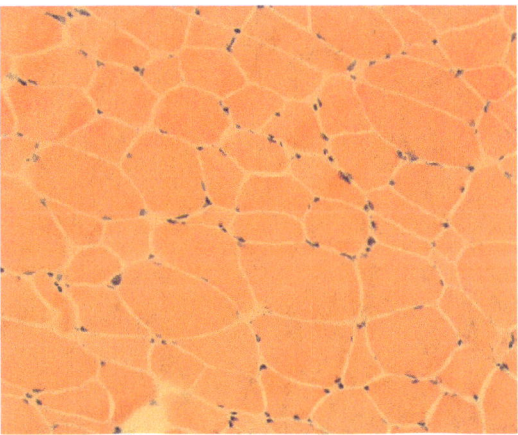

Figure 35.1 Muscle biopsy showing a mildly increased variation in fibre size on the H&E stain, but no other abnormalities, especially no cores or rodlike structures.

leg (Fig. 35.2A). Qualitative muscle MRI of the shoulder and hip girdle and upper and lower arms and legs also did not show any increased signal on both T1 (compatible with absent fatty replacement) and T2 STIR sequences (compatible with absent oedema or inflammation) (Fig. 35.2B). A clinically weak muscle with a normal appearance on muscle imaging suggested the possibility of myasthenic weakness. This could not be confirmed by repetitive nerve stimulation (RNS) of the right ulnar nerve and of the left facial nerve with recording electrodes on the hypothenar and nasalis muscles, respectively. Stimulated single-fibre EMG of the right frontal muscle also yielded a normal mean jitter of 14 microseconds (ref < 20) and no blocking. Based on the clinical phenotype of predominant limb girdle muscle weakness and asymmetric endorotation of the leg during walking, it was decided to perform sequencing of the *DOK7* gene that revealed compound heterozygosity for a nonsense mutation in exon 5 (c.601C>T, p. Arg201X) and a duplication in exon 7, leading to a frame shift (c.1124_1127dupTGCC, p.Ala378fs).

Follow-Up

Treatment with oral salbutamol was initiated up to 4 mg tid. This led to significant improvement after one month. She was able to walk faster and longer and could alternate steps when climbing stairs. Increase in muscle strength continued, and after one year she was able to run and hop on both legs (**Video 35.2**). At the age of 18, she experienced no

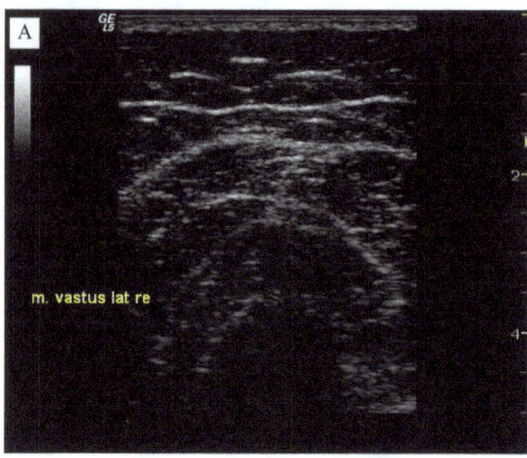
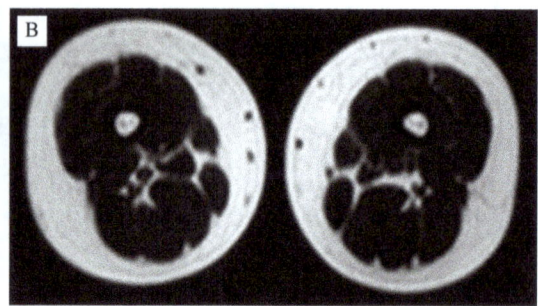

Figure 35.2 (A,B) Normal muscle ultrasound (A) and T1-weighted MRI (B) in affected muscles in the upper leg.

limitation when playing tennis. Facial weakness, however, had not improved since the first presentation.

General Remarks

Congenital myasthenic syndromes (CMS) are neuromuscular diseases caused by genetic variants that affect the function of proteins involved in the neuromuscular signal transmission. No less than 35 genes have been associated with CMS, although there is a wide variety of prevalence and regional variation due to founder variants in some of the genes involved, and some genes are only described in individual cases or families.

In general, variations involving one of the subunits of the acetylcholine receptor (AChR) are most prevalent, followed by Collagen Q, Rapsyn, and Dok7. Most syndromes have an autosomal recessive inheritance. Proteins can be involved in presynaptic acetylcholine release, synaptic breakdown of acetylcholine, postsynaptic signal transmission, structural formation of the neuromuscular synapse, or protein glycosylation (Fig. 35.3). The increased knowledge of structural and intramuscular pathways has led to an overlap between CMS and congenital myopathies, as many of these genes also lead to structural changes in striated muscle. In recent years, congenital syndromes like *PURA*-related CMS with intellectual disability, and Pierson syndrome with a nephrotic syndrome due to *LAMB2* variants have been added to this spectrum.

Clinical Features

Clinical symptoms can be very variable, ranging from severe neonatal weakness with respiratory insufficiency and feeding difficulties to more milder phenotypes with an onset in infancy or even in (early) adulthood. Fatigability of muscle is a key symptom, but fluctuations can also occur over a longer period, with exacerbations triggered by fever or infections. Contractures and scoliosis are frequent in the severe phenotypes. Cardiac muscle is not affected. CMS should be distinguished from neonatal myasthenia due to maternal antibodies, and from (seronegative) autoimmune myasthenia gravis, especially in young adults. Clinical clues for CMS are a positive family history, the early onset, and a lack of response to immunosuppressive therapy.

Variants in the *CHRNE* gene encoding the epsilon subunit of the AChR, and in the *RAPSN* gene both lead to a deficiency of AChRs in the endplate. Clinical symptoms resemble those of autoimmune myasthenia gravis (MG) with fluctuating ptosis and muscle weakness, although ptosis is more symmetric and ophthalmoparesis is often more fixed. Diplopia is far less prominent than in autoimmune MG. Congenital contractures and episodic apnoeas are at the more severe end of the spectrum of *RAPSN* variants. Variants in *COLQ* cause a deficiency of acetylcholinesterase. Neonatal weakness with external ophthalmoplegia and initial respiratory insufficiency is later complicated by the development of scoliosis, although most patients become ambulant, and respiratory

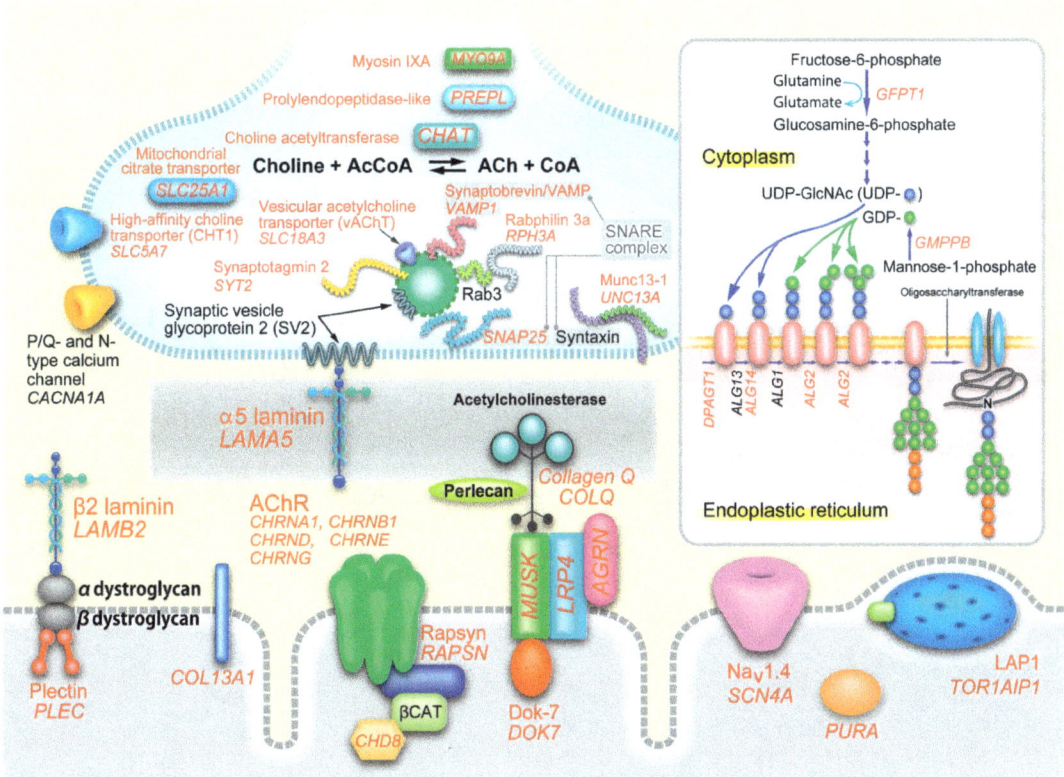

Figure 35.3 Thirty-five genes involved in CMS indicated in red. From Ohno et al., *Int J Mol Sci* 2023;13:3730, with permission.

difficulties may become less prominent. Milder phenotypes may present with proximal weakness in adulthood. A slow or delayed pupillary response can be observed in a proportion of patients. Dok7 CMS is also hallmarked by a wide variability in clinical severity with neonatal weakness, respiratory insufficiency, and inspiratory stridor up to a later presentation with limb girdle weakness and a waddling gait as in the presented case. Ptosis and bulbar weakness are common, but eye movements are preserved.

Diagnosis

The underlying disturbance of the neuromuscular transmission can be confirmed by electromyography where RNS shows 10% or more decremental response of the compound muscle action potential (CMAP). However, depending on the genotype, this decrement may only occur upon high-frequency stimulation or after exercise. Similar to Lambert–Eaton myasthenic syndrome, high-frequency RNS may yield an increment in the CMAP in presynaptic CMS. Single-fibre EMG has a higher sensitivity and lower specificity than RNS. Muscle imaging has become increasingly important in the diagnosis of neuromuscular disease using pattern recognition. In the presented case, a severely weak muscle with a normal appearance on ultrasound and MRI pointed towards the diagnosis of a CMS. However, a higher degree of replacements by fat has been reported in many CMS subtypes, especially in the older population. The introduction of next-generation sequencing panels has highly facilitated the diagnosis of CMS, and this would now be the most obvious first choice of ancillary investigation, often replacing complicated EMG recordings.

Treatment

A clinical and genetic diagnosis of CMS is important because in many cases weakness can improve with treatment, as shown in the described patient. Symptomatic treatment includes drugs also used in autoimmune MG, such as pyridostigmine, which blocks the acetylcholinesterase, amifampridine, which enhances presynaptic acetylcholine release, and adrenergic agonists such as ephedrine and salbutamol. However, the choice of medication entirely depends on the underlying genetic defect and electrophysiological characteristics. Drugs that are effective in a specific CMS subtype can be without benefit in another, or even increase weakness. For example, whereas both salbutamol and ephedrine are used in Dok7 CMS, pyridostigmine can lead to worsening of symptoms that can be potentially life-threatening. For this reason, a neostigmine test is not recommended as part of the diagnostic work-up of a CMS that is not genetically characterized.

Suggested Reading

Finlayson S, Morrow JM, Rodriguez Cruz PM, et al. Muscle magnetic resonance imaging in congenital myasthenic syndromes. *Muscle Nerve* 2016;54(2):211–219. doi: 10.1002/mus.25035. Epub 2016 Feb 22. PMID: 26789134; PMCID: PMC4982021.

Kao JC, Milone M, Selcen D, et al. Congenital myasthenic syndromes in adult neurology clinic: a long road to diagnosis and therapy. *Neurology* 2018;91(19):e1770–e1777. doi: 10.1212/WNL.0000000000006478. Epub 2018 Oct 5. PMID: 30291185; PMCID: PMC6251603.

Ohno K, Ohkawara B, Shen XM, Selcen D, Engel AG. Clinical and pathologic features of congenital myasthenic syndromes caused by 35 genes-a comprehensive review. *Int J Mol Sci* 2023;24(4):3730. doi: 10.3390/ijms24043730. PMID: 36835142; PMCID: PMC9961056.

Ramdas S, Beeson D. Congenital myasthenic syndromes: where do we go from here? *Neuromuscul Disord* 2021;31(10):943–954. doi: 10.1016/j.nmd.2021.07.400. PMID: 34736634.

Myopathies

CASE 36 — Duchenne Muscular Dystrophy (DMD)

Clinical History
A boy was referred at the age of 2 years and 8 months because of frequent falls. This occurred several times per day and he had hurt his head on multiple occasions. Earlier major motor milestones had been delayed by several months. He had achieved rolling over at 9 months, crawling at 15, and independent walking just before his second birthday. Speech and language development were also behind as his first word had been heard around the age of 2 and he now mastered no more than ten. He was friendly in his behaviour and made good eye contact. Pregnancy and birth had been unremarkable. His mother was 5 months pregnant with her second child. Family history was unremarkable.

Examination
He made a friendly and interactive impression and appeared interested in his surroundings. He spoke a few words that were difficult to understand. There was hypertrophy of both calves (Fig. 36.1A), and probably also of the quadriceps femoris muscles. He was able to walk, but not to gain speed. Upon rising from a sitting position, he pushed himself up with both hands on his knees (positive Gowers sign) (Fig. 36.1B).

Diagnostic Considerations
A positive Gowers sign is a manifestation of proximal muscle weakness, even in young children. Together with muscle hypertrophy, this is highly suggestive of a muscular dystrophy. Within the spectrum of muscular dystrophies with a limb girdle distribution, Duchenne muscular dystrophy (DMD) is by far the most prevalent form in boys. More global developmental delay is common in this condition and could also have been the primary reason for referral, as illustrated by the clinical history.

Ancillary Investigations
Serum CK was more than 10 × ULN (18,534 U/L). Multiplex ligation-dependent probe amplification analysis of the *DMD* gene revealed a deletion of exons 18 to 44, predicting a shift in the mRNA reading frame (Fig. 36.2). Therefore, a diagnosis of DMD was made.

Follow-Up
The boy underwent neuropsychological evaluation at the age of three years and seven months, showing a nonverbal IQ of 60 and a global developmental delay of approximately one year. At the age of four, he was admitted to special education. Because of

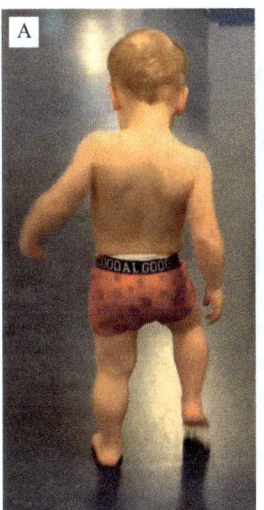
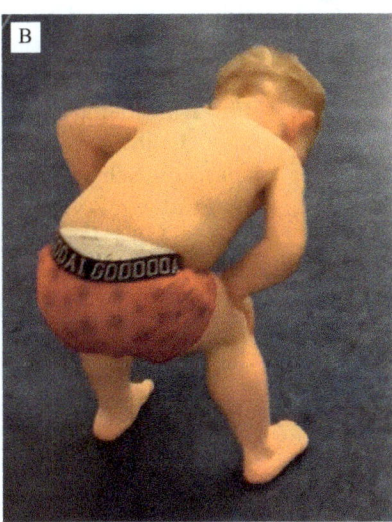

Figure 36.1 (A,B) Calf hypertrophy with the inability to run (A), and a positive Gowers sign compatible with proximal muscle weakness (B).

DMD, he was treated with chronic corticosteroids from the age of five years using an intermittent scheme of 10 days on and 10 days off prednisone 0.75 mg/kg/day. Upon the diagnosis, his mother was seen by a clinical geneticist and proved to be the carrier of the *DMD* gene mutation. She was then referred to a cardiologist for periodic screening. A few months later, she gave birth to a son who unfortunately also carried the same mutation.

General Remarks

DMD is the most common genetic muscle-wasting disease in children. It is an X-linked recessive disease, thus affecting males, although female carriers can be symptomatic. DMD is caused by variants in the *DMD* gene, located on Xp21. These include not only larger deletions of one or more exons (60–70%) and duplications (5–15%), but also small deletions or insertions or point mutations (20%). They usually cause out-of-frame variants and lead to the near absence of functional dystrophin, a key protein connecting the sarcolemma and the cytoskeleton that among others protects muscle fibres from contraction-induced damage. Clinical presentation is typically with proximal muscle weakness, most prominent in the legs, leading to difficulty standing up and frequent falls, although many parents in hindsight report concerns about early motor development. Muscle hypertrophy can be seen in the calves, and occasionally also in the upper legs, arms, and shoulders. Independent walking is achieved, but generally the ability to run (i.e., to clear both feet from the ground) is impaired. Due to maturation, muscle function increases in the first years, but then plateaus around the age of five, followed by inevitable decline. This leads to wheelchair dependency in all patients, most commonly between the ages of 10 and 12. This is followed by progressive respiratory insufficiency, scoliosis, and cardiomyopathy, resulting in premature death.

Becker muscular dystrophy (BMD) is the allelic disorder in which reduced levels of partially functional dystrophin are produced, generally as a result of in-frame deletions in the *DMD* gene (see **Case 37**). BMD is hallmarked by a milder and far more variable phenotype ranging from adult-onset muscle cramps with normal life expectancy to an overlap with DMD and loss of ambulation before the age of 20. There are no sharp boundaries between DMD and BMD, and therefore the dystrophinopathies are being considered a spectrum of phenotypes.

Neuropsychological comorbidity in DMD is frequent, including autism spectrum disease, obsessive compulsive behaviour, and attention deficit. One-third of patients have cognitive impairment and learning difficulties. Cognitive involvement in DMD is related to the expression of multiple dystrophin isoforms in the brain (Dp427, Dp140, and Dp71), and thus depends partly on the location of the variant (Fig. 36.2). Global developmental delay can also be the presenting symptom, as illustrated in this case. Therefore, determination of serum CK is an essential part of the work-up in these children. This increase in CK is accompanied by an increase in aspartate aminotransferase (ASAT) and alanine aminotransferase (ALAT). Whereas these are generally considered as liver enzymes, they derive from muscle as well. In presymptomatic children, incidentally discovered ASAT and ALAT elevation can lead to unnecessary liver studies, even up to a biopsy, before CK activity is assessed.

Genetic counselling is essential for family planning and screening of female carriers for cardiomyopathy as well as for muscle involvement. The present case illustrates that a diagnostic delay can have major implications. Newborn screening is an important topic of debate, but currently not implemented in routine healthcare because of the absence of early treatment consequences. This could change with emerging therapies that include adeno-associated virus-mediated transfer of a significantly shortened microdystrophin construct, as well as antisense oligonucleotide (AON)-mediated exon skipping, of which the first compounds have now gained conditional approval by the FDA. Exon skipping is achieved through binding of an AON to a specific target exon in the pre-mRNA that hides it from the splicing machinery and thus prevents the inclusion in the mRNA. Although the deletion is then enlarged, the reading frame is restored, allowing the production of partially functional dystrophin similar to that seen in BMD patients (Fig. 36.2). The percentage of variants that can be treated with a single AON, however, is limited, with four different compounds developed for the most common genotypes targeting exons 51, 53, 45, and 44 being applicable to approximately one-third of the population.

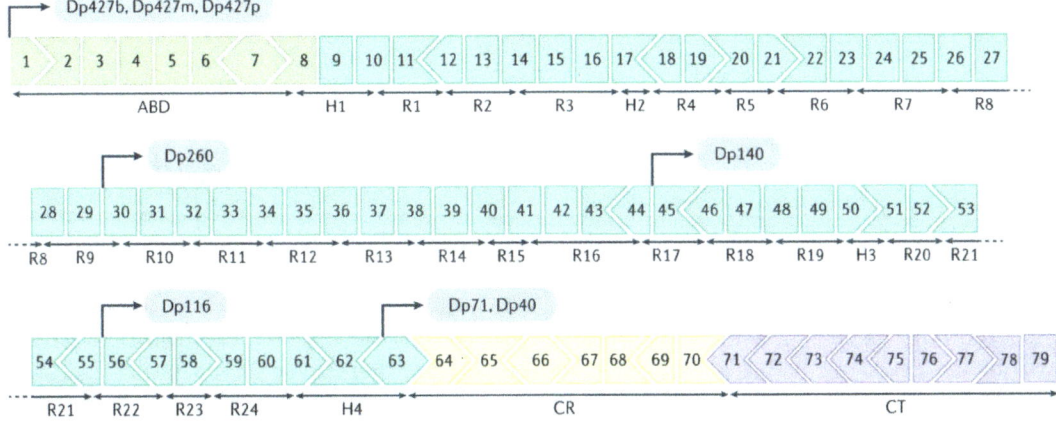

Figure 36.2 Schematic representation of the *DMD* gene including four internal promotor sites for the various dystrophin (Dp) isoforms (from Duan et al., *Nat Rev Dis Primers* 2021;7(1):13, with permission). In the present case, the deletion of exons 18 to 44 disrupts the reading frame and is classified as out of frame. Skipping of exon 45 in the splicing process would lead to a restoration of the reading frame by linking exons 17 and 46.

Current treatment for DMD consists of chronic corticosteroids applied daily or in intermittent regimens and usually initiated around the age of four or five, and before decline in motor functioning occurs. Steroids are thought to reduce inflammation and increase muscle mass and force. This has led to a significant delay in important disease milestones such as loss of ambulation by approximately one to three years depending on the use of daily or intermittent regimens. Corticosteroids also delay the onset of noninvasive respiratory support and cardiomyopathy and reduce the incidence of scoliosis surgery. On the other hand, corticosteroids cause significant side effects including behaviour and mood changes, weight gain, growth reduction, delayed puberty, and reduced bone mineral density. The use of ACE inhibitors is now recommended as prophylaxis when boys approach the age of 10 and prior to the onset of cardiomyopathy. Multidisciplinary supportive care is essential and, in combination with the aforementioned interventions, has increased the life expectancy up to 20 to 40 years. Cardiac and respiratory insufficiencies are the main causes of mortality.

Suggested Reading

Birnkrant DJ, Bushby K, Bann CM, et al.; DMD Care Considerations Working Group. Diagnosis and management of Duchenne muscular dystrophy, part 1: diagnosis, and neuromuscular, rehabilitation, endocrine, and gastrointestinal and nutritional management. *Lancet Neurol* 2018;17(3):251–267. doi: 10.1016/S1474-4422(18)30024-3. Epub 2018 Feb 3. Erratum in: Lancet Neurol. 2018 Apr 4: PMID: 29395989; PMCID: PMC5869704.

Birnkrant DJ, Bushby K, Bann CM, et al.; DMD Care Considerations Working Group. Diagnosis and management of Duchenne muscular dystrophy, part 2: respiratory, cardiac, bone health, and orthopaedic management. *Lancet Neurol* 2018;17(4):347–361. doi: 10.1016/S1474-4422(18)30025-5. Epub 2018 Feb 3. PMID: 29395990; PMCID: PMC5889091.

Birnkrant DJ, Bushby K, Bann CM, et al.; DMD Care Considerations Working Group. Diagnosis and management of Duchenne muscular dystrophy, part 3: primary care, emergency management, psychosocial care, and transitions of care across the lifespan. *Lancet Neurol* 2018;17(5):445–455.

Duan D, Goemans N, Takeda S, Mercuri E, Aartsma-Rus A. Duchenne muscular dystrophy. *Nat Rev Dis Primers* 2021;7(1):13. doi: 10.1038/s41572-021-00248-3. PMID: 33602943.

Case 37 Becker Muscular Dystrophy (BMD)

Clinical History

A 23-year-old man gradually noticed slowly progressive difficulty running and climbing stairs and therefore he was referred. In retrospect, he had a hollow back since age 10, and when running, he had had difficulty keeping up with his peers. He had a younger brother with similar complaints. Serum CK activity was elevated (15 × ULN). EMG, which had been carried out by the referring neurologist, showed small motor unit action potentials.

Examination

He had hypertrophy of the calf muscles (Fig. 37.1) and weakness of the proximal muscles of the upper and lower limbs. There was a positive Gowers sign (**Video 37.1**) and a bilateral positive Trendelenburg sign consistent with weakness of the gluteal muscles and the quadriceps femoris.

Diagnostic Considerations

The presentation of proximal muscle weakness led to a differential diagnosis of a slowly progressive limb girdle syndrome (Chapter 3, Box 3.7). Spinal muscular atrophy type 3 or 4 may be considered (**Case 7**), congenital myasthenic syndrome, hereditary myopathies (e.g., limb girdle muscular dystrophies (LGMD), Becker muscular dystrophy (BMD), Pompe disease, mitochondrial myopathies, myotonic dystrophy type 2). Given the > 10 × elevated CK and the 'myopathic' EMG, a diagnosis of BMD or LGMD was most likely. First, a muscle biopsy was performed; given the weakness of the leg muscles, imaging was done to select the most suitable site for a muscle biopsy.

Ancillary Investigations

Muscle imaging demonstrated widespread abnormalities of muscles of the legs (Fig. 37.2). A skeletal muscle biopsy showed dystrophic changes (Fig. 37.3). Reduced dystrophin was observed on a Western blot (Fig. 37.4). Multiplex ligation-dependent probe amplification (MLPA) of the dystrophin gene later revealed a deletion of exons 45–47.

Follow-Up

The patient was referred to the cardiology department where he was found to have a dilation of the left ventricle with a reduced function. He was prescribed an ACE inhibitor, but over the years the ejection fraction slowly decreased. He had slowly progressive muscle weakness but was still ambulatory after a 17-year follow-up.

After the patient was diagnosed, his brother was referred at age 20 years. He had been a keen baseball player until two years before, although he experienced muscle cramps on exertion and he was not as fast as his peers while running. On examination, he was found to have a similar clinical picture as his brother.

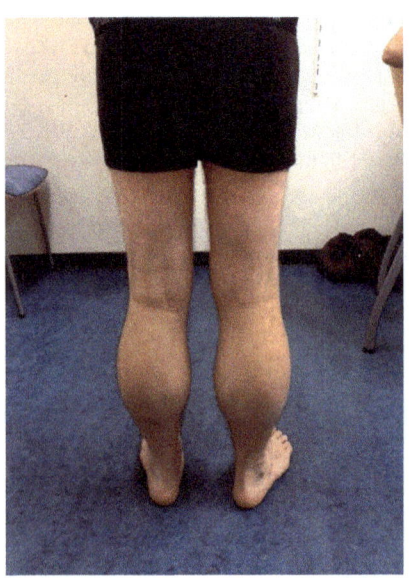

Figure 37.1 Hypertrophy of the calf muscles of the described patient.

Case 37 Becker Muscular Dystrophy

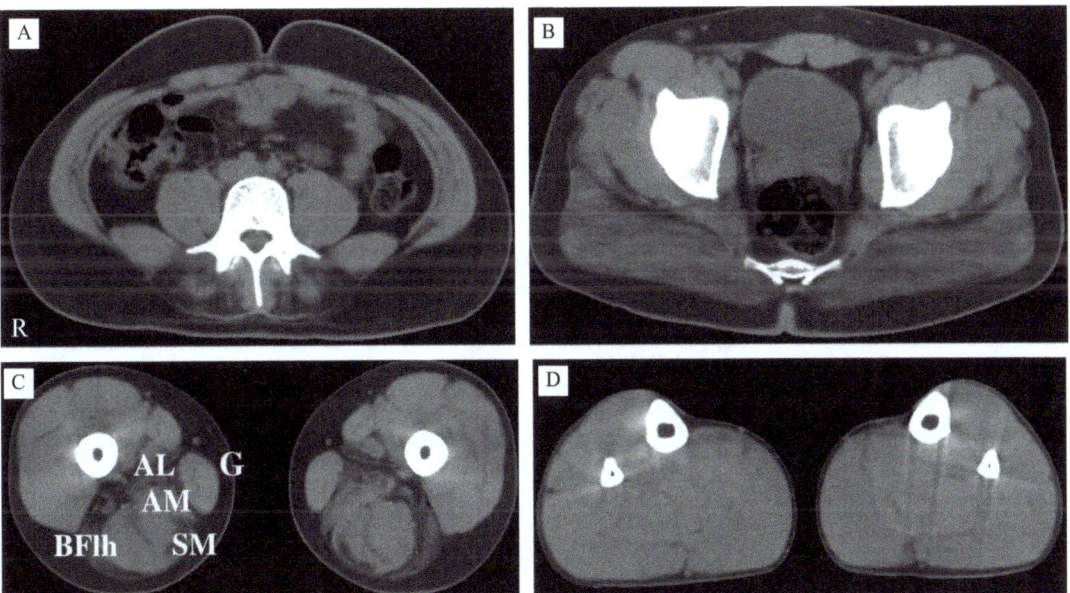

Figure 37.2 (A–D). CT scan of the described patient showing replacement by fat of the paraspinal muscles at the lumbar level (A). At the pelvic girdle level, there is lower attenuation of the gluteus maximus muscles (B), and at the thigh level of the adductor longus (AL), adductor magnus (AM), semimembranosus (SM), and long head of the biceps femoris muscles (BFlh), with compensatory hypertrophy of the gracilis (G) muscles (C). The gastrocnemius muscles are hypertrophic (D).

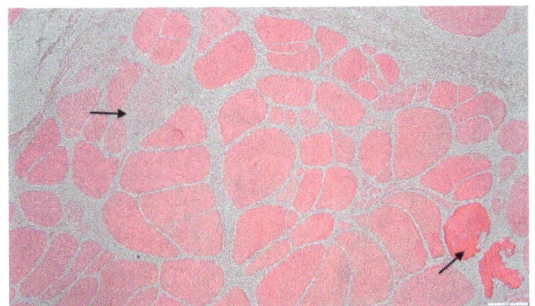

Figure 37.3 Muscle biopsy. Marked variation in the size of the muscle fibres. Various necrotic muscle fibres (arrows), fibre splitting, increase in connective tissue consistent with a dystrophic pattern.

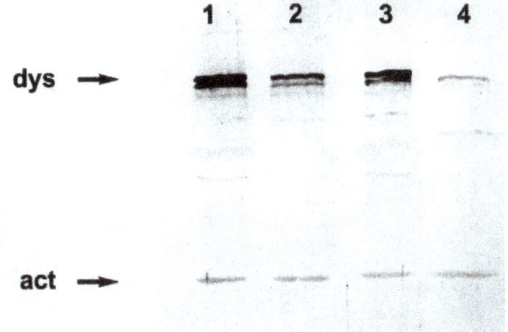

Figure 37.4 Lanes from a Western blot of skeletal muscle extract from three control subjects with normal dystrophin (dys, 1–3) and a patient with BMD showing reduced dystrophin (4). Actin (act) is present in equal amounts. Courtesy Dr Ieke Ginjaar.

General Remarks

BMD is an X-linked recessive disease caused by a variant in the *DMD* (dystrophin) gene. Together with Duchenne muscular dystrophy (DMD) BMD is the main phenotype of dystrophinopathy. In Table 37.1 all phenotypical variants of dystrophinopathies are depicted.

The incidence of BMD is one-third that of DMD: 1 in 2,500 to 3,500 live male births.

Approximately 80% of the DMD/BMD patients have a deletion of one of more exons, in 5–10% of the patients a duplication is found, and in a similar percentage point mutations and insertions/deletions within exons or splice sites. Rarely, no variant is detected. The variants in BMD are usually in-frame, that is, the reading frame of the dystrophin gene is preserved and not disrupted, so

Table 37.1 Phenotypical spectrum of dystrophinopathies

Phenotype	Age at onset	Muscle weakness	Heart involvement	Cognitive/ behavioural impairment	Prognosis	CK
Duchenne MD (DMD)	Early childhood (< 5 years)	Progressive symmetric proximal > distal weakness, starting in proximal leg muscles; calf hypertrophy	Dilated cardiomyopathy (DCM) starts in teenage years and > 18 years all patients have DCM	Intellectual disability (ID) up to 30%, autism spectrum disorder (ASD) 0–21%; isolated cognitive impairment extremely rare	Wheelchair-dependent < 13 years; death in 3rd or 4th decade (improved prognosis due to treatment with corticosteroids, scoliosis surgery, and noninvasive ventilation)	> 10 × ULN
Becker MD (BMD)	3–21 years, mean 11 years; later onset (up to 7th decade) also reported	Variable: very mild to severely progressive, symmetric proximal > distal, starting in proximal leg muscles; often calf hypertrophy	Similar to DMD, later onset. Severity of cardiac disease does not correlate with skeletal muscle weakness	ID may be present; prevalence unknown ASD 0–1.4%	Wheelchair-dependency (> 16 years); some remain ambulatory into 30s, 40s, and beyond. Mean life expectancy 40–50 years. Cause of death mostly cardiac.	> 5 × ULN
X-linked dilated cardiomyopathy (DCM) (in men)	1st–2nd decade	Mostly absent. Sometimes myalgia, cramps, calf hypertrophy	DCM main phenotype	Unknown	Rapidly progressive (1–2 years)	Normal to slightly elevated
(Manifesting) carriers	1st–7th decade	Weakness in 14–16%; if present, mostly asymmetric proximal weakness legs > arms	In DMD or BMD carrier DCM in 9%; subclinical DCM (gadolinium enhancement on MRI) in 48%	May also have ID/ ASD	Dependent on presence of DCM and muscle weakness	2–10 × ULN; significantly higher at age < 20 years
Myalgia and cramps syndrome	Childhood	Mostly absent	May be present	Not known	Dependent on presence of DCM	> 10 × ULN

ULN = upper limit of normal

some dystrophin protein can be made and this leads to an altered, partially functional dystrophin. However, approximately 15% do not follow the reading frame rule. In general, the severity of the phenotype correlates to the reading frame rule.

An X-linked dilated cardiomyopathy (DCM) is mostly caused by variants in the region from the muscle promoter to muscle exon 1 or the 'hot spot' region from exons 45–55. There is no relation between site of variant and presence of weakness or DCM in manifesting carriers.

Cardiac involvement is similar to that in DMD – degeneration of cardiac muscle fibres leading to rhythm disturbances and dilated cardiomyopathy – and is ultimately present in all BMD patients. Severe dilated cardiomyopathy – requiring heart transplantation – may be the presenting symptom in BMD.

CK is usually more than five times elevated. BMD may present with hyperCKaemia without significant clinical symptoms, or rarely with rhabdomyolysis. EMG usually does not contribute to the diagnosis, especially if CK is markedly elevated (> 10 × ULN). Muscle imaging may be helpful in showing early fatty replacement of the adductor magnus muscle, semimembranosus muscle, and long head of the biceps femoris muscle as the first manifestations that are specific findings in BMD.

For accurate genetic classification, there is a variety of sequencing and genetic diagnostic methodologies, including multiplex PCR and/or MLPA for large deletions/duplications identification and Sanger sequencing for known point mutations. MLPA is mostly used for diagnosis, albeit in most laboratories next-generation sequencing is able to capture the smaller deletions and duplications as well.

A muscle biopsy with dystrophin staining can still be useful in cases with negative genetic analysis. In BMD, muscle immunohistochemistry may show that dystrophin is distributed normally but globally reduced or that the staining is discontinuous with either a normal or reduced intensity. However, Western blot analysis, which is a semi-quantitative measurement of dystrophin, is more sensitive, showing abnormal amounts of dystrophin and/or dystrophin with a different molecular weight.

The disease course is slowly progressive but shows considerable heterogeneity. Usually in due course the upper limbs become affected as well. The clinical distinction between DMD and BMD is historically based on the age of wheelchair dependency: before age 13 in DMD in untreated cases and after age 16 years in BMD. An intermediate group is also recognized and a clear distinction based on loss of ambulation is cumbersome with the chronic use of corticosteroids, which have a significant effect on disease progression of DMD. In BMD, corticosteroids are not routinely used, mainly due to insufficient evidence and the long-term side effects.

At the time of diagnosis, evaluation for cardiomyopathy by electrocardiography, cardiac echocardiography, and/or cardiac MRI should take place and consultation with a clinical geneticist and/or genetic counsellor if relevant. Monitoring of the cardiac status is recommended biannually unless findings dictate otherwise. Treatment of cardiological manifestations includes ACE inhibitor and/or beta blockers. Heart transplantation can be considered in BMD cases with severe dilated cardiomyopathy and little clinical evidence of skeletal muscle damage. Dependent on the extent of muscle involvement, referral to a rehabilitation physician who usually operates in a multidisciplinary team is recommended.

Contractures are less common in BMD compared with DMD, but Achilles tendon contractures may occur. Scoliosis is also less common but should be monitored with referral to an orthopaedic surgeon for spinal fusion if necessary.

Suggested Reading

Darras BT, Urion DK, Ghosh PS. Dystrophinopathies. 2000 Sep 5 [updated 2022 Jan 20]. In Adam MP, Mirzaa GM, Pagon RA, et al., editors. *GeneReviews®* [Internet]. Seattle, WA: University of Washington; 1993–2023. PMID: 20301298.

Fratter C, Dalgleish R, Allen SK, et al. EMQN best practice guidelines for genetic testing in dystrophinopathies. *Eur J Hum Genet* 2020;28(9):1141–1159. doi: 10.1038/s41431-020-0643-7. Epub 2020 May 18. PMID: 32424326; PMCID: PMC7608854.

Papa AA, D'Ambrosio P, Petillo R, Palladino A, Politano L. Heart transplantation in patients with dystrophinopathic cardiomyopathy: review of the literature and personal series. *Intractable Rare Dis Res* 2017;6(2):95–101. doi: 10.5582/irdr.2017.01024. PMID: 28580208; PMCID: PMC5451754.

Straub V, Guglieri M. An update on Becker muscular dystrophy. *Curr Opin Neurol* 2023;36(5):450–454. doi: 10.1097/WCO.0000000000001191. Epub 2023 Aug 21. PMID: 37591308; PMCID: PMC10487383.

Tasca G, Iannaccone E, Monforte M, et al. Muscle MRI in Becker muscular dystrophy. *Neuromuscul Disord* 2012;22 Suppl 2:S100-6. doi: 10.1016/j.nmd.2012.05.015. PMID: 22980760.

CASE 38: Facioscapulohumeral Muscular Dystrophy (FSHD)

Clinical History

In her early forties, a 51-year-old woman first noticed fatigue when walking. She attributed this to hollowing of her back and a tendency to push her tummy forward. Later, she noticed difficulty and pain in lifting her right arm. She had never been able to whistle properly. Her parents and sisters did not have muscle complaints.

Examination

When attempting to pout the lips, there was a slight inability to contract the lower lip completely on one side (Fig. 38.1A). There was a scapula alata on the right side (Fig. 38.1B). She could not stand on her heels. When walking, there was lumbar hyperlordosis.

Diagnostic Considerations

The phenotype is typical for facioscapulohumeral muscular dystrophy (FSHD). Many patients with FSHD present with unilateral shoulder and arm pain, probably as result of chronic overuse. Facial weakness is often unnoticed but becomes apparent upon physical examination. In 95% of patients with a typical FSHD phenotype, the diagnosis can be confirmed relatively easily by showing a deletion in the D4Z4-repeat on chromosome 4qter.

Ancillary Investigations

Serum CK activity was slightly elevated (2 × ULN). DNA analysis showed a normal EcoRI/BlnI fragment as detected by the P13E-11 probe, indicating a normal D4Z4 repeat size. This made FSHD type 1 highly unlikely. Subsequent methylation-sensitive Southern blot analysis (performed in a research setting) revealed a loss of D4Z4 methylation levels, confirming the clinical diagnosis of FSHD, albeit the much rarer FSHD type 2.

Follow-Up

In the course of five years, walking became more difficult, forcing her to use a walker for longer distances.

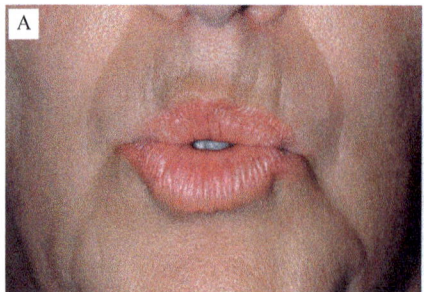
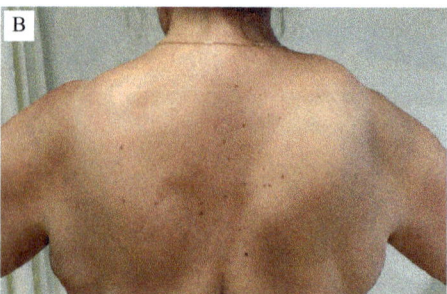

Figure 38.1 (A,B) Subtle asymmetric weakness of the orbicularis oris muscle (A) and asymmetric winging of the scapulae (B) in the described patient.

General Remarks

FSHD is one of the most common hereditary myopathies. Inheritance is autosomal dominant in most cases (FSHD1). Up to 30% of cases are due to a *de novo* mutation. The disease is caused by an aberrant expression of the transcription factor DUX4, which is normally repressed. This is caused by hypomethylation of the D4Z4 region of chromosome 4q35, allowing transcription of the *DUX4* gene located in this region. The toxic effects of inappropriate *DUX4* expression are not fully understood yet. Type 1 FSHD (95% of cases) and type 2 FSHD (5% of cases) are clinically indistinguishable. In FSHD1, hypomethylation of the D4Z4 region of chromosome 4q35 is caused by a reduction in the number of repeats (< 10 units) in the D4Z4 region, in the presence of a specific 4qter background (the A haplotype). In FSHD2, hypomethylation of the D4Z4 region is caused by mutation in a chromatin-modifier gene on another chromosome, the *SMCHD1* gene in most cases, in the presence of a semi-shortened D4Z4 repeat (8–10 units) and the A haplotype. FSHD1 is inherited as an autosomal dominant repeat disorder with incomplete penetrance. FSHD2 is a digenic disorder, and its inheritance pattern is complex.

Genetic testing for FSHD is complex and should be done in a specialized laboratory. It includes assessment of the number of repeats in the D4Z4 region, distinguishing a reduced length (contraction) of the D4Z4 region on chromosome 4 from a homologous (and nonpathogenic) region on chromosome 10, 4q haplotype testing, and, in FSHD2, mutation analysis of the *SMCHD1*, *LRIF1* and *DNMT3B* genes or assessment of the methylation status of the 4q35 subtelomeric region.

Disease severity and age at onset vary widely, even within sibships, but the distribution and weakness evolution are characteristic, see Table 38.1 (although sometimes atypical, see Table 38.2). Facial muscles, especially the orbicularis oris muscle and to a lesser extent orbicularis oculi muscles, and scapular fixators are the first to become weak. Many patients recall that they have never been able to drink through a straw. Orbicularis oris weakness may be subtle and only apparent on the patient's attempt to whistle. Weakness is typically asymmetric, and asymmetric lip closure and winging scapulae allow for a spot diagnosis. In 25% of patients other orofacial muscles are also weak, leading to difficulties in swallowing and in verbal and social communication.

Patients with a classic phenotype have problems with fixation of the shoulder to the trunk while abducting the arms. This causes considerable overuse pain in the shoulder, which often is the first symptom. Winging of the scapulae is not always visible at rest and will become more evident on anteflexion or abduction of the upper arm. Usually, the deltoid muscle is relatively spared, but its function is hampered by the loose scapula. Wasting of the pectoral muscles can be seen as an extra-axillary fold. Progression of weakness subsequently involves the upper arm muscles (biceps and triceps muscles), foot dorsiflexors, lower abdominal muscles, and proximal leg muscles. Approximately 20% of patients become wheelchair bound.

There is no cardiac involvement. One-third of wheelchair-dependent patients have mild to moderate weakness of respiratory muscles, but only rarely is there a need for ventilator support and life expectancy is normal. Severe disease is sometimes associated with retinal vasculopathy and hearing loss (Coats syndrome), in particular in early-onset disease (10 years). In FSHD1, the number of repeats partially explains the variability in disease severity and progression. Ten percent of patients have an early onset (< 10 years of age) and severe, rapidly progressive disease. These patients have the shortest D4Z4 repeats. Atypical

Table 38.2. Atypical phenotypes of facioscapulohumeral dystrophy (FSHD)

- Facial sparing with scapular winging
- Limb girdle syndrome
- Axial myopathy with bent spine syndrome
- Distal myopathy with frequently asymmetric foot drop, rarely calf weakness
- Initially, exclusive involvement of the calves

Table 38.1 Main features of facioscapulohumeral muscular dystrophy (FSHD)

- Variable age at onset
- Onset with asymmetric weakness of orbicularis oris muscle and asymmetric winging scapula
- Slow progression with weakness of biceps and triceps brachii muscles, foot dorsiflexors, lower abdominal muscles, and proximal leg muscles.
- Moderately increased CK
- No cardiac involvement
- Autosomal dominant inheritance. Genetic analysis and counselling may be complex.

phenotypes of FSHD have been recognized (see Table 38.2).

Management of patients with FSHD includes genetic counselling, which is complex in FSHD2 because of the digenic nature of the disease, and rehabilitation care with special attention for reduction of pain. Surgical scapular fixation has been reported to be successful in patients with preserved deltoid muscle strength, but no consensus exists. Ankle-foot orthoses are helpful if there is foot drop.

Suggested Reading

Goselink RJM, Mul K, van Kernebeek CR, et al. Early onset as a marker for disease severity in facioscapulohumeral muscular dystrophy. *Neurology* 2019;92(4):e378–e385. doi: 10.1212/WNL.0000000000006819. Epub 2018 Dec 19. PMID: 30568007; PMCID: PMC6345117.

Mul K, Berggren KN, Sills MY, et al. Effects of weakness of orofacial muscles on swallowing and communication in FSHD. *Neurology* 2019;92(9):e957–e963. doi: 10.1212/WNL.0000000000007013. Epub 2019 Jan 25. PMID: 30804066; PMCID: PMC6404471.

Mul K. Facioscapulohumeral muscular dystrophy. *Continuum (Minneap Minn)* 2022;28(6):1735–1751. doi: 10.1212/CON.0000000000001155. PMID: 36537978.

Vincenten SCC, Van Der Stoep N, Paulussen ADC, et al. Facioscapulohumeral muscular dystrophy-Reproductive counseling, pregnancy, and delivery in a complex multigenetic disease. *Clin Genet* 2022;101(2):149–160. doi: 10.1111/cge.14031. Epub 2021 Aug 1. PMID: 34297364; PMCID: PMC9291192.

CASE 39 Myotonic Dystrophy Type 1 (DM1)

Clinical History

A 54-year-old man was referred by his GP. He had lived with his mother until her death when he was 47 years old. He then moved into an assisted living facility. His father had died in his early 30s in a car accident. A sister was said to have died of a muscle disease and a brother had reportedly died of a heart attack at age 35 years. A niece from his father's side was also reported to have a muscle disease. Apart from having difficulties opening his hands since childhood (upon request) he had had no complaints until his late thirties, when he experienced muscle weakness. This hampered him during his full-time work as a groundskeeper in public gardens, but he continued working. Two months ago, however, he had to give up this job because of severe fatigue and increasing generalized weakness. Speaking clearly had also become difficult. He slept restlessly, with early awakenings, and sometimes had morning headaches. He experienced shortness of breath, in particular when lying flat. During the day, he watched TV and often dozed off.

Examination

On examination, there was a loss of facial expression due to weakness of facial muscles and bilateral ptosis (Fig. 39.1). Coughing was weak. There was bulbar dysarthria, frontotemporal baldness, atrophy of temporal muscles, distal more than proximal muscle wasting and weakness, MRC grade 4. Action myotonia could be easily elicited.

Diagnostic Considerations

The combination of a mild intellectual disability, generalized muscle weakness, respiratory insufficiency, bilateral ptosis, bulbar dysarthria, premature balding, action myotonia, and a family history compatible with autosomal dominant inheritance leaves no other diagnosis than myotonic dystrophy type 1 (DM1). Genetic confirmation is relatively straightforward. Of note, repeat expansions cannot be found using a next-generation sequencing gene panel analysis.

Ancillary Investigations

Instructing the patient for the measurement of the forced vital capacity using a facial mask was

Case 39 Myotonic Dystrophy Type 1

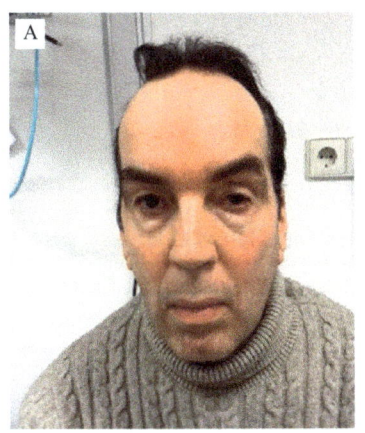 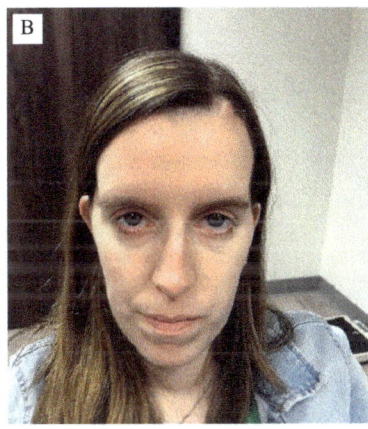

Figure 39.1 (A,B) Described patient (A) and another patient, both with myotonic dystrophy type 1 (DM1) (B) showing ptosis, myopathic face, atrophy of temporal muscles, and, in the male patient, frontal balding. Note the similarity in appearance.

unsuccessful. Capillary blood gasses showed daytime hypercapnia: pCO2 57 mmHg /7.6 kPa (normal range pCO2 35–45 mmHg)/4.7–6.0 kPa), bicarbonate 33.2 mmol/L (normal range 22–29), base excess 8.0 mmol/L (normal range −3 to +3). Long-range PCR and triplet primed PCR showed a cytosine–thymine–guanine (CTG) repeat expansion (120–1000; normal range 4–34) in the dystrophia myotonica protein kinase (DMPK) gene on chromosome 19. ECG showed a right bundle branch block; 24-hour registration of the cardiac rhythm revealed no disturbances. No cataract was found on split-lamp examination.

Follow-Up

He started noninvasive ventilation at night without difficulties and felt much fitter during the day. He subsequently received yearly standardized check-ups by a specialized nurse who coordinates multidisciplinary care by his GP, neurologist, cardiologist, pulmonologist, ophthalmologist, gastroenterologist, and rehabilitation services. Atrium flutter developed and was treated by medication and, later, atrium fibrillation was treated by electrocardioversion. He was treated for pneumonia, probably following choking, albeit he did not specifically complain about it. He was instructed to use air-stacking because of decreased coughing force in order to prevent further infections. Weakness increased fairly quickly. Walking devices secured ambulation. Modafinil was prescribed for daytime sleepiness. He remained fairly well-humoured and enjoyed playing checkers with his housemates.

General Remarks

DM1 is autosomal dominantly transmitted with almost full penetrance. It is the most prevalent muscular dystrophy. There may be a considerable delay in patient diagnosis, since patients with this disorder in general do not readily express any complaints, possibly due to a combination of apathy and inertia, mood disorder, and excessive daytime sleepiness. They often assume that certain traits, such as ptosis or a steppage gait, are peculiarities that just 'run in the family'. A late diagnosis may impede the timely recognition of cardiac conduction, rhythm disturbances, and respiratory failure due to early diaphragm weakness, which are preventable causes of unexpected and premature death. A late diagnosis also impedes timely genetic counselling. A 'spot diagnosis' is often possible based on the appearance of ptosis, frontal balding in men, a sluggish presentation, partly due to facial weakness, and foot drop.

DM1 is a multisystem disease, and many other organs and tissues may be involved (see Table 39.1). Since many manifestations of DM1 can be alleviated with the appropriate treatment, and patients do not readily themselves alert their doctor, it is important to provide a scheduled and comprehensive check-up, coordinated by a specialized nurse, and involving social worker, psychologist, neurologist, cardiologist, pulmonologist, ophthalmologist, gastroenterologist, rehabilitation services such as occupational therapy, and home ventilation services. A social worker can also relieve the often considerable burden experienced by a partner and other family members. Special care should be taken to avoid perioperative

Part II Neuromuscular Cases: Myopathies

Table 39.1 Main features in the spectrum of myotonic dystrophy type 1 (DM1); selected management recommendations

Number of CTG repeats (normal 4–34)	Major symptoms and signs
Mild DM1 50–150 repeats	Posterior subcapsular cataract < 40 years of age
	Mild myotonia (sustained muscle contraction)
	Diabetes mellitus
Classic DM1 100–1000 repeats	Onset 2nd or 3rd decade
	Wasting and weakness of facial muscles (temporal muscles), bulbar muscles (dysarthria, dysphagia),[a] neck flexors, distal limb muscles (e.g., foot drop (**Video 39.1**)) and later on also proximal limb muscles. CK is mildly elevated. Moderate intensity exercise is recommended.
	Weakness of diaphragm, which may require noninvasive nocturnal ventilation. Vaccination for pneumonia and flu is recommended.
	Grip myotonia (**Videos 39.2 and 39.3**). Mexiletine can be used if needed, but is contraindicated in cardiac involvement.
	Irritable bowel-like symptoms: diarrhoea (high-fibre diet, loperamide), (pseudo-)obstruction (increased water intake, laxatives); gallstones
	Frequently cardiac conduction abnormalities and arrhythmia requiring pacemaker or cardioverter-defibrillator implantation, less often cardiomyopathy. Sudden death in 1/3. Prophylactic permanent pacing may decrease sudden death substantially.
	Frontal balding in men
	Excessive daytime sleepiness (EDS) due to central sleep apnoea, obstructive sleep apnoea, nocturnal hypoventilation. Modafinil may be effective.
	Central nervous system involvement: mood disorders, anxiety, mildly decreased IQ, frontal lobe dysfunction
	Posterior subcapsular cataract. Surgery if troublesome.
	Diabetes mellitus, calcium dysregulation, testicular atrophy, subfertility
	Fatigue
	Increased risk of obstetric complications: miscarriage rate 33%, pre-eclampsia ~10%, placenta praevia, preterm labour 31–50%. Increase of weakness (30%).
	Succinylcholine is contraindicated. Local anaesthesia is preferred. Serious complications in the postanaesthesia period, also due to hypersomnolence and cognitive impairment, adverse effects of opioids and anaesthesia.
	Life expectancy is decreased (median age at death 55.4 years)
Congenital or childhood DM1 > 1000 repeats	Present at birth or onset in 1st decade
	Polyhydramnios and reduced fetal movement in congenital type, perinatal death ~15%
	Hypotonia, severe generalized progressive weakness, including facial weakness, respiratory insufficiency, club foot
	Intellectual disability (50% of congenital type)
	Excessive daytime sleepiness
	Early respiratory death (25% of patients die before 18 months of age and 50% die before their mid 30s).

[a] Dysphagia often goes unnoticed and should be asked about (increased duration of mealtime, coughing while drinking, choking on foods, nasal regurgitation, piecemeal deglutition, weight loss, aspiration pneumonia).

complications. Preoperative checks of respiratory function and heart are especially important. Women with DM1 are at increased risk of various complications in pregnancy and labour, and special surveillance is warranted (see also Part I, Table 8.1).

DM1 is caused by the expansion of the CTG trinucleotide repeat in the 3′ non-coding region of the *DMPK* gene. This repeat expansion is unstable and increases with subsequent generations, which is accompanied by earlier onset and increased severity (known as 'anticipation'). Thus, the affected father of a patient with 'classic' DM1, such as the patient described here, may have a short repeat expansion and the characteristic cataract as the sole clinical manifestation. Severe congenital myotonic dystrophy is usually transmitted by the mother with classic DM1. Genetic counselling should be offered to all patients and their families. Pre-implantation diagnosis is one of the available options for a patient desiring to become pregnant.

Suggested Reading

Ashizawa T, Gagnon C, Groh WJ, et al. Consensus-based care recommendations for adults with myotonic dystrophy type 1. *Neurol Clin Pract* 2018;8(6):507–520. doi: 10.1212/CPJ.0000000000000531. PMID: 30588381; PMCID: PMC6294540.

Bird TD. Myotonic dystrophy type 1. 1999 Sep 17 [updated 2021 Mar 25]. In Adam MP, Mirzaa GM, Pagon RA, et al., editors. *GeneReviews*® [Internet]. Seattle, WA: University of Washington; 1993–2023. PMID: 20301344

Wahbi K, Furling D. Cardiovascular manifestations of myotonic dystrophy. *Trends Cardiovasc Med* 2020;30(4):232–238. doi: 10.1016/j.tcm.2019.06.001. Epub 2019 Jun 13. PMID: 31213350.

Myotonic Dystrophy Type 2 (DM2)

Clinical History

A 60-year-old woman was referred because from the age of 50 years onwards she experienced muscle weakness that led to increasing difficulty in climbing stairs. In addition, she complained about exercise-induced myalgia.

History included cataract surgery at the age of 58 years, and lately, unexpected and unexplained falls. Family history revealed early-onset cataract in several paternal family members. Her father and brother had died suddenly and unexpectedly despite a pacemaker.

Examination

There was mild muscle weakness with a limb girdle distribution, slightly atrophic thighs, and firm calf muscles. Gowers sign was positive. No facial weakness was noted. Myotonia could not be elicited. Reflexes were normal and there were no contractures.

Diagnostic Considerations

The combination of late-onset proximal muscle weakness, cataract, and sudden death in family members due to a cardiac cause is consistent with a diagnosis of myotonic dystrophy type 2 (DM2; previously called proximal myotonic myopathy, PROMM).

Ancillary Investigations

Serum CK activity was two times the upper limit of normal. EMG showed signs of myopathy, but no myotonia. DNA analysis showed a heterozygous pathogenic CCTG repeat expansion in intron 1 of the *CNBP* (formerly *ZNF9*) gene. Cardiac evaluation was normal.

Follow-Up

Once the diagnosis had been established, the cardiologist implanted a reveal cardiac monitor because of previous syncopes.

General Remarks

DM2 is an autosomal dominantly inherited myopathy. The mutation that underlies DM2 is a CCTG repeat expansion (normal < 30) in intron 1 of the *CNBP* gene on chromosome 3q. A toxic gain-of-function effect of the abnormally expanded RNA that accumulates in the muscle nuclei is suggested to be responsible for the pathological features common to both DM1 and DM2.

The number of CCTG repeats in a pathogenic expansion ranges from approximately 75 to more than 11,000, with a mean of approximately 5,000 repeats.

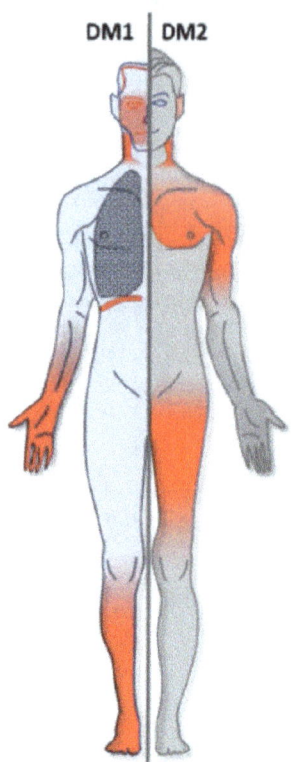

Figure 40.1 Regions of weakness and atrophy (highlighted in red) in DM1 and DM2. From Wenninger et al., Core clinical phenotypes in myotonic dystrophies. *Front Neurol* 2018;9:303, with permission.

Table 40.1 Features that discriminate myotonic dystrophy type 2 (DM2) from type 1 (DM1)

- Milder disease course
- More prominent myalgia, stiffness, and fatigue
- Proximal muscle weakness
- Less weakness of the face, no ptosis, and less bulbar weakness
- Frequent calf hypertrophy
- Cognitive abnormalities are present but less severe as compared with DM1
- Similar cardiac manifestations as in DM1, but with a lower prevalence, later age of onset, and lower risk of sudden death
- Apparent lack of mental retardation in juvenile cases
- Congenital DM2 rare
- No anticipation

Repeat size has not been found to correlate with specific phenotypes, such as proximal muscle weakness, cardiac arrhythmias, and cognitive decline. However, this is likely in part due to the relative paucity of studies measuring these correlations.

The detection rate of a *CNBP* CCTG expansion is more than 99% with the combination of conventional PCR (which detects normal-sized alleles but not abnormal-sized alleles), Southern blot analysis, and the PCR repeat-primed assay. The latter two tests are performed if routine PCR analysis detects only one allele, which occurs in 15% of unaffected individuals who are homozygous and in all affected individuals.

The onset of DM2 is usually in the third to fourth decade of life, with muscle weakness being the most common presenting symptom. Weakness in DM2 typically affects proximal and axial muscles, including the neck flexors, and long flexors of the fingers. Facial muscles are usually not involved. Most DM2 patients also complain about muscle pain. Calf hypertrophy is found in a proportion of patients. Symptoms may worsen during pregnancy.

Other clinical features include cardiac conduction defects (atrioventricular and intraventricular), dysrhythmias, left ventricular dysfunction, dilated cardiomyopathy, and sudden death. Posterior subcapsular cataracts can be found as early as the second decade. Endocrine features are insulin-insensitive diabetes mellitus type 2, thyroid dysfunction, and hypogonadism in adult males. Gastrointestinal complications are common and mostly include constipation, swallowing difficulty, and acid reflux. Cognitive manifestations such as problems with organization, concentration, and word-finding, as well as excessive daytime sleepiness are present in DM2.

The phenotype of DM2 resembles adult-onset DM1, but differences exist (Table 40.1). Clinical myotonia is rarely present in DM2 and, if so, mainly present in the proximal leg muscles. On EMG, myotonic discharges are found in only two-thirds of the patients. Serum CK is normal or mildly elevated. Muscle biopsy shows rather nonspecific myopathic and 'denervation-like' changes and is therefore not useful for diagnosis.

Care considerations for DM2 have been published by a Consortium of Experts aimed at monitoring and management of cardiac and respiratory complications, pain control, muscle weakness, and gastrointestinal complications. Genetic counselling is paramount for those who have clinical symptoms and signs indicative of DM2 and at-risk family members.

Suggested Reading

Meola G. Myotonic dystrophy type 2: the 2020 update. *Acta Myol* 2020;39(4):222–234. doi: 10.36185/2532-1900-026. PMID: 33458578; PMCID: MC7783423.

Schoser B, Montagnese F, Bassez G, et al.; Myotonic Dystrophy Foundation. Consensus-based care recommendations for adults with myotonic dystrophy type 2. *Neurol Clin Pract* 2019;9(4):343–353. doi: 10.1212/CPJ.0000000000000645. PMID: 31583190; PMCID: PMC6745739.

Wenninger S, Montagnese F, Schoser B. Core clinical phenotypes in myotonic dystrophies. *Front Neurol* 2018;9:303. doi: 10.3389/fneur.2018.00303. PMID: 29770119; PMCID: PMC5941986.

CASE 41 Limb Girdle Muscular Dystrophy (LGMD) R1, Calpain-Related

Clinical History

In his late twenties, a 30-year-old man reported difficulty with raising his arms and running, which had progressed over subsequent years. During his teens he had been a very good soccer player.

Examination

There was bilateral symmetric scapular winging (Fig. 41.1), hypertrophy of the calves, and symmetric MRC grade 4 weakness of elbow flexion, hip flexion, and hip adduction. He had a pronounced lumbar lordosis and a waddling gait (**Video 41.1**). Contractures were not found.

Diagnostic Considerations

The patient had onset of symptoms in early adulthood, symmetric scapular winging, weakness predominantly of elbow flexion more than extension and of hip adduction more than abduction, and normal respiratory function. Progression over years points to a genetic disease. The most frequent neuromuscular disorder presenting with a scapula alata is facioscapulohumeral dystrophy, but in this disease, the winging scapula is asymmetric and usually there also is facial weakness. If serum CK is strongly elevated, an autosomal recessive limb girdle muscular dystrophy (LGMD) is more likely. Winging scapula is a characteristic feature of LGMD type R1, caused by mutations in the calpain3 (*CAPN3*) gene.

Ancillary Investigations

Respiratory and cardiac functions were normal. Serum CK activity was 40 × ULN. CT imaging was similar to the pattern found in LGMD R1: in the arms, involvement of biceps more than triceps and deltoid muscles; lateral paraspinal muscles more affected than medial paraspinal muscles; involvement of hip adductors and biceps femoris with sparing of quadriceps muscles (Fig. 42.2). Analysis of the *CAPN3* gene revealed two pathogenic variants: c.551C>T, p.Thr184Met, and c.2464T>C, p.X822Argext62X.

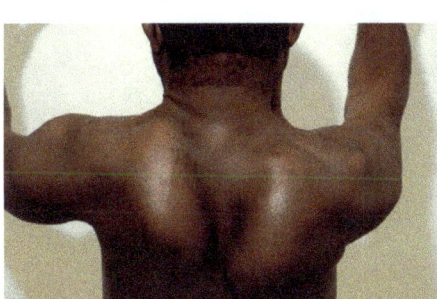
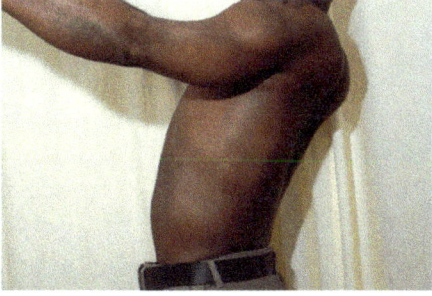

Figure 41.1 Symmetric scapular winging in the described patient.

General Remarks

Limb Girdle Muscular Dystrophies (LGMDs)

Limb girdle muscular dystrophies are defined as genetically inherited conditions that primarily affect skeletal muscle, leading to progressive, predominantly proximal muscle weakness at presentation caused by a loss of muscle fibres. Patients by definition achieve independent walking. Cardiac involvement and/or clinically relevant respiratory weakness is a feature of some but not all LGMDs. Muscle imaging demonstrates fatty substitution of muscle, typically involving the hip adductors and hamstrings, and muscle histology shows dystrophic changes. LGMDs are classified according to the mode of inheritance: autosomal dominant or autosomal recessive (excluding X-linked recessive Duchenne and Becker muscular dystrophies), and the affected protein (Tables 41.1 and 41.2).

Limb girdle muscular dystrophies are very rare, much rarer than other muscular dystrophies, that is, Duchenne muscular dystrophy, myotonic dystrophies, and facioscapulohumeral muscular dystrophy. The recessive forms together make up about 90% of all LGMDs. They have a younger age at onset, faster progression, and more severe weakness than the dominant forms. Serum CK is markedly elevated in recessive forms and may be normal in dominant forms. The proteins involved are located in the extracellular space, the sarcolemma, or in the intracellular compartments (Fig. 41.3). Next-generation sequencing (NGS) gene

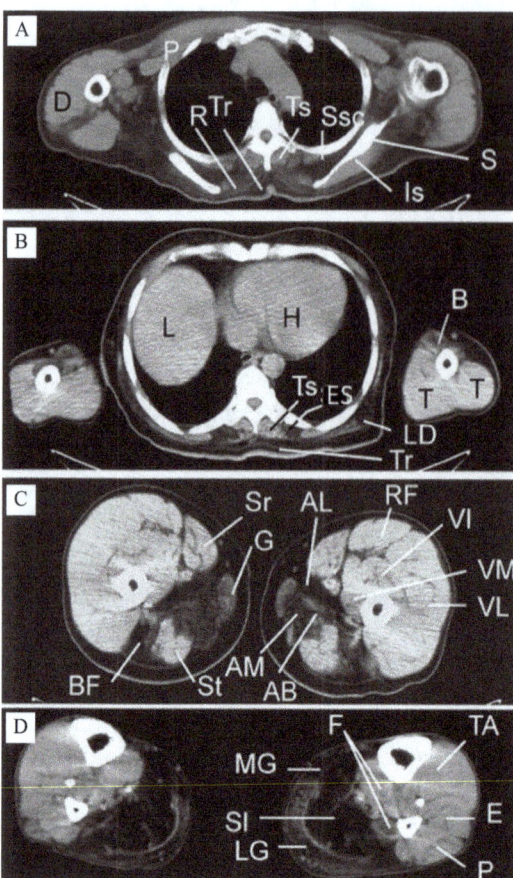

Figure 41.2 (A–D) CT imaging in the described patient showing replacement of various muscles (light grey) by fat (black): at the shoulder girdle and mid-thoracic levels (A,B): subscapular (Ssc), infraspinatus (Is), rhomboid (R), trapezius (Tr), latissimus dorsi (LD), sacrospinal (Ss), erector spinae (ES), and biceps brachii (B) muscles. At the upper and lower leg level (C,D): biceps femoris (BF), adductor magnus (AM), adductor brevis (AB), lateral and medial head of the gastrocnemius (LG, MG), soleus (Sl) muscles. Not shown: fatty replacement of gluteus minimus and medius muscles. Relatively preserved muscles: deltoid (D), pectoral (P), transversospinalis (TS), triceps brachii (T), lateral vastus (VL), medial vastus (VM), intermedius vastus (VI), rectus femoris (RF), gracilis (G), sartorius (Sr), semitendinosus (St), anterior tibial (TA), peroneal (P) muscles, toe flexors (F), and toe extensors (E). H = heart; L = liver; S = scapula.

Follow-Up

Fifteen years after onset of symptoms, there was total loss of elbow flexion that – together with the loss of scapular fixation – made it almost impossible for him to use his arms. With great effort, he could walk for a few minutes. Cycling was impossible because of the tendency to fall when getting off the bike. Respiratory function, as measured by means of vital capacity, was slightly decreased (78% of expected).

Table 41.1 Autosomal dominant limb girdle muscular dystrophy (LGMD) subtypes identified so far (old subtype nomenclature in parentheses)

Subtype	Gene	Protein
LGMD D1 (1D)	DNAJB6	DNAJB6
LGMD D2 (1F)	TNPO3	Transportin 3
LGMD D3 (1G)	HNRNPDL	Heterogeneous nuclear ribonucleoprotein D-like
LGMD D4 (1I)	CAPN3	Calpain 3
LGMD D5	COL6A1, COL6A2, COL6A3	Collagen 6α1, 6α2, 6α3

Table 41.2 Autosomal recessive limb girdle muscular dystrophy (LGMD) subtypes identified so far (old subtype nomenclature in parentheses)

Subtype	Gene	Protein
LGMD R1 (2A)	CAPN3	Calpain 3
LGMD R2 (2B)	DYSF	Dysferlin
LGMD R3 (2D)	SGCA	α-Sarcoglycan
LGMD R4 (2E)	SGCB	β-Sarcoglycan
LGMD R5 (2C)	SGCG	γ-Sarcoglycan
LGMD R6 (2F)	SGCD	δ-Sarcoglycan
LGMD R7 (2G)	TCAP	Telethonin
LGMD R8 (2H)	TRIM32	TRIM32
LGMD R9 (2I)	FKRP	Fukutin-related protein
LGMD R10 (2 J)	TTN	Titin
LGMD R11 (2 K)	POMT1	Protein O-mannosyltransferase 1
LGMD R12 (2L)	ANO5	Anoctamin5
LGMD R13 (2 M)	FKTN	Fukutin
LGMD R14 (2 N)	POMT2	Protein O-mannosyltransferase 2
LGMD R15 (2O)	POMGnT1	Protein O-linked mannose N-acetylglucosaminyltrans-ferase 1
LGMD R16 (2P)	DAG1	Dystroglycan 1
LGMD R17 (2Q)	PLEC	Plectin
LGMD R18 (2S)	TRAPPC11	Trafficking protein particle complex 11
LGMD R19 (2T)	GMPPB	GDP-mannose pyrophosphorylase B
LGMD R20 (2U)	ISPD/CRPPA	CDL-L-ribitol pyrophosphorylase A
LGMD R21 (2Z)	POGLUT1	Protein O-glucosyltransferase 1
LGMD R22	COL6A1, COL6A2, COL6A3	Collagen 6α1, 6α2, 6α3
LGMD R23	LAMA2	Laminin α2
LGMD R24	POMGNT2	Protein O-linked mannose N-acetylglucosaminyltransferase 2
LGMD R25 (2X)	POPDC1/BVES	Popeye domain-containing protein 1
LGMD R26	POPDC3	Popeye domain-containing protein 1

panel analysis is the first diagnostic step, but currently enables a diagnosis in only a minority of patients. There is no causal treatment.

Limb Girdle Muscular Dystrophy R1, Calpain-Related

In most regions of the world, LGMD type R1, caused by homozygous or compound heterozygous mutations in the gene for calpain 3, is the most frequent LGMD (about 20% of all LGMDs). A much rarer dominant form with similar but milder phenotype exists (LGMD type D4). The function of calpain 3, a sarcomeric cysteine protease, is as yet unknown. Severity and age at onset are variable, partly corresponding to specific genotypes, but many patients show a clinical classic pattern, summarized in Table 41.3. Typically, patients report completely normal muscle function prior to the first symptoms of upper leg weakness, which usually presents in their teens. Gait is waddling with increased lumbar lordosis and sometimes tiptoeing with ankle contractures.

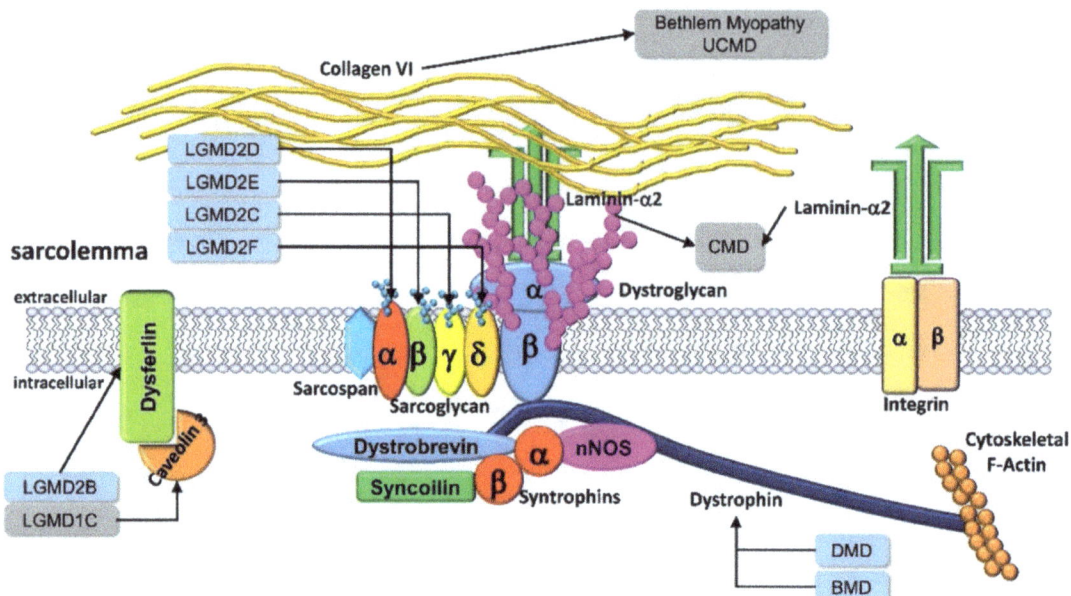

Figure 41.3 Schematic representation of dystrophin–glycoprotein complex (DGC) and of other sarcoplasmic associated proteins involved in muscular dystrophies.
From Nigro and Piluso, Spectrum of muscular dystrophies associated with sarcolemmal-protein genetic defects. *Biochim Biophys Acta* 2015;1852:585–593, with permission.
BMD = Becker muscular dystrophy; CMD = congenital muscular dystrophy; DMD = Duchenne muscular dystrophy; UCMD = Ullrich congenital muscular dystrophy.

Table 41.3 Main features of limb girdle muscular dystrophy R1, calpain-related

- Onset in late childhood or adolescence with difficulty running and sometimes tendency to walk on tiptoe
- Symmetric scapular winging
- Sometimes contractures: ankle dorsiflexion, finger flexion, wrist flexion, elbow flexion
- Specific pattern of muscle involvement with predominant and early weakness of hip adductors, extensors, and knee flexors
- Relative preservation of elbow extension, knee extension, and distal muscles
- Normal or mildly decreased respiratory function, preserved cardiac function
- (Very) high CK activity

Mean time to loss of ambulation is 12–15 years after disease onset. Winging of the scapula, usually symmetric, is a distinctive feature. The diagnosis is made by NGS gene panel analysis. If this results in the finding of a variant of uncertain significance, MR imaging can be useful. Western blotting of muscle biopsy material is not always helpful, because calpain 3 expression may appear normal, or may be decreased secondary to another protein defect. Rehabilitation therapy and genetic counselling should be offered to all patients.

Suggested Reading

Barp A, Laforet P, Bello L, Tasca G, et al. European muscle MRI study in limb girdle muscular dystrophy type R1/2A (LGMDR1/LGMD2A). *J Neurol* 2020;267(1):45-56. doi: 10.1007/s00415-019-09539-y. Epub 2019 Sep 25. PMID: 31555977.

Johnson NE, Statland JM. The limb-girdle muscular dystrophies. *Continuum (Minneap Minn)* 2022;28(6):1698–1714. doi: 10.1212/CON.0000000000001178. PMID: 36537976.

Liewluck T, Milone M. Untangling the complexity of limb-girdle muscular dystrophies. *Muscle Nerve* 2018;58(2):167–177. doi: 10.1002/mus.26077. Epub 2018 Feb 7. PMID: 29350766.

Lostal W, Urtizberea JA, Richard I ; Calpain 3 study group. 233rd ENMC International Workshop: clinical trial readiness for calpainopathies, Naarden, the Netherlands, 15-17 September 2017. *Neuromuscul Disord* 2018;28(6):540–549. doi:

10.1016/j.nmd.2018.03.010. Epub 2018 Mar 28. PMID: 29655529.

Spinazzi M, Poupiot J, Cassereau J, et al. Late-onset camptocormia caused by a heterozygous in-frame CAPN3 deletion. *Neuromuscul Disord* 2021;31 (5):450–455. doi: 10.1016/j.nmd.2021.02.012. Epub 2021 Feb 14. PMID: 33741228.

Straub V, Murphy A, Udd B ; LGMD workshop study group.229th ENMC International Workshop: limb girdle muscular dystrophies – nomenclature and reformed classification Naarden, the Netherlands, 17-19 March 2017. *Neuromuscul Disord* 2018;28 (8):702–710. doi: 10.1016/j.nmd.2018.05.007. Epub 2018 May 24. PMID: 30055862.

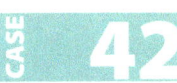

Limb Girdle Muscular Dystrophy (LGMD) R9, FKRP-Related

Clinical History

A 41-year-old man was referred because of persistent backache. When questioned, he recalled that he had had firm calves since childhood. Once, after strenuous exercise, he had experienced black coffee-coloured urine. At the time, he did not consult his GP.

Examination

He had hypertrophic calves and MRC grade 4 weakness of the hip flexors. Gowers sign was positive due to weakness of the gluteus maximus muscles. Otherwise, neurological examination was normal.

Diagnostic Considerations

The presence of limb girdle distribution of muscle weakness and calf hypertrophy since childhood points to a genetic myopathy. The finding of an elevated serum CK can restrict the differential diagnosis to a limb girdle muscular dystrophy (LGMD, see **Case 41**, Tables 41.1 and 41.2) or Becker muscular dystrophy. The latter was considered less likely because of the distribution of weakness (e.g., early weakness of the iliopsoas muscles). At the time, the patient first visited the neuromuscular outpatient department, Next-generation sequencing (NGS) gene panel testing was not yet available. It was decided to perform muscle imaging, followed by examination of a muscle biopsy.

Ancillary Investigations

Serum CK activity was 15 × ULN. Cardiac examination was normal. A muscle CT scan showed wasting and fatty replacement of the pelvic girdle (gluteus, psoas, and iliac muscles) and upper leg muscles. A muscle biopsy showed moderate variation in muscle fibre size and scattered necrotic and regenerating fibres. Dystrophin and other membrane markers were normally present, but alpha-dystroglycan was reduced. Later, mutation analysis of the fukutin-related protein (FKRP) gene revealed a common homozygous missense variant (c.826C>A), which was consistent with a diagnosis of LGMD type 2I at the time (type R9 in the present classification).

Follow-Up

The patient had no cardiac involvement at presentation, but two years later he was found to have developed left ventricular dysfunction. He died while waiting for implantation of a cardioverter defibrillator.

General Remarks

Dystroglycanopathies

Dystroglycanopathies result from abnormal O-glycosylation (the attachment of a sugar molecule to an oxygen atom) of alpha (α)-dystroglycan. Alpha-dystroglycan is part of the dystrophin-associated protein complex (DAPC: dystrophin, α- and β- dystroglycan, sarcoglycan complex, see **Case 41**, Fig. 41.3), which links the intracellular cytoskeleton with the extracellular matrix and thus provides structural stability. O-Glycosylation is dependent on several proteins, for example fukutin-related protein (FKRP), fukutin (FKTN), protein O-mannosyl transferase (POMT1), and like-acetylglucosaminyltransferase (LARGE1), among many others. Pathogenic variants in the genes coding for these proteins give rise to (secondary) dystroglycanopathies (primary dystroglycanopathies being caused by variants in the dystrophin-associated glycoprotein (DAG)1 gene, which encodes the dystroglycan precursor protein).

The spectrum of clinical phenotypes of the dystroglycanopathies is wide: infants with the most severe α-dystroglycan-related congenital muscular dystrophies (Walker Warburg syndrome (WWS), muscle–eye–brain diseases (MEB), Fukuyama CMD (FCMD)) present with hypotonia at birth and various cerebral anomalies. Infants with a congenital muscular dystrophy (CMD) phenotype without severe involvement of brain or eye (MDC1C) present at birth or in the first few months of life with severe muscle weakness and wasting of shoulder girdle muscles, hypertrophy, and weakness of leg muscles, and have high CK. Respiratory failure and cardiac involvement are frequent. These children do not achieve independent ambulation and can be severely cognitively impaired, also with normal MRI. In the milder LGMDs, onset is later in childhood or adulthood and patients achieve ambulation (by definition). Of the latter, the FKRP-related LGMD type R9 is the most frequent.

Limb Girdle Muscular Dystrophy Type R9 (Table 42.1)

Limb girdle muscular dystrophy type R9 accounts for about 10% of all LGMDs and is more common in certain parts of northern Europe (Denmark and parts of England). Onset is usually in childhood or adolescence and sometimes at adult age, as in this case. The most frequently reported presenting symptom is proximal muscle weakness in the lower limbs. Calf hypertrophy is found in a majority of the cases, which can cause confusion with Becker muscular dystrophy. The same holds true for exertional pain and muscle cramps. Serum CK is usually moderately to markedly elevated, and exertion-induced myoglobinuria is found in 25% of cases. Rhabdomyolysis may be the initial presentation. Cardiomyopathy develops in about one-third of patients, including children as young as three years,

Table 42.1 Main features of limb girdle muscular dystrophy type R9, FKRP-related

- Onset in late childhood or adolescence, sometimes at adult age with proximal weakness in the legs
- Calf hypertrophy, exertional muscle pain, cramps
- Loss of ambulation in ~40% of the patients
- Cardiomyopathy in one-third
- Early diaphragm weakness requiring noninvasive ventilation in early adulthood in 25% of patients
- Markedly elevated CK
- Rhabdomyolysis may be first manifestation

and may be the presenting feature. Cognitive impairment has been reported, but is usually not a clinically relevant feature. The clinical course is slowly progressive. About 40% of patients lose ambulation, and in one-quarter of the patients noninvasive ventilation is initiated in early adulthood. Management includes rehabilitation therapy and monitoring of respiratory and cardiac function. There is no causative treatment that cures this disease or slows down progression.

Suggested Reading

Bönnemann CG, Wang CH, Quijano-Roy S, et al.; Members of International Standard of Care Committee for Congenital Muscular Dystrophies. Diagnostic approach to the congenital muscular dystrophies. *Neuromuscul Disord* 2014;24(4):289–311. doi: 10.1016/j.nmd.2013.12.011. Epub 2014 Jan 9. PMID: 24581957; PMCID: PMC5258110.

Ten Dam L, Frankhuizen WS, Linssen WHJP, et al. Autosomal recessive limb-girdle and Miyoshi muscular dystrophies in the Netherlands: The clinical and molecular spectrum of 244 patients. *Clin Genet* 2019;96(2):126–133. doi: 10.1111/cge.13544. Epub 2019 May 6. PMID: 30919934.

Murphy LB, Schreiber-Katz O, Rafferty K, et al. Global FKRP registry: observations in more than 300 patients with limb girdle muscular dystrophy R9. *Ann Clin Transl Neurol* 2020;7(5):757–766. doi: 10.1002/acn3.51042. Epub 2020 Apr 28. PMID: 32342672; PMCID: PMC7261761.

Ortiz-Cordero C, Azzag K, Perlingeiro RCR. Fukutin-related protein: from pathology to treatments. *Trends Cell Biol* 2021;31(3):197–210. doi: 10.1016/j.tcb.2020.11.003. Epub 2020 Dec 1. PMID: 33272829; PMCID: PMC8657196.

Bethlem Myopathy, a Collagen VI-Related Myopathy (LGMDD5); Ullrich Congenital Muscular Dystrophy

Clinical History

A 55-year-old man had had muscle complaints for as long as he could remember. He could not stretch his arms or walk without shoes due to deformities of the feet. Proximal muscle weakness was mild and slowly progressive over years, and contractures had always been prominent. His stamina was low, but he still worked full-time as a manual worker. He was otherwise healthy.

Family history revealed that his father was similarly affected. In addition, a half-brother and half-sister not only had contractures but also had muscle weakness. The latter underwent surgery for torticollis in the neonatal period.

Examination

There were flexion contractures of the elbows (Fig. 43.1), contractures of the wrists and knees, and shortening of the Achilles tendons. He had pes cavus and claw toes.

Atrophy of the sternocleidomastoid muscles was observed, and there was MRC grade 4 weakness of the neck flexors, infraspinatus, triceps brachii, and iliopsoas muscles.

Diagnostic Considerations

The combination of slowly progressive proximal muscle weakness, contractures, and the probably autosomal dominant inheritance suggests Bethlem myopathy caused by pathogenic variants in the *COL6A1*, *COL6A2*, and *COL6A3* genes or Emery–Dreifuss muscular dystrophy (EDMD) due to a pathogenic variant in the *LMNA* (lamin A/C) gene. The only distinctive features between collagen VI-related Bethlem myopathy and EDMD is the presence of torticollis in the former and heart involvement in EDMD. No heart involvement was found in our patient, and torticollis had been found in a sibling.

Ancillary Investigations

Serum CK activity was normal. Genetic testing was performed and a heterozygous pathogenic variant (c.739-1G>A) was found in the *COL6A1* gene and confirmed the clinical diagnosis of Bethlem myopathy.

General Remarks

The *COL6A1–COL6A2* cluster on chromosome 21q and the *COL6A3* gene on chromosome 2q encode for the three α-chains of collagen type VI, a ubiquitous extracellular matrix protein capable of forming an interstitial and pericellular microfibrillar network. As this network is closely associated with the basement membrane around skeletal muscle fibres, collagen VI plays a role in the integrity and function of the skeletal muscle. This notion of extracellular dysfunction explains why contractures form an early and predominant part of the spectrum of Bethlem myopathy (Table 43.1).

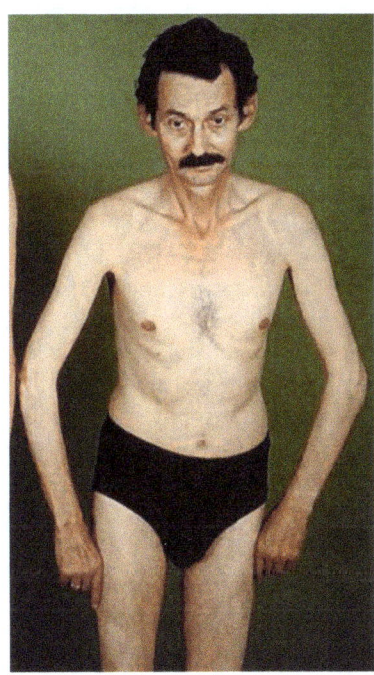

Figure 43.1 Contractures of the elbows in a patient with Bethlem myopathy.

Table 43.1 Main features of collagen VI-related myopathies

Autosomal recessive or autosomal dominant. Genes: *COL6A1*, *COL6A2*, or *COL6A3*

Ullrich congenital muscular dystrophy (UCMD):
- Congenital weakness and hypotonia, contractures, and distal hyperlaxity
- Severe and progressive weakness with early kyphoscoliosis and respiratory insufficiency
- Usually autosomal recessive

Bethlem myopathy:
- Usually childhood or adult onset. Onset with mild hypotonia and weakness at birth and extension contractures of the feet does occur
- Contractures: finger flexors, elbows, shoulders, Achilles tendons, torticollis (10%), proximal weakness
- Milder disease course than UCMD. Normal life expectancy
- Usually autosomal dominant.

Common features:
- Proximal joint contractures
- Skin abnormalities (keratosis pilaris or follicular keratosis, along the extensor surfaces of arms and legs, and keloid scars)
- Relative sparing of the central part of the vastus lateralis muscle on MRI (more prominent in Bethlem myopathy)
- No cardiac involvement

Bethlem Myopathy

There is considerable variation in the manifestation of Bethlem myopathy, even within families. In our patient, muscle contractures were predominant and in his half-sister muscle weakness and torticollis were the most prominent features. Patients may have had diminished fetal movements, or have been born as floppy babies with extension contractures of the feet which resolved spontaneously. Children with limb girdle distribution of muscle weakness with hyperlaxity of the knee joints have also been reported. In the classic type of Bethlem myopathy, characterized by proximal weakness and contractures of the elbows, Achilles tendons, and long finger flexors and the presence of follicular hyperkeratosis and keloid formation, life expectancy is usually normal. After the age of 60 years, a fair proportion of patients have to use walking aids or a wheelchair for outdoor transportation. In about 10% of the cases, respiratory insufficiency occurs due to involvement of the diaphragm. The heart is not affected.

CK activity can vary from normal to 10 × ULN. Muscle biopsy is usually nonspecific. Muscle imaging is characteristic, showing that the vastus muscles, which appear to be the most frequently and most strikingly affected thigh muscles, have a rim of abnormal signal at the periphery of each muscle and relative sparing of the central part. Another frequent finding is involvement of the rectus femoris with a central area of abnormal signal within the muscle (Fig. 43.2).

The diagnosis of Bethlem myopathy (also called collagen VI-related myopathy or limb girdle muscular dystrophy (LGMD)D(ominant)2) can be established in patients with the characteristic clinical and muscle imaging by identifying a heterozygous or bi-allelic pathogenic variant(s) in *COL6A1*, *COL6A2*, or *COL6A3* identified by molecular genetic testing.

When the phenotype is suggestive of Bethlem myopathy, one should perform sequence analysis first to detect small intragenic deletions/insertions and missense, nonsense, and splice site variants; If no pathogenic variant is found, gene-targeted deletion/duplication analysis to detect intragenic deletions or duplications is carried out. An additional recurrent dominant-negative pathogenic variant consists of a deep-intronic change in intron 11 of *COL6A1* due to its deep intronic location; this pathogenic variant may be missed on exon-only-based platforms. When the phenotype is indistinguishable from many other inherited disorders characterized by a myopathy or muscular dystrophy, comprehensive genomic testing (exome sequencing, genome sequencing) is the best option.

Ullrich Congenital Muscular Dystrophy

The combination of muscle weakness, hyperlaxity of distal joints (Fig. 43.3), and proximal contractures is also present in Ullrich congenital muscular dystrophy (UCMD), which runs a more progressive course with early kyphoscoliosis and

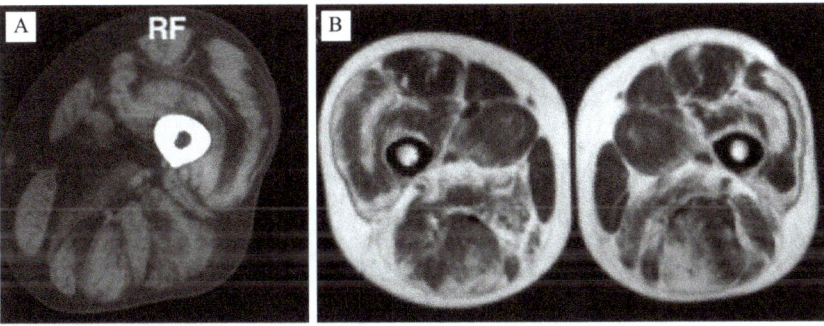

Figure 43.2 (A,B) CT scan of the left thigh of the patient showing a rim of abnormal signal (black) at the periphery of the vastus muscles and the rectus femoris (RF) (A). MRI of another patient with a similar picture, showing a central area of abnormal signal (white) within the rectus femoris muscle and at the periphery of the lateral vastus muscle (B).

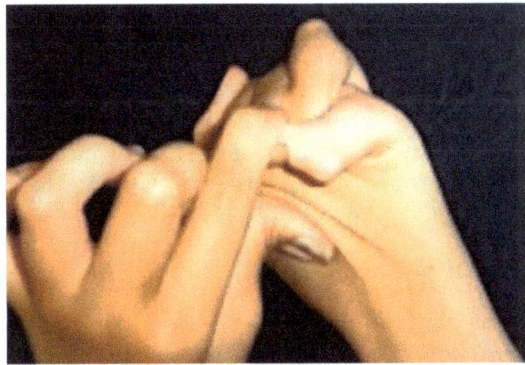

Figure 43.3 Hyperlaxity of the left thumb and the right little finger of a patient with Ullrich congenital muscular dystrophy.

respiratory insufficiency. The resemblance to Bethlem myopathy led to the discovery that collagen VI mutations were also the culprit in this condition, whose inheritance was long considered to be autosomal recessive. Genetic counselling is not, however, straightforward, since severe cases with autosomal dominant inheritance and relatively mild cases of autosomal recessive inheritance (intermediate collagen VI-related myopathy) have been described. The majority of patients with UCMD – except the severely affected patients – achieve ambulation but lose it by an average age of 10 years. Decline in pulmonary function is early and invariable: 2.6% per year with an average age of onset of noninvasive ventilation of 11 years in the severe UCMD patients. In the intermediate cases, decline in pulmonary function starts slightly later than in classic UCMD, but proceeds at a similar rate: 2.3% per year with an average age of onset of noninvasive ventilation of 21 years. In Bethlem myopathy, decline in pulmonary function is variable and does not occur until adulthood (typically after age 40 years), which necessitates respiratory surveillance including annual pulmonary function tests in the upright and supine positions.

A rare disease with distal joint hypermobility in combination with proximal joint contractures, scoliosis or kyphosis, and abnormal scarring caused by *COL12A1* variants has many commonalities with collagen VI myopathies and Ehlers–Danlos syndrome. In addition, (congenital) muscle hypotonia with variable delay in gross motor development may occur. Other features include mild dysmorphic facial features (light blue sclerae, micrognathia, and/or high arched palate), congenital torticollis, bilateral hip dislocation, scoliosis, kyphosis, pectus excavatum, and hyperkeratosis pilaris.

Suggested Reading

Delbaere S, Dhooge T, Syx D, et al. Novel defects in collagen XII and VI expand the mixed myopathy/Ehlers-Danlos syndrome spectrum and lead to variant-specific alterations in the extracellular matrix. *Genet Med*. 2020 Jan;22(1):112–123. doi: 10.1038/s41436-019-0599-6. Epub 2019 Jul 5. PMID: 31273343.

Foley AR, Quijano-Roy S, Collins J, et al. Natural history of pulmonary function in collagen VI-related myopathies. *Brain*. 2013 Dec;136(Pt 12):3625–3633. doi: 10.1093/brain/awt284. Epub 2013 Nov 22. PMID: 24271325; PMCID: PMC3859224.

Foley AR, Mohassel P, Donkervoort S, Bolduc V, Bönnemann CG. Collagen VI-related dystrophies. 2004 Jun 25 [updated 2021 Mar 11]. In Adam MP, Mirzaa GM, Pagon RA, et al., editors. *GeneReviews*® [Internet]. Seattle, WA: University of Washington; 1993–2023. PMID: 20301676.

Jöbsis GJ, Boers JM, Barth PG, de Visser M. Bethlem myopathy: a slowly progressive congenital muscular dystrophy with contractures. *Brain*. 1999 Apr;122 (Pt 4):649–655. doi: 10.1093/brain/122.4.649. PMID: 10219778.

Salim R, Dahlqvist JR, Khawajazada T, et al. Characteristic muscle signatures assessed by quantitative MRI in patients with Bethlem myopathy. *J Neurol*. 2020 Aug;267(8):2432–2442. doi: 10.1007/s00415-020-09860-x. Epub 2020 May 3. PMID: 32363432.

Oculopharyngeal Muscular Dystrophy (OPMD)

Clinical History

A 68-year-old woman was referred because of slowly progressive difficulty climbing stairs. Four years earlier, she had had ptosis surgery of both eyes. Her mother had been diagnosed with progressive external ophthalmoplegia at the age of 69 years. She denied having swallowing difficulties, but her daughter stressed that eating biscuits took her much longer than others.

Examination

There was symmetric ptosis and a minor limitation of eye movements without diplopia. This did not worsen with sustained looking upward or sideways. There was no dysarthria and no weakness of neck muscles. Hip abductors and flexors and foot dorsal flexors were slightly weak (MRC grade 4+). She had no problems getting up from a chair. Gait was slightly waddling.

Diagnostic Considerations

Initially, difficulties with swallowing were denied, probably because she had unconsciously adapted by chewing her food thoroughly. The combination of symmetric ptosis, dysphagia, and familial occurrence makes oculopharyngeal muscular dystrophy (OPMD) a likely diagnosis. In oculopharyngodistal myopathy (OPDM), another triplet repeat disease, even rarer than OPMD, limb weakness is distal rather than proximal. Mitochondrial disease and myotonic dystrophy type 1 are alternative diagnoses in a patient with slowly progressive, symmetric external ophthalmoplegia without diplopia. Myasthenia gravis may manifest with ptosis without extraocular muscle involvement, but is less likely because in myasthenia, ptosis is asymmetric and fluctuating. In amyotrophic lateral sclerosis/motor neuron disease and inclusion body myositis, dysphagia may be prominent at onset, but ptosis does not occur.

Ancillary Investigations

Analysis of *PABPN1* gene showed an expansion of the number of (GCG) trinucleotide repeats in exon 1 ($n = 16$, normal $n = 6$–10). This finding is diagnostic for OPMD.

General Remarks

OPMD is a rare, slowly progressive disease of skeletal muscles featured by ptosis, dysphagia, and weakness of proximal leg muscles. Inheritance is autosomal dominant with complete penetrance at older age in most families. In 90% of patients, the cause is a heterozygous GCN (GCA/GCC/GCG/or GCT) trinucleotide repeat expansion of 11 to 18 repeats in exon 1 of the *PABPN1* gene, which encodes an RNA-binding protein. The triplet repeat expansion results in lengthening of the *PABPN1* N-terminal polyalanine tail. Pathogenetic mechanisms are as yet not fully understood. Autosomal recessively inherited biallelic GCN repeat expansions are found in 10% of patients. Patients with longer repeats and patients with biallelic repeat expansions have an earlier disease onset. The triplet repeat expansion in *PABPN1* is stable in contrast to other (polyglutamine) triplet expansion disorders. Anticipation

Table 44.1 Main features of oculopharyngeal muscular dystrophy (OPMD)

- Onset in 5th decade with symmetric ptosis soon followed by dysphagia
- In more advanced stage proximal limb weakness
- CK normal or mildly elevated
- Autosomal dominantly inherited repeat expansion disease: cannot be captured by gene panel analysis

(earlier age of onset in successive generations) does probably not occur in OPMD.

The clinical manifestations are fairly uniform (Table 44.1). Onset is usually in the fifth decade with weakness of the levator palpebrae muscles leading to ptosis, and with weakness of pharyngeal muscles. Ptosis may be severe and can hamper daily life activities. Dysphagia is the first symptom in one-third of patients and manifests with solid food getting stuck in the throat. This may cause choking, aspiration pneumonia, or malnutrition. Mild speech difficulties (nasal speech and hypophonia) may also occur. Facial muscles, extraocular muscles, and the tongue may become weak eventually. Some years after disease onset walking becomes difficult in a quarter of patients due to weakness of pelvic girdle and proximal leg muscles. At older age, about 10% of patients become dependent on a wheelchair for outdoor transportation. Shoulder girdle weakness and more distal weakness may occur in the course of the disease. Many patients experience fatigue. Median survival is 20–30 years after the onset of ptosis. Death is relatively often due to aspiration pneumonia. Clinically relevant weakness of the diaphragm usually does not occur and there is no cardiac involvement. Serum CK activity is normal or mildly increased. A muscle biopsy will show dystrophic features, sparse rimmed vacuoles, and nuclear inclusions, but is not indicated for making the diagnosis. In the setting of a typical clinical presentation, the diagnosis is made by single-gene testing for the number of GCN repeats in exon 1 of the *PABPN1* gene.

Oculopharyngeal distal myopathy (OPDM) shares with OPMD clinical and histopathological features except for the distribution of limb weakness. Onset of OPDM is typically in late adolescence or early adulthood. About 50% of patients manifest first with ptosis and ophthalmoplegia. Around a third of patients will present with limb weakness. As the diseas progresses, the involvement of the distal limb muscles becomes apparent. Respiratory function deteriorates in the late stages of the disease in one-third to two-thirds of patients. Cardiac involvement has been described. OPDM is a worldwide condition, but mainly found in Asian families with autosomal dominant inheritance and is caused by repeat expansions in *LRP12*, *GIPC1*, *NOTCH2NLC*, and *RILP1*.

A severe, progressive early-onset disorder similar to OPMD has been reported to be caused by heterozygous frameshift variants in the *hnRNPA2B1* gene, which also encodes for an RNA-binding protein. Pathogenetic mechanisms probably differ from missense variants in this gene, which cause a multisystem proteinopathy, phenotypically very different from OPMD.

Management may include ptosis surgery and advice on swallowing technique and diet modifications. Cricopharyngeal myotomy or dilation can be beneficial if dysphagia leads to choking or is socially disabling, and percutaneous gastrostomy may be considered if there is more than 10% weight loss. Patients with proximal leg weakness can benefit from physiotherapy. All patients should be offered genetic counselling. No causative treatment exists as yet.

Suggested Reading

Argov Z, de Visser M. Dysphagia in adult myopathies. *Neuromuscul Disord* 2021;31(1):5–20. doi: 10.1016/j.nmd.2020.11.001. Epub 2020 Nov 13. PMID: 33334661.

Brisson JD, Gagnon C, Brais B, Côté I, Mathieu J. A study of impairments in oculopharyngeal muscular dystrophy. *Muscle Nerve* 2020;62(2):201–207. doi: 10.1002/mus.26888. Epub 2020 May 22. PMID: 32270505.

Eura N, Noguchi S, Ogasawara M, et al.; OPDM/OPMD Image Study Group. Characteristics of the muscle involvement along the disease progression in a large cohort of oculopharyngodistal myopathy compared to oculopharyngeal muscular dystrophy. *J Neurol* 2023 Dec;270(12):5988–5998. doi: 10.1007/s00415-023-11906-9. Epub 2023. PMID: 37634163.

Kim HJ, Mohassel P, Donkervoort S, et al. Heterozygous frameshift variants in HNRNPA2B1 cause early-onset oculopharyngeal muscular dystrophy. *Nat Commun* 2022;13(1):2306. doi: 10.1038/s41467-022-30015-1. PMID: 35484142; PMCID: PMC9050844.

Richard P, Trollet C, Stojkovic T, et al.; Neurologists of French Neuromuscular Reference Centers CORNEMUS and FILNEMUS. Correlation between

PABPN1 genotype and disease severity in oculopharyngeal muscular dystrophy. *Neurology* 2017;88(4):359–365. doi: 10.1212/WNL.0000000000003554. Epub 2016 Dec 23. PMID: 28011929; PMCID: PMC5272966.

Trollet C, Boulinguiez A, Roth F, et al. Oculopharyngeal muscular dystrophy. 2001 Mar 8 [updated 2020 Oct 22]. In Adam MP, Mirzaa GM, Pagon RA, et al., editors. *GeneReviews®* [Internet]. Seattle, WA: University of Washington; 1993–2023. PMID: 20301305.

Emery–Dreifuss Muscular Dystrophy (EDMD)

Clinical History

A 24-year-old man is the youngest of five children and of Turkish origin, who since the age of five years had noticed that he was not able to fully extend his arms. Furthermore, his Achilles tendons were taut. His previous history was unremarkable. An older brother had similar symptoms. Both had no cardiac symptoms. His parents were not affected.

Examination

He had a rigid spine and neck, contractures at the elbows, shortening of the Achilles tendons, scoliosis, and increased lumbar lordosis. Atrophy of the muscles of the lower arms and legs and scapulae alatae was noted. There was an MRC grade 4 weakness of the triceps brachii and iliopsoas muscles. Generalized areflexia was also noted.

Diagnostic Considerations

Contractures and muscle weakness can be found in a number of neuromuscular conditions. However, mild scapuloperoneal muscle weakness, contractures, and an inheritance pattern compatible with an X-linked recessive trait is indicative of Emery–Dreifuss muscular dystrophy (EDMD) caused by pathological variant in the *EMD* or *FHL1* gene.

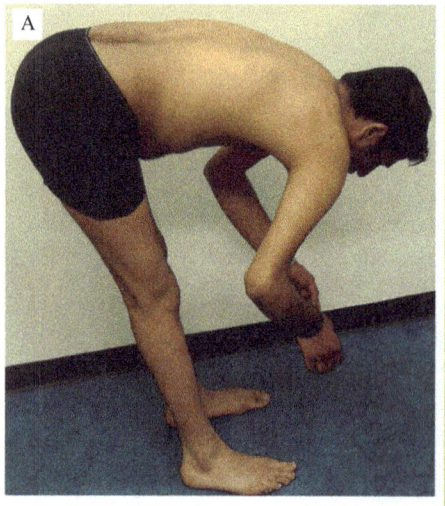
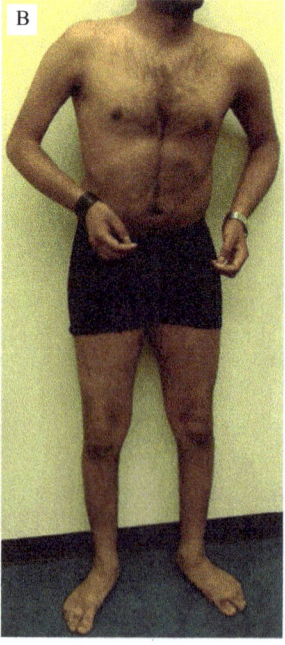

Figure 45.1 (A,B) Rigid spine (A) and elbow contractures and atrophy of the muscles of the lower arms and legs (B).

Table 45.1 Main features of X-linked and autosomal dominant (AD) Emery–Dreifuss muscular dystrophy (EDMD)

	X-linked EDMD	AD-EDMD
Onset	Neonatal to 3rd decade, mean 5–10 years	Childhood
Contractures (Achilles tendons, elbows, spine)	Contractures appear, often *preceding* muscle weakness	Contractures appear, often *after* muscle weakness
Distribution of weakness	Humeroperoneal, rarely leading to wheelchair dependency	Humeroperoneal, within families also limb girdle distribution of weakness ('LGMD'); loss of ambulation may occur
Cardiac involvement	Cardiomyopathy and conduction defects, sudden death	Cardiomyopathy and conduction defects, sudden death; isolated dilated cardiomyopathy associated with cardiac conduction defects may occur
Most frequent genes	*EMD*, *FHL1*	*LMNA*
Affected females	Rarely manifesting	Yes

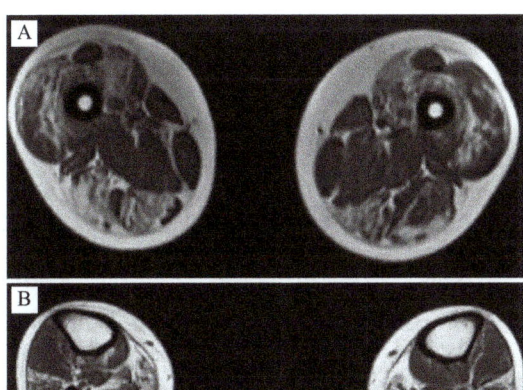

Figure 45.2 (A,B) Muscle MRI in the described patient showing preferential involvement of the vastus muscles and the hamstrings in the upper legs (A), and in the lower legs mainly the peroneus muscle and the medial head of the gastrocnemius muscle were afflicted (B).

Ancillary Investigations

Cardiological examination showed a first-degree AV block. Serum CK activity was 715 IU/L (normal < 171). MRI of the legs showed preferential involvement of the vastus muscles and the hamstrings in the upper legs, and in the lower legs the peroneal muscle and the medial head of the gastrocnemius muscle were mainly affected (Fig. 45.2A,B). Genetic testing revealed a pathogenic variant (c.3G>A) in the *STA/EDM* gene on chromosome Xq28.

Follow-Up

Over the years (last follow-up visit at age 36 years), he complained about buckling of the knees, sometimes leading to falls. On examination, there was progression of weakness of the shoulder girdle (MRC grade 4+) and upper arm (MRC 2) muscles, and leg muscles (proximal MRC 4, distal MRC 4+). Cardiac situation was stable.

General Remarks

Onset of X-linked EDMD may vary from the neonatal period to third decade, mean age between 5 and 10 years. Contractures – often preceding muscle weakness – may occur at the Achilles tendons, elbows, and posterior cervical muscles (rigid neck). Limitation of forward flexion of the thoracic and lumbar spine (rigid spine) occurs later. In contrast, in autosomal dominantly (AD) inherited EDMD, contractures usually appear after muscle weakness (Table 45.1). Muscle weakness is slowly progressive with a humeroperoneal distribution rarely leading to wheelchair dependency, whereas in AD-EDMD loss of ambulation may occur. Dilated cardiomyopathy and atrioventricular conduction defects are almost invariably present and usually appear after the second decade of life, irrespective of contractures or muscle weakness. Even complete heart block can occur. Occasional sudden death without preceding cardiac symptoms warrants preventive pacemaker implantation.

There is considerable inter- and intrafamilial variation, but even more so in AD-*LMNA*. Within the same family the same pathogenic variant can lead to AD-EDMD, 'LGMD1B' (myopathy manifesting with limb girdle distribution of muscle weakness), or isolated DCM-CD (dilated cardiomyopathy associated with cardiac conduction defects).

Routine ancillary investigations are usually noncontributory. Serum CK is slightly to markedly elevated (up to 20 × ULN). The muscle biopsy shows a dystrophic picture with absent emerin staining. However, diagnosis is usually established by molecular genetic testing. Given the differential diagnosis of myopathies associated with contractures, targeted next-generation sequencing should be performed. An EDMD phenotype can be caused by a hemizygous pathogenic variant in *EMD* (emerin) or *FHL1* (four-and-a-half-LIM), a heterozygous pathogenic variant in *LMNA* (lamin A/C), or (more rarely) biallelic pathogenic variants in *LMNA*, and the collagen VI genes. The likelihood of identifying a causative variant in *EMD*, *FHL1*, or *LMNA* is dependent on the known or suspected mode of inheritance. In cases of X-linked inheritance, *EMD*-related disease is most likely, followed by *FHL1*. In cases of autosomal dominant or recessive inheritance, *LMNA*-related disease is more likely. In the absence of a clear inheritance pattern, *LMNA*-related disease is most likely followed by *EMD*- and then *FHL1*-related disease. Affected females are much more likely to have AD-EDMD since X-linked EDMD carriers are rarely manifesting.

Emerin and lamins code for nuclear envelope proteins. Emerin is an inner nuclear membrane protein, essential for the structural integrity of the nucleus. Lamins are proteins that form nuclear lamina and anchor inner nuclear membrane proteins. They thus help to provide a mechanical, resistant meshwork. *FHL1* localizes to sarcomere and sarcolemma, and collagen VI is localized in the extracellular matrix.

Laminopathies also include *LMNA*-related congenital muscular dystrophy, axonal Charcot–Marie–Tooth disease, and autosomal dominant Dunnigan-type partial lipodystrophy.

Timely cardiac evaluation and monitoring should be part of the clinical management. Management of contractures is difficult. Stretching was proven not to have clinically important short-term effects on joint mobility, was uncertain regarding pain, and has not been investigated for quality of life. Surgery of elbow contractures is complicated and very often the effect is only temporary.

Suggested Reading

Bonne G, Leturcq F, Ben Yaou R. Emery-Dreifuss muscular dystrophy. 2004 Sep 29 [updated 2019 Aug 15]. In Adam MP, Mirzaa GM, Pagon RA, et al., editors. *GeneReviews*® [Internet]. Seattle, WA: University of Washington; 1993–2023. PMID: 20301609.

Heller SA, Shih R, Kalra R, Kang PB. Emery-Dreifuss muscular dystrophy. *Muscle Nerve* 2020;61(4):436–448. doi: 10.1002/mus.26782. Epub 2019 Dec 28. PMID: 31840275; PMCID: PMC7154529.

Caveolinopathy, Rippling Muscle Disease

Clinical History

Since early childhood, a 22-year-old-man had difficulty keeping up with his peers at gym class activities. He noticed increasing weakness in his leg muscles when getting up the stairs, and gradually his arm muscles were also involved. He had noticed rolling movements of his thigh muscles triggered by exercise and squeezing the muscles.

Family history was positive: his brother, mother, maternal grandfather, maternal aunt, and nephew had similar complaints.

Examination

There was MRC grade 4 muscle weakness with a limb girdle pattern. He had noticed rippling muscles, especially the thigh muscles, which worsened when he squeezed his thighs (**Video 46.1**). There was mild calf hypertrophy.

Diagnostic Considerations
The autosomal dominant inheritance pattern and the combination of muscle weakness with a limb girdle pattern and rippling muscles are consistent with a diagnosis of caveolinopathy.

Ancillary Investigations
Serum CK activity was 17 × ULN. DNA analysis revealed a pathogenic variant in the caveolin-3 gene.

His mother and brother were also investigated and showed a similar clinical picture; both had calf hypertrophy and pes cavus. Serum CK was elevated (7 × ULN) in his mother and not assessed in his brother. In both, the same variant was found in the *CAV3* gene.

Follow-Up
There was very little increase in muscle weakness over the years, and he remained ambulatory.

General Remarks
CAV3 encodes caveolin-3, a muscle-specific plasma membrane protein involved in several processes related to the formation of caveolae, invaginations of the plasma membrane. Autosomal dominant – and, less frequently, recessive – *CAV3* mutations have been implicated in hyperCKaemia, manifestations of muscle hyperirritability (rippling muscle movements and percussion-induced rapid contractions – PIRCs or percussion-induced muscle mounding (PIMMs; local contraction)), rhabdomyolysis, and proximal and, rarely, distal muscle weakness. These phenotypes can appear on their own or in combination. There may be intrafamilial variation. Rippling muscle disease also exists as an acquired autoimmune disease with AChR and MURC/Cavin-4 antibodies, associated with thymoma and myasthenia gravis.

Many patients with a caveolinopathy present with myalgia and elevated CK without weakness (Table 46.1). PIRCs or mounding can easily be elicited by exercise, tapping, or stretching. PIRCs/PIMMs and rippling muscle contraction are important clinical clues for caveolinopathies and should be assessed for in patients presenting with exercise intolerance, myalgia, and rhabdomyolysis, even if other features suggestive of a caveolinopathy are absent. If there is proximal or distal myopathy, muscle weakness is mild or moderate. There is usually muscle hypertrophy, especially of the calves. Cardiac abnormalities (hypertrophic or dilated cardiomyopathy, long Q-T syndrome) can occur and may even be the first manifestation of caveolinopathy. Age at onset ranges from early childhood (myalgia and toe walking) to the eighth decade. Proximal muscle weakness due to *CAV3* variants was long considered a limb girdle muscular dystrophy (LGMD), but after a reform of the LGMD classification in 2017 this diagnosis no longer holds because the main clinical features are rippling muscles and myalgia, and the muscle biopsy does not comply with the picture of a muscular dystrophy, which should consist of muscle fibre necrosis, regeneration, and an increase in fibrosis and adipose tissue.

Table 46.1 Main features of caveolinopathy

- Mostly autosomal dominantly inherited; *CAV3* gene
- Onset at any age. Young children often present with toe-walking
- Often presentation with myalgia and hyperCKaemia, can cause rhabdomyolysis
- Muscle hypertrophy often present (in particular the calves)
- Manifestations of muscle hyperexcitability (rippling muscle)
- Mild to moderate mostly proximal weakness; rarely distal muscle weakness
- Cardiac abnormalities can occur, may even be the first manifestation

Suggested Reading
Dubey D, Beecher G, Hammami MB, et al. Identification of caveolae-associated protein 4 autoantibodies as a biomarker of immune-mediated rippling muscle disease in adults. *JAMA Neurol* 2022;79(8):808–816. doi: 10.1001/jamaneurol.2022.1357. PMID: 35696196; PMCID: PMC9361081.

Scalco RS, Gardiner AR, Pitceathly RD, et al. CAV3 mutations causing exercise intolerance, myalgia and rhabdomyolysis: Expanding the phenotypic spectrum of caveolinopathies. *Neuromuscul Disord* 2016;26(8):504–510. doi: 10.1016/j.nmd.2016.05.006. Epub 2016 May 11. PMID: 27312022.

Case 47: Distal Myopathies: Miyoshi Myopathy, Dysferlinopathy; Anoctaminopathy

Clinical History

A 24-year-old man complained of instability of his feet since the age of 16 years. From the age of 19 years onwards, he could no longer stand on tiptoe, and he experienced difficulties when playing basketball. At 20 years of age, his calves appeared to be thin. Gradually, he had some difficulty running, whereas he could climb the stairs and rise from a chair normally. He had no symptoms in his arms. The parents did not have similar problems.

Examination

He had normal posture and the musculature of his arms, trunk, and upper legs was well developed and of normal strength. There were no contractures or scoliosis. Both calves, but also the anterior muscles of the lower legs, were thin (Fig. 47.1). There was weakness of the calf and flexor digitorum muscles, MRC grade 4. Sensation was normal. Achilles tendon reflexes were absent. He had difficulty tiptoeing. To compensate for the calf muscle weakness, he could walk only on his toes while bending his knees. He could also not walk on his heels

Diagnostic Considerations

The main clinical abnormalities were predominant atrophy and weakness of both calf muscles, gradual onset in adolescence, and a family history compatible with autosomal recessive inheritance. Although rare, Miyoshi myopathy and distal anoctaminopathy fit this phenotype. Other distal myopathies with posterior weakness are autosomal dominantly transmitted. A strongly elevated serum CK further differentiates these diagnoses from other distal myopathies, distal spinal muscular atrophy (SMA) (hereditary motor neuropathy (HMN)), and a conus-cauda tumour. The diagnosis is made by next-generation sequencing (NGS) gene panel analysis for distal myopathies or single gene tests for the dysferlin (*DYSF*) and anoctamin-5 (*ANO5*) genes.

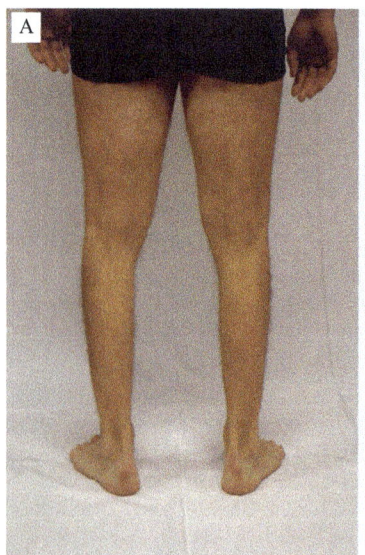
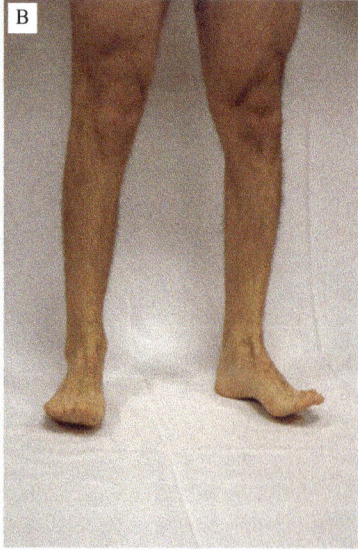

Figure 47.1 (A,B) Atrophy of posterior (A) and anterior distal (B) leg muscles in the described patient. He cannot stand on tiptoes or on heels.

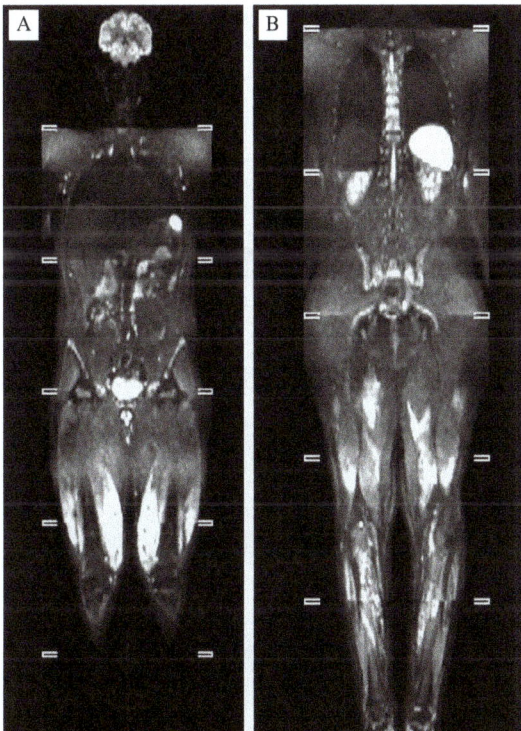

Figure 47.2 (A,B) T2 STIR coronal sections show oedema in anterior upper leg muscles (A) and posterior muscles of the upper and lower legs (B) in the described patient.

Ancillary Investigations

Serum CK activity was 15,820 IU/L (> 90× ULN). ECG was normal. MRI showed oedema in the calves and in clinically unaffected muscles of both upper legs (Fig. 47.2), and complete replacement of the gastrocnemius muscles by fat. Targeted gene panel NGS showed two pathogenic variants (c.4765C>T and c.1106T>C) in the *DYSF* gene. Both parents carried one of these variants, confirming the trans-position of both mutations (i.e., both alleles harbouring one mutation, proving compound heterozygosity).

Follow-Up

The complaints remained stable during the following three years.

General Remarks

Distal Myopathies

Distal myopathies feature predominant or exclusive distal weakness. This contrasts with myopathies that show distal weakness in the course of the disease, such as facioscapulohumeral muscular dystrophy, myotonic dystrophy type 1, and oculopharyngeal distal myopathy. In distal myopathies, weakness may occur early or predominantly in the hands, the ankle dorsiflexors, or the ankle plantar flexors. Table 47.1 lists the disorders that are, or can be, featured by muscle atrophy and weakness of the ankle plantar flexors.

Most distal myopathies are genetic in origin. In the most frequent acquired distal myopathy, inclusion body myositis, muscle wasting and weakness are typically asymmetric in the hands. In many distal myopathies, CK is only mildly increased or even normal. In these cases, and especially if there is marked muscle atrophy, a neurogenic disorder should also be considered in the differential diagnosis. In patients with distal weakness, it is notoriously difficult to differentiate neurogenic from myopathic disease by EMG and muscle biopsy. The same may hold true for genetic analysis, since some genes have been recognized as causing disease with both neurogenic and myopathic features (e.g., *HSPB8*, which led to the concept of neuromyopathy). There is no known cure for inherited distal myopathies.

Many genes are now known to be associated with distal myopathy, some with early-onset disease, others with late-onset disease. Still, many patients remain undiagnosed as to date. Many distal myopathies are allelic to a range of other phenotypes, especially in autosomal dominantly (AD) inherited disorders (e.g., *CAV3*, *VCP*, *POLG*, *RYR1*, *TTN*). Distal myopathies may be AD, AR, or X-linked inherited. Distal myopathies are commonly caused by single nucleotide variants, but copy number variants (deletions) occur in titinopathies. Digenic distal myopathy, caused by pathogenic variants in two different genes, has also been reported. Some distal myopathies show histopathological features such as rimmed vacuoles or myofibrillar disorganization. These features can be useful in 'reverse phenotyping', in case genetic testing yields difficult to interpret results.

Dysferlinopathy; Anoctaminopathy

Some distal myopathies, notably those caused by variants in *DYSF* and *ANO5*, are allelic disorders of a limb girdle muscular dystrophy (LGMDR2 and LGMDR12, respectively), and both manifestations may occur within the same family. In individual families, the distal and proximal phenotypes generally merge with progression of the disease. Some patients show only myalgia and hyperCKaemia (Fig. 47.3). Age of onset, age at loss of ambulation,

Part II Neuromuscular Cases: Myopathies

Table 47.1 Neuromuscular disorders with early or prominent weakness of foot plantar flexors

	Gene Inheritance	Age at onset	Presenting signs	Muscle biopsy
Miyoshi myopathy type 1 (MMD1)	*DYSF* AR Allelic disorder LGMD R2	Adolescence or early adulthood	Asymmetric atrophy and weakness. Prone to rhabdomyolysis. CK markedly elevated.	May show mononuclear cell infiltrates and amyloid
ANO5 distal myopathy (MMD3)	*ANO5* AR Allelic disorder LGMD R12	Onset decade later than Miyoshi myopathy	Asymmetric atrophy and weakness. Prone to rhabdo-myolysis. CK markedly elevated.	May show mononuclear cell infiltrates and amyloid
DNAJB6 distal myopathy	*DNAJB6* AD Allelic disorder LGMD D1	Adulthood	Symmetric weakness of posterior or anterior distal leg muscles	May show rimmed vacuoles
Distal myopathy with myotilin defect	*MYOT* AD	Late adulthood	Early calf involvement, later weakness of foot dorsal flexors	Shows myofibrillar changes
Distal filaminopathy	*FLNC* AD	Adulthood	Flinger flexion at onset, followed by calf weakness	Shows myofibrillar changes
VRK1 dSMA/HMN	*VRK1* AR	Early adulthood	Posterior distal wasting and weakness	Neurogenic and myopathic features

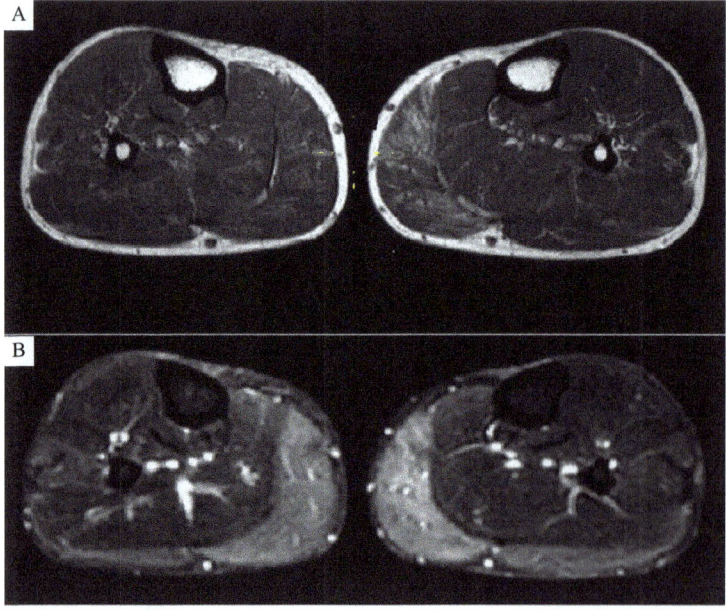

Figure 47.3 Muscle oedema in both gastrocnemius muscles (T2 STIR, A) and fatty replacement of the left medial gastrocnemius muscle (T1, B) in a 43-year-old man with activity-induced myalgia in the anterior upper legs. No weakness. CK 450–2000 U/L. Gene panel analysis showed heterozygosity for one probable pathogenic and another pathogenic variant in the *ANO5* gene, compatible with bi-allelic variants (compound heterozygosity).

and CK do not differ between the distal and proximal phenotypes. Weakness in shoulder girdle muscles is less frequent than in proximal leg muscles, in contrast to, for example, in LGMDR1. The biceps brachii muscle may have a ball-like appearance caused by the selective atrophy of the distal half of the muscle (Fig. 47.4). Involvement of diaphragm and the heart are not features of these disorders, but cardiac complications have occasionally been described in anoctaminopathy. Anoctaminopathy is probably more frequent than dysferlinopathy.

Genetic analysis shows many different missense, nonsense, and splice site variants, but (large) deletions and duplications have also been reported. The diagnosis is made by NGS and, if needed, multiplex ligation-dependent probe amplification (MLPA) analysis. Immunohistochemical analysis and Western blotting of a muscle biopsy specimen can be useful in case of diagnostic uncertainty (Fig. 47.5), but dysferlin interacts with other sarcolemmal proteins, notably caveolin-3 and calpain-3, which may cause secondary reductions, complicating interpretation.

Dysferlin and anoctamin 5 both probably play a role in membrane repair. The muscle fibre plasma membrane (sarcolemma) acts as a biological barrier between extracellular and intracellular environments and maintains cell integrity. Minor physiological disruptions occur frequently in active skeletal muscle cells. Active membrane repair mechanisms aimed at resealing these lesions are essential for normal muscle function.

Treatment is symptomatic with a prominent role for rehabilitation.

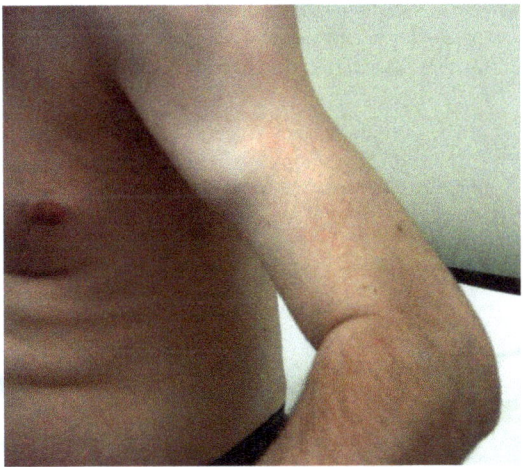

Figure 47.4 A biceps lump is observed in an ambulatory patient with dysferlinopathy. The ball-like appearance is caused by the selective atrophy of the distal half of the biceps brachii muscle.

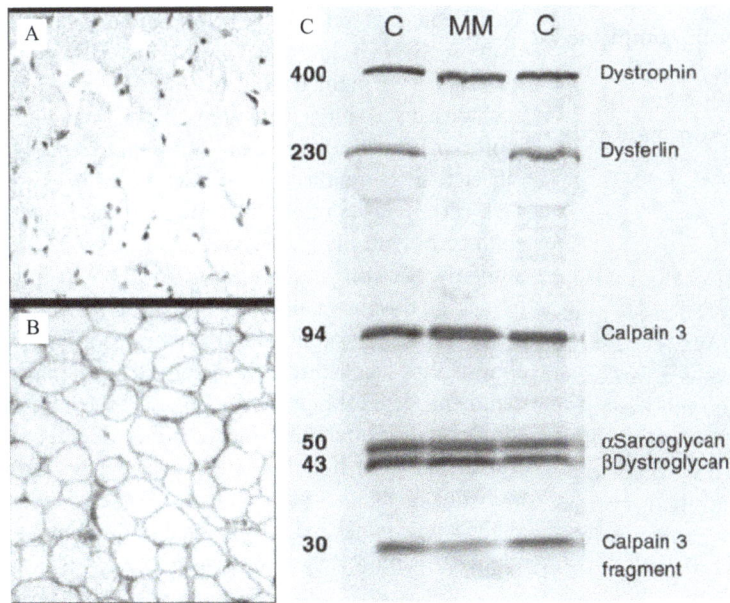

Figure 47.5 (A–C) Absent dysferlin (A, as compared with a control, B) on a dysferlin stain. Near-absent dysferlin in a Western blot (C) in a patient with Miyoshi myopathy (MM).

Suggested Reading

Bugiardini E, Morrow JM, Shah S, et al. The diagnostic value of MRI pattern recognition in distal myopathies. *Front Neurol* 2018;9:456. doi: 10.3389/fneur.2018.00456. PMID: 29997562; PMCID: PMC6028608.

El Sherif R, Hussein RS, Nishino I. 'Boule du biceps' in dysferlinopathy. *Neurology* 2020;94(2):83–84. doi: 10.1212/WNL.0000000000008782. Epub 2019 Dec 10. PMID: 31822577.

Milone M, Liewluck T. The unfolding spectrum of inherited distal myopathies. *Muscle Nerve* 2019;59 (3):283–294. doi: 10.1002/mus.26332. Epub 2018 Nov 28. PMID: 30171629.

Moore U, Gordish H, Diaz-Manera J, et al.; Jain COS Consortium.Miyoshi myopathy and limb girdle muscular dystrophy R2 are the same disease. *Neuromuscul Disord* 2021;31(4):265–280. doi: 10.1016/j.nmd.2021.01.009. Epub 2021 Jan 21. PMID: 33610434.

Pegoraro E, Mendell JR, Straub V, Díaz-Manera J. Expanding the muscle imaging spectrum in dysferlinopathy: description of an outlier population from the classical MRI pattern. *Neuromuscul Disord* 2023;33(4):349–357. doi: 10.1016/j.nmd.2023.02.007. Epub 2023 Mar 2. PMID: 36972667.

Savarese M, Sarparanta J, Vihola A, et al. Panorama of the distal myopathies. *Acta Myol* 2020;39(4):245–265. doi: 10.36185/2532-1900-028. PMID: 33458580; PMCID: PMC7783427.

ten Dam L, Frankhuizen WS, Linssen WHJP, et al. Autosomal recessive limb-girdle and Miyoshi muscular dystrophies in the Netherlands: the clinical and molecular spectrum of 244 patients. *Clin Genet* 2019;96(2):126–133. doi: 10.1111/cge.13544. Epub 2019 May 6. PMID: 30919934.

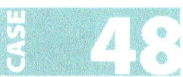

CASE 48 Distal Myopathies: GNE Myopathy

Synonyms: distal myopathy with rimmed vacuoles (DMRV), hereditary inclusion body myopathy (h-IBM, HIBM, IBM2), Nonaka myopathy, quadriceps sparing myopathy (QSM)

Clinical History

A 21-year-old man had for some years complained of diffuse pain and weakness of the legs. His sister was reported to have a severe disorder of the nerves or muscles. Their parents were reportedly not related.

Examination

There was mild symmetric atrophy of the anterior tibial muscles and the medial gastrocnemius muscles and a hammer toe deformity. We found normal strength of both arms. There was a weakness MRC grade 4+ of the hip adductors, and weakness MRC grade 4+ of the foot dorsal flexors and MRC 3–4 of the toe dorsal flexor muscles. Quadriceps muscles were well developed and had normal strength. Walking on heels was not possible. Sensation and tendon reflexes were normal.

Diagnostic Procedures

This patient presented with anterior, distal more than proximal weakness of both legs that had existed for years. This pointed to a hereditary distal myopathy, or a distal spinal muscular atrophy (hereditary motor neuropathy), probably autosomal recessive (affected sister, unaffected parents). In distal disorders, serum CK is often only mildly or moderately elevated in both myopathic and neurogenic disease. Similarly, electromyography is often not very helpful in making this distinction. The muscle biopsy in his affected sister was reported to show only nonspecific abnormalities, no rimmed vacuoles, and also no evident neurogenic abnormalities. Muscle imaging can show specific patters of muscle involvement in several myopathies, but this is not always helpful in individual patients. In this patient, it was decided to apply a gene panel analysis directed at distal myopathies early in the diagnostic process.

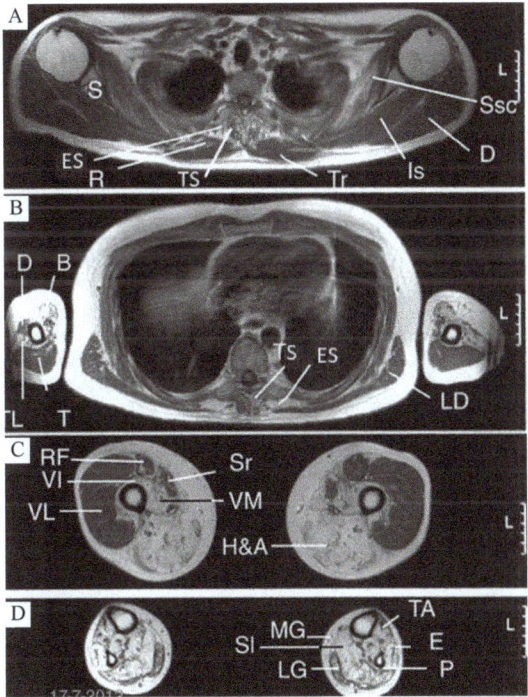

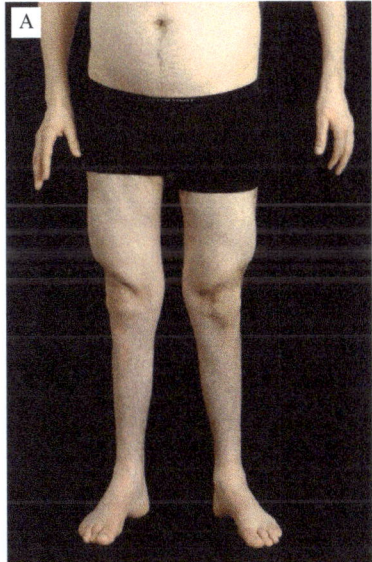

Figure 48.1 (A–D) T1-weighted section at the level of the shoulders (A), proximal upper arms (B), proximal upper legs (C), and mid-lower legs (D) showing prominent symmetric atrophy and fatty replacement (white) of the biceps brachii (B), the lateral head of the triceps brachii (TL), the erector spinae (ES) muscles, the complete medial and posterior compartment of the upper leg (with relative sparing of the sartorius muscle (Sr)), the medial vastus muscle (VM), the vastus intermedius muscle (VI), and all muscles of the lower leg. D = deltoid muscle; E = toe extensors; H&A = hamstrings and adductor muscles; Is = infraspinatus muscle; LD = latissimus dorsi muscle; LG and MG = lateral and medial head of the gastrocnemius muscle; P = peroneal muscles; R = rhomboid muscle; RF = rectus femoris muscle; S = scapula; Ssc = subscapular muscle; Sl = soleus muscle; T = triceps brachii muscle; TA = anterior tibial muscle; Tr = trapezius muscle; TS = transversospinal muscle; VL = lateral vastus muscle.

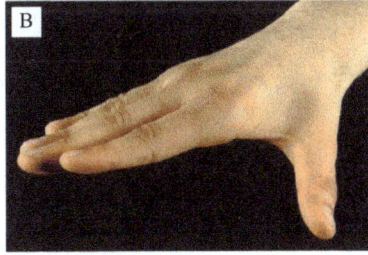

Figure 48.2 (A,B) Severe muscle atrophy of anterior lower leg muscles with sparing of the quadriceps muscles (A), and atrophy of the first dorsal interosseus muscle (B) in the described patient.

Ancillary Investigations

Serum CK was elevated (6 × ULN). Muscle MRI nine years after initial presentation showed severe abnormalities, with sparing of the quadriceps muscles (Fig 48.1), suggesting a GNE-distal myopathy. Next-generation sequencing (NGS) gene panel analysis showed a homozygous pathogenetic variant (c.172C>T) of the *GNE* gene.

Follow-Up

Nine years after presentation, he had difficulty climbing stairs and holding heavy objects. He tried ankle-foot orthoses because of foot drop, but this did not suit him. Forced vital capacity was 108% of expected and there were no cardiac abnormalities. He had symmetric atrophy of distal leg muscles and hand muscles. There was weakness MRC grade 4 of biceps brachii and finger flexor muscles; weakness MRC grade 3 of the iliopsoas and toe plantar flexors; and weakness MRC grade 2 of the hamstrings and ankle plantar flexor muscles. Hip adductors and all other distal leg muscles MRC 0. Figure 48.2 shows the patient nine years after presentation.

General Remarks

The epimerase–kinase enzyme that is encoded by the *GNE* gene is thought to be involved in the sialic acid modification of components of the sarcolemma, but the relation between dysfunctional protein and muscle disease is as yet not understood. Sialic acid supplementation has been shown to be ineffective in improving muscle function in a phase 3 clinical trial. Muscle biopsies show scattered atrophic fibres, subsarcolemmal rimmed vacuoles

Table 48.1 Neuromuscular disorders typically showing rimmed vacuoles in a muscle biopsy

Disorder	Gene	Inheritance	Age at onset	First signs
GNE-myopathy	GNE	AR	Early adulthood	Anterior distal leg muscles
Welander distal myopathy	TIA1 TIA1+ SQSTM1	AD	Late adulthood	Finger and wrist extensors
Oculopharyn-geal muscular dystrophy (OPMD)	GCA/GCC/GCG or GCT expansion in PABPN1	AD	Adulthood	Ptosis, dysphagia, ext. ophthalmoplegia, facial weakness, proximal leg muscles
Oculopharyn-geal distal myopathy (OPDM)	CGG/GGC expansions in LRP12, NOTCH2NLC, GIPC1, RILPL1	Mostly AD	Adulthood	Ptosis and ext. ophthalmoplegia, facial weakness, dysphagia, anterior distal leg muscles Mainly patients from Asia
VCP distal myopathy [a]	VCP	AD	Adulthood	Anterior distal leg muscles
DNAJB6 and PLIN4 distal myopathies	DNAJB6, PLIN4	AD	Adulthood	Anterior or posterior distal leg muscles
Myofibrillar myopathies	e.g., MYOT, LDB3, BAG3, HSPB8	Mostly AD	Adulthood	Weakness axial, proximal, distal, and respiratory muscles, cardiac involvement
SMPX distal myopathy	SMPX	X-linked	Adulthood	Anterior distal leg muscles
Inclusion body myositis (IBM)	Acquired		(Late) adulthood	Asymmetric deep finger flexors, dysphagia, quadriceps

RVs are not specific for the disorders listed here. RVs have also been described not only in distal myopathies such as MYH7 myopathy and Udd myopathy, but also in Becker muscular dystrophy and various limb girdle muscular dystrophies.

[a] VCP is a highly pleiotropic gene: mutations cause a multisystem proteinopathy (MSP), which can include amyotrophic lateral sclerosis, frontotemporal dementia, Charcot–Marie–Tooth disease type 2, hereditary motor neuropathy, or Paget disease of bone.

(RVs) on hematoxylin and eosin, and modified Gomori trichome staining, intranuclear inclusion on electron microscopy, and dystrophic changes in advanced disease. RVs are thought to result from abnormal autophagy, probably as a secondary phenomenon, but the pathogenic mechanism of RV formations remains ill understood. RVs are not specific for GNE-myopathy. They can be found in many inherited distal myopathies, mostly with autosomal dominant inheritance and adult onset, as well as in other myopathies. Table 48.1 lists a selection of neuromuscular disorders featured by RVs.

GNE-myopathy (Table 48.2) is also called distal myopathy with rimmed vacuoles, Nonaka myopathy; and hereditary inclusion body myopathy. It has an autosomal recessive inheritance pattern. It usually presents in early adulthood with progressive symmetric weakness of foot and toe dorsiflexors, causing

Table 48.2 Main features of GNE myopathy

- Onset mostly in 2nd/3rd decade with symmetric foot drop
- Progression may be relatively rapid
- Sparing of quadriceps muscles
- Weakness in arms starts in intrinsic hand muscles and deep finger flexors
- No cardiac involvement; respiratory impairment uncommon
- CK normal or mildly elevated
- Bi-allelic pathogenic variants in the GNE gene
- Muscle biopsy may show rimmed vacuoles

notable foot drop and steppage gait. Weakness shows distal to proximal progression with relative sparing of the quadriceps muscles. Half the patients have lost ambulation 20 years after disease onset. Arm and hand muscles become weak over time. The pattern of evolving weakness is fairly uniform, but age at onset and rate of progression vary. This is only partly explained by the GNE genotype, but mutations associated with severe, respectively mild disease have been identified. There is no weakness of respiratory muscles until late stages of the disease, and routine respiratory function testing for an ambulant patient is not required. Cardiac involvement is usually not seen, and routinely assessment is not recommended. Rarely, GNE myopathy is associated with congenital thrombocytopenia. Serum CK activity is normal or moderately increased. The diagnosis is made by targeted sequencing or NGS gene panel analysis. A muscle biopsy may be helpful if genetic testing yields uncertain results, but the absence of RVs does not exclude GNE myopathy. Standards of care are based on expert opinion and include foremost rehabilitation and occupational treatment. Genetic counselling may include preconceptional carrier screening in regions with a high concentration of patients, such as Middle Eastern countries.

Suggested Reading

Mullen J, Alrasheed K, Mozaffar T. GNE myopathy: history, etiology, and treatment trials. *Front Neurol* 2022;13:1002310. doi: 10.3389/fneur.2022.1002310. PMID: 36330422; PMCID: PMC9623016.

Savarese M, Sarparanta J, Vihola A, et al. Panorama of the distal myopathies. *Acta Myol* 2020;39(4):245–265. doi: 10.36185/2532-1900-028. PMID: 33458580; PMCID: PMC7783427.

Yoshioka W, Nishino I, Noguchi S. Recent advances in establishing a cure for GNE myopathy. *Curr Opin Neurol* 2022;35(5):629–636. doi: 10.1097/WCO.0000000000001090. Epub 2022 Aug 11. PMID: 35959526.

Myofibrillar Myopathies: Desminopathy

Clinical History

A 36-year-old woman was concerned about being affected with a disease that ran in the family in an autosomal dominant (AD) manner. A few years before presentation, she noticed difficulty when walking in the mountains and this had gradually progressed to problems climbing stairs and an inability to run. She also noted that she could no longer lift her head when in supine position. Her mother had died of this disease in her early forties. She mentioned that many affected family members had been diagnosed with cardiac problems in addition to muscle weakness. Some were treated with an implantable cardioverter defibrillator. In elderly family members, cardiac enlargement was not uncommon.

Examination

On examination, there was a slight dysarthria, and an MRC grade 4+ weakness of neck flexors and hip and knee flexors. There were positive Gowers and Trendelenburg signs, and she could not walk on her heels.

Diagnostic Considerations

In a patient with AD inherited weakness in an axial–proximal–distal distribution, including cardiac involvement, it is justified to start the diagnostic work-up with a gene panel analysis directed at myofibrillar myopathies.

Ancillary Investigations

Forced vital capacity (FVC) was 81% of expected in sitting position. Serum CK activity was mildly increased. Light and electron microscopic examination of earlier muscle biopsies in this family had shown disruption of the myofibrillar organization and accumulation of granulofilamentous material (Fig. 49.1). In our patient a next-generation sequence (NGS) gene panel analysis showed the pathogenic p.Asn342Asp variant in the *DES* gene.

Follow-Up

Five years after presentation, she could only just walk without support. FVC had decreased to 70% in the sitting position and 52% when lying down. A year later, she experienced frequent, frightening night-time awakenings and headaches on

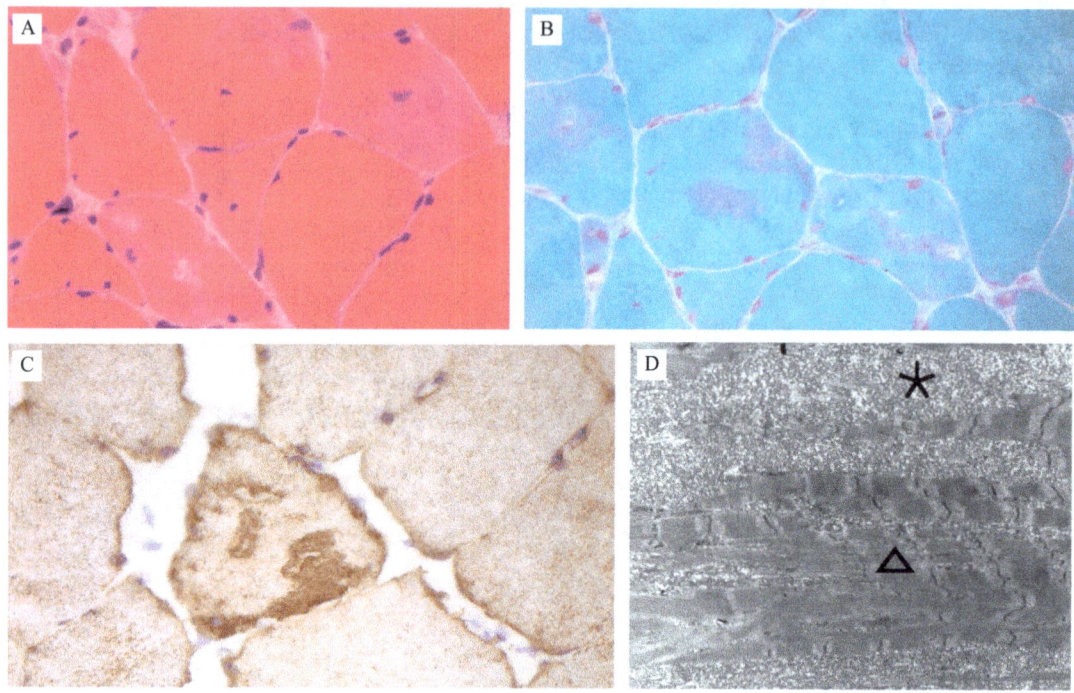

Figure 49.1 (A–D) Muscle biopsy showing variation in muscle fibre size with small vacuoles and accumulation of eosinophilic material on the H&E stain (A), more pronounced on the modified Gomori trichrome stain (B). Inclusions contain desmin (C). Electron microscopic image shows granulofilamentous material (asterisk) that is interspersed between disorganized myofibrils (arrow head) (D).

awakening in the morning. During the day, she felt tired. Nocturnal measurements of pCO2 showed hypercapnia. Subsequently, nocturnal noninvasive ventilatory support was initiated, making her feel much better. Asymptomatic ventricular tachycardia and right bundle branch block were found. Four years later, at age 45, she became completely wheelchair dependent.

General Remarks

Myofibrillar Myopathies (MFMs)

The myofibrillar myopathies (MFMs) are defined based on their histopathological abnormalities. The most characteristic feature is best identified on electron microscopy and consists of disorganization of the sarcomere, starting at the Z-disk. Degraded granulofilamentous material accumulations between myofibrils and membranous organelles and glycogen aggregates in autophagic vacuoles are characteristic findings. Accumulating proteins include desmin, dystrophin, and beta-amyloid precursor protein. Despite these distinctive features, it can be difficult to make a diagnosis of myofibrillar myopathy, because at the light microscopic level, these abnormalities may be difficult to recognize or can be overlooked if not abundantly present. Light microscopic examination of a muscle biopsy specimen can show many rather nonspecific features, such as degeneration and regeneration, necrosis and increased fibrosis (suggesting muscular dystrophy), vacuoles and grouped atrophy, and abnormal protein aggregates appearing as amorphous, granular, or hyaline deposits in various shapes, colours, and localizations (in frozen sections).

In addition, the clinical presentation is variable. Progressive distal muscle weakness of the legs is often the first symptom, but patients can also show a limb girdle or scapuloperoneal distribution of weakness. Respiratory insufficiency, axial weakness, facial weakness, dysphagia, and dysarthria also occur. Cardiac involvement is frequent and cardiac evaluation should thus be part of the diagnostic work-up of any myopathy with dystrophic features or intrafibre structural abnormalities (Table 49.1).

Myofibrillar myopathies have their onset in adulthood in most patients and are usually transmitted in an autosomal dominant manner. At the molecular genetic level, mutations found to cause myofibrillar myopathy involve Z-disk-associated

Table 49.1 Main features of myofibrillar myopathies

- Defined by myofibrillar changes in a muscle biopsy
- Adult onset
- Variable distribution of weakness, often distal onset
- Diaphragm weakness
- Cardiac conduction abnormalities, arrhythmias, dilated and hypertrophic cardiomyopathy
- CK mildly elevated
- Mostly autosomal dominantly inherited
- Desmin most frequent gene, but many other genes have been identified

proteins, in particular desmin (*DES*), and also myotilin (*MYOT*), alpha B-crystallin (*CRYAB*), *ZASP/LDB3*, filamin C (*FLNC*), and *Bag3*. Many other genes have recently been recognised to be associated with MFM-like disease (among other clinical and histopathological manifestations), for instance *TTN*, *FHL1*, *DNAJB6*, *PLEC*, *ACTA1*, *HSPB8*, and *LMNA*. These genes should be included in gene panels. Still, about 40% of patients with a myopathy that can be classified as MFM histopathologically remain undiagnosed at the DNA level.

Desminopathy

Desmin is a tissue-specific type III intermediate filament expressed in skeletal and cardiac myocytes. It surrounds the Z-discs and links the myofibrillar structure to the sarcolemma, the nucleus, and cytoplasmic organelles. In most patients with a desminopathy, symptoms start in their teens or adulthood with progressive distal weakness. Others present with simultaneous distal and proximal weakness, or with scapuloperoneal or axial weakness, or incidentally with isolated facial weakness. Weakness of respiratory muscles occurs frequently. There is no phenotype–genotype correlation. Different phenotypes can coexist within one family.

Skeletal muscle weakness in desminopathy is often accompanied by cardiac involvement, including conduction abnormalities, arrhythmias, dilated and hypertrophic cardiomyopathy, and sudden death. Cardiac involvement may be the presenting sign of desminopathy.

The inheritance pattern of desminopathy is usually AD but can also be autosomal recessive. Many sporadic cases are caused by *de novo* mutations. The diagnosis is made by NGS gene panel testing. If negative, a diagnosis of an MFM can made by means of a muscle biopsy.

Whole-body MRI may show relatively specific findings in some of the MFMs. In DES-related MFM, early fatty degeneration of the leg muscles, particularly in the long fibular, then the tibialis anterior and the muscles of the posterior leg, is found. At a later stage, there is involvement of the thighs with predominant involvement of the gracilis, sartorius, and semitendinosus as well as involvement of the shoulder muscles.

In case of an established genetic diagnosis, genetic counselling should be offered promptly, as patients may be planning to start a family at the time of presentation.

Management of a patient with a desminopathy includes regular cardiac examinations for timely placement of a pacemaker or implantable cardioverter defibrillator. Respiratory function should also be monitored. A drop of more than 10–15 percentage points of the FVC in supine as compared with the sitting position indicates diaphragm weakness. Nocturnal noninvasive assisted ventilation is often beneficial in case hypercapnia has developed. Rehabilitation treatment should always be offered.

Suggested Reading

Carroll LS, Walker M, Allen D, et al. Desminopathy presenting as late onset bilateral facial weakness, with diagnosis supported by lower limb MRI. *Neuromuscul Disord* 2021;31(3):249–252. doi: 10.1016/j.nmd.2020.12.013. Epub 2021 Jan 8. PMID: 33546848.

Carvalho AAS, Lacene E, Brochier G, et al. Genetic mutations and demographic, clinical, and morphological aspects of myofibrillar myopathy in a French cohort. *Genet Test Mol Biomarkers* 2018;22 (6):374–383. doi: 10.1089/gtmb.2018.0004. PMID: 29924655

Fichna JP, Maruszak A, Żekanowski C. Myofibrillar myopathy in the genomic context. *J Appl Genet* 2018;59(4):431–439. doi: 10.1007/s13353-018-0463-4. Epub 2018 Sep 10. PMID: 30203143.

Jungbluth H. Myopathology in times of modern imaging. *Neuropathol Appl Neurobiol* 2017;43(1):24–43. doi: 10.1111/nan.12385. PMID: 28111795.

Venturelli N, Tordjman M, Ammar A, et al. Contribution of muscle MRI for diagnosis of myopathy. *Rev Neurol (Paris)* 2023;179(1-2):61–80. doi: 10.1016/j.neurol.2022.12.002. Epub 2022 Dec 21. PMID: 36564254.

Wahbi K, Béhin A, Charron P, et al. High cardiovascular morbidity and mortality in myofibrillar myopathies due to DES gene mutations: a 10-year longitudinal study. *Neuromuscul Disord* 2012;22(3):211–218. doi: 10.1016/j.nmd.2011.10.019. Epub 2011 Dec 5. PMID: 22153487.

CASE 50 Skeletal Muscle Channelopathies: Non-Dystrophic Myotonia; Myotonia Congenita (Becker)

Clinical History

A 35-year-old man complained about muscle stiffness and weakness, especially when initiating a movement. He had experienced these symptoms for as long as he could remember. They were present in his eyes, jaws, tongue, and limb muscles. He had noticed that cold weather had a negative influence. He was not able to run and did not participate in team sport activities. In spite of these symptoms, he experienced no limitations in activities of daily living. He was referred because he had been informed elsewhere about possible treatment. The family history revealed similar symptoms in a sister and a brother, but not in the parents. His father's grandparents were cousins.

Examination

The patient had an athletic appearance. In particular, there was hypertrophy of the calf muscles and of the quadriceps femoris muscles. When asked to open his eyes after first firmly closing them, we observed action myotonia of the orbicularis oculi muscles that consisted of not being able to open the eyes promptly (Fig. 50.1). He had action myotonia of the hand muscles after making a fist. There was percussion myotonia of various limb muscles.

When setting off, his gait was stiff; this gradually improved as the muscles 'warmed up'. Similarly, he noticed weakness of the neck flexors and of various arm and leg muscles, which also improved after sustained contraction of the muscles. He was found to have a lumbar hyperlordosis and slight contractures at the elbows and wrists. Arm reflexes were normal, whereas the knee jerks were decreased and Achilles tendon reflexes absent.

Diagnostic Considerations

The patient had two key features that led to the diagnosis of non-dystrophic myotonia: attacks

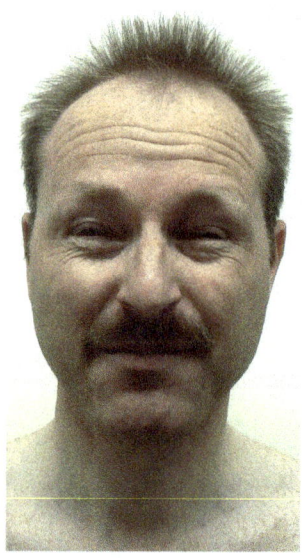

Figure 50.1 When asked to open his eyes after first firmly closing them, action myotonia of the orbicularis oculi muscle was observed, which resulted in not being able to open the eyes properly.

of transient weakness elicited by movement after rest and a 'warm-up' phenomenon. Given the apparent absence of symptoms in the parents and the involvement of his two siblings, an autosomal recessive trait was likely. The suspected diagnosis was Becker myotonia, a non-dystrophic myotonia. Therefore, EMG was not performed.

Ancillary Investigations

Genetic testing revealed heterozygosity for one pathogenic variant in the chloride channel (*CLCN1*) gene, a missense variant (c.854G>A; p.Gly285Glu), and an unclassified variant (c.1938G>A; p.Met646Ile). We established a diagnosis of autosomal recessive congenital myotonia (Becker myotonia), a muscle chloride channelopathy.

Table 50.1 Skeletal muscle channelopathies[a]

Disease Gene[a]	Age at onset	Clinical features	Triggers	Management
Myotonia congenita (MC) *CLCN1*	Autosomal dominant (AD) (Thomsen disease): infancy–early childhood Autosomal recessive (AR) (Becker disease): 4–10 years, or as late as 3rd or 4th decade	Legs > arms, face; in AR MC episodic weakness improves with repeated movement; calf hypertrophy, often generalized; 'warming up' characteristic. Pain is common. AR MC more severe than AD.	Prolonged rest (after activity); extreme temperature	Adjust triggers. Relieving factor: Warm environment. Mexiletine; lamotrigine
Paramyotonia congenita (PMC) *SCN4A*	Early childhood	Face and hands > legs; prolonged weakness; paradoxical myotonia characteristic	Cold environment	Adjust triggers. Mexiletine; lamotrigine
Sodium channel myotonia (SCM) *SCN4A*		Either pattern of muscle involvement; 'warming up' and paradoxical myotonia can occur (AD MC mimic). Painful myotonia common.	Prolonged rest (after activity); extreme temperature	Adjust triggers. Relieving factor: Warm environment
Hyperkalaemic periodic paralysis (hyperPP) *SCN4A*	Early childhood (~50% first attack < 10 years) to 4th decade; 60% < 16 years	Episodes of weakness (hips, shoulders, back) with concomitant high serum potassium, lasting minutes to hours. Patients may also show paratonia (muscle stiffness or inability to relax muscles).	Period of rest following physical activity, potassium-rich diet, stress	Frequent carbohydrate-rich meals, thiazide diuretic, or carbonic anhydrase inhibitor
Hypokalaemic periodic paralysis (hypoPP) *CACNA1S* (60%) *SCN4A* (20%)	Early teens	Episodes of weakness (legs first, proximal > distal) with concomitant low serum potassium, lasting hours to days. *CACNA1S* variants that cause primary hypoPP differ from those causing malignant hyperthermia syndrome.	Period of rest after physical activity, carbohydrate-rich evening meal followed by nocturnal rest, cold, salt intake, stress	Prevention: carbonic anhydrase inhibitor (acetazolamide or dichlorphenamide)
Andersen–Tawil syndrome (ATS) *KCNJ2*	1st or 2nd decade with either cardiac symptoms (palpitations and/or syncope) or weakness	Classical syndrome is a triad of periodic paralysis, cardiac conduction defects and dysmorphic features (the latter may be subtle).	Prolonged rest, rest following physical activity	Annual cardiac review. Treat if arrhythmias are found, also in asymptomatic patients. Carbonic anhydrase inhibitor. Flecainide for ventricular arrhythmia. Implantable ICD if tachycardia-induced syncope.
Thyrotoxic hypokalaemic periodic paralysis (TPP), most commonly associated with Graves disease. *KCNJ18* (about 1/3)	Onset in adulthood, Most prevalent in men of East Asian ancestry	Episodes of mainly proximal leg weakness, myalgia, hypokalaemia and thyreotoxicosis. Weakness may progress, including respiratory muscles.	High carbohydrare meals, vigorous exercise, alcohol, trauma, inffection, stress and medication (e.g., insuline, diuretics).	Potassium supplementation with close monitoring. Weakness resolves with correction of thyrotoxicosis.

Adapted from Matthews et al., *Pract Neurol* 2021;21:196–205, and Patel M, Ladak K, *Clin Med Res* 2021;19(3):148–151.

[a] All disorders listed here are autosomal dominantly (AD) inherited, apart from autosomal recessive (AR) myotonia congenita (Becker).

Part II Neuromuscular Cases: Myopathies

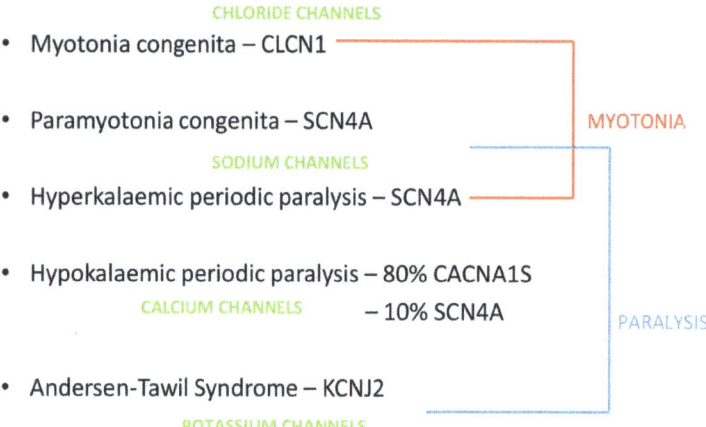

Figure 50.2 The skeletal muscle channelopathies - causative genes, dysfunctional ion channel and resultant clinical symptom. From: Matthews E, Holmes S, Fialho D. Skeletal muscle channelopathies: a guide to diagnosis and management. Pract Neurol. 2021;21:196–204, with permission

Table 50.2 Conditions associated with secondary periodic paralysis

Low potassium	High potassium
Thyrotoxic	Addison disease
Primary hyperaldosteronism	Hpoaldosteronism
Renal tubular acidosis	Potassium-sparing diuretics
Juxtaglomerular apparatus hyperplasia	Excessive potassium suppplementation
Gastrointestinal potassium wastage	
Laxative abuse	
Licorice consumption	
Corticosteroids	
Potassium depleting diuretics	

Adapted from: Trivedi JR. Muscle Channelopathies. Continuum (Minneap Minn). 2022 28:1778-1799

Follow-Up

Mexiletine 200 mg bid considerably reduced muscle stiffness. Increasing the dosage to 600 mg per day caused significant side effects (nausea and abdominal pain).

General Remarks

Skeletal Muscle Channelopathies

Skeletal muscle channelopathies are a group of rare episodic genetic disorders caused by dysfunction of sarcolemmal ion channels that are critical for muscle membrane excitability. Skeletal muscle channelopathies can be divided into the non-dystrophic myotonias, the primary periodic paralyses and Andersen-Tawil syndrome (Table 50.1, Fig. 50.2), and based on whether the predominant clinical symptom is muscle weakness or myotonia (delayed muscle relaxation after voluntary contraction, which is usually described as muscles 'locking', 'sticking', or 'cramping') (**Videos 39.2 and 39.3**). The hallmark of a skeletal muscle channelopathy is that symptoms occur in an episodic or paroxysmal fashion, causing acute disability.

Non-Dystrophic Myotonic Syndromes

Non-dystrophic myotonic syndromes comprise a heterogeneous group of skeletal muscle disorders caused by mutations in genes encoding the skeletal muscle chloride (*CLCN1*) or sodium channel (*SCN4A*, Table 50.1)

Myotonia congenita is characterized by muscle stiffness present from childhood; all striated muscle groups including the extrinsic eye muscles, facial muscles, tongue, and limb muscles may be involved. Stiffness is relieved by repeated contractions of the muscle (the 'warm-up' phenomenon). In contrast, in paramyotonia congenita there is paradoxical myotonia, meaning that myotonia increases with repetition. Generalized muscle hypertrophy is common in all congenital myotonic syndromes.

Serum creatine kinase activity may be normal but is usually slightly elevated (≤ 3–4 × ULN). Conventional needle electromyography shows myotonic bursts, which in itself is not specific and is currently no longer routinely performed. Diagnosis requires genetic testing, which is done with a gene panel including all genes relevant to skeletal muscle channelopathies, including the periodic paralyses, non-dystrophic myotonias, and Anderson-Tawil syndrome.

It is important to provide advice regarding the avoidance of precipitating factors such as exposure to cold or strenuous exercise. Mexiletine and lamotrigine have been shown to be efficacious with no or acceptable side effects.

Primary Periodic Paralyses

The primary periodic paralyses (PP) are autosomal dominantly inherited disorders characterized by episodes of flaccid paralysis (**Case 51, Table 50.1**). Hypokalaemic periodic paralysis and hyperkalaemic periodic paralysis relate to episodes of muscle weakness with concomitant low or high serum potassium concentrations, respectively. Weakness often presents during a period of rest following physical activity, and may be task-specific or affecting only one limb. The severity of weakness can vary from dramatic with tetraparesis requiring presentation to the emergency department to modest weakness in most patients.

It is important to exclude secondary causes of hypokalemia or hyperkalemia as these can mimic primary periodic paralysis in their clinical presentation (Table 50.2)

Andersen–Tawil Syndrome

Andersen–Tawil syndrome is the only skeletal muscle channelopathy to affect systems other than skeletal muscle – namely, cardiac muscle and bone development. The classic syndrome is a triad of periodic paralysis (usually mirroring the hypokalaemic periodic paralysis variety), cardiac conduction defects, and dysmorphic features. In many cases, the dysmorphic features are subtle and overlooked, and muscle features or cardiac symptoms may be the predominant features. Sudden cardiac death may occur but is generally considered rare. Twenty percent of patients require an implantable cardiac defibrillator. Therefore, patients should have an annual cardiac review with ECG and Holter monitoring.

Suggested Reading

Dunø M, Vissing J. Myotonia congenita. 2005 Aug 3 [updated 2021 Feb 25]. In Adam MP, Mirzaa GM, Pagon RA, et al., editors. *GeneReviews®* [Internet]. Seattle, WA: University of Washington; 1993–2023. PMID: 20301529.

Matthews E, Holmes S, Fialho D. Skeletal muscle channelopathies: a guide to diagnosis and management. *Pract Neurol* 2021;21(3):196–204. doi: 10.1136/practneurol-2020-002576. Epub 2021 Feb 9. PMID: 33563766.

Sekhon DS, Vaqar S, Gupta V. Hyperkalemic periodic paralysis. 2023 May 8. In *StatPearls* [Internet]. Treasure Island, FL: StatPearls Publishing; 2023 Jan–. PMID: 33231989.

Siddamreddy S, Dandu VH. Thyrotoxic *periodic paralysis*. 2022 Jul 25. In *StatPearls* [Internet]. Treasure Island, FL: StatPearls Publishing; 2023 Jan–. PMID: 32809505.

Statland JM, Fontaine B, Hanna MG, et al. Review of the diagnosis and treatment of periodic paralysis. *Muscle Nerve* 2018;57(4):522–530. doi: 10.1002/mus.26009. Epub 2017 Nov 29. PMID: 29125635; PMCID: PMC5867231.

Veerapandiyan A, Statland JM, Tawil R. Andersen-Tawil syndrome. 2004 Nov 22 [updated 2018 Jun 7].

In Adam MP, Mirzaa GM, Pagon RA, et al., editors. *GeneReviews®* [Internet]. Seattle, WA: University of Washington; 1993–2023. PMID: 20301441.

Vicart S, Franques J, Bouhour F, et al. Efficacy and safety of mexiletine in non-dystrophic myotonias: a randomised, double-blind, placebo-controlled, cross-over study. *Neuromuscul Disord* 2021;31(11):1124–1135. doi: 10.1016/j.nmd.2021.06.010. Epub 2021 Jun 27. PMID: 34702654.

Weber F, Lehmann-Horn F. Hypokalemic periodic paralysis. 2002 Apr 30 [updated 2018 Jul 26]. In Adam MP, Mirzaa GM, Pagon RA, et al., editors. *GeneReviews®* [Internet]. Seattle, WA: University of Washington; 1993–2023. PMID: 20301512.

CASE 51 Skeletal Muscle Channelopathies: Hypokalaemic Periodic Paralysis

Clinical History

A 33-year-old man was referred by his nephrologist who treats him with potassium supplementation for a hypokalaemic periodic paralysis, which had been diagnosed by the finding of heterozygosity for the missense mutation c.1853 G->A; p.Arg528His in the voltage-gated calcium channel (*CAGNA1S*) gene. He now visited our department in search of an explanation and treatment for an apparently fixed (permanent) weakness in his upper legs, which hampered climbing stairs.

The attacks of flaccid weakness had begun when he was 13 years old. The frequency had been increasing starting a few years ago. He now experiences mild attacks four to five times a week, with a heavy feeling in the affected limb during hours or a whole day. Heavy attacks with more severe flaccid weakness occur every few weeks. Moving around then is very difficult. Severe weakness is triggered by more than normal physical activity such as sports, but sometimes generalized weakness is present at awakening. Weakness can occur in the arms or the legs, or can affect only one limb, and the fingers may become affected when using the computer. Sometimes he cannot move his feet at all, while the strength in the upper legs remains unchanged. Coughing always becomes weak during a heavy attack, as well as holding his head up, but speech, swallowing, and breathing are never affected. At the start of an attack, he takes oral potassium chloride 50–100 mg (75 mg/mL; 1 mmol/mL), which seems to alleviate the attack somewhat. He has a low-carbohydrate diet.

Examination

There was weakness MRC grade 4+ of both iliopsoas muscles. There was no Gowers sign, but getting to a standing position from kneeling on one knee was not possible. The examination was otherwise normal, apart from an absent Achilles tendon reflex on the left side.

Diagnostic Considerations

Permanent weakness due to a myopathy of proximal leg muscles is known to develop in many patients with periodic paralysis, apparently unrelated to the frequency or severity of the episodic weakness. Although permanent weakness usually occurs later in life, we saw no reason to do ancillary investigations into an alternative explanation.

Ancillary Investigations

A whole-body muscle MRI showed marked symmetric fatty replacement of several pelvic girdle and proximal leg muscles, as well as of the medial head of the gastrocnemius muscle on the left side (Fig. 51.1). Potassium levels in between attacks were 3.3–3.8 mmol/L (normal 3.8–5.0).

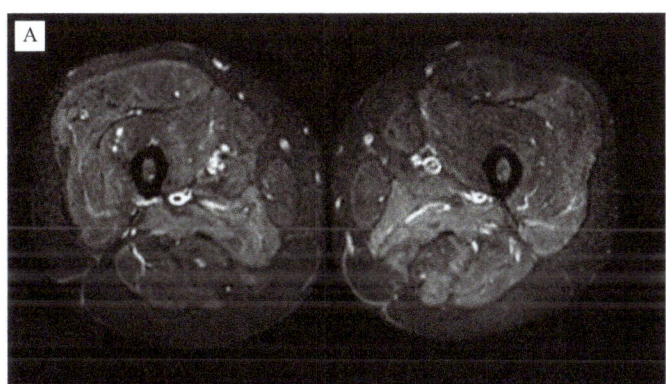
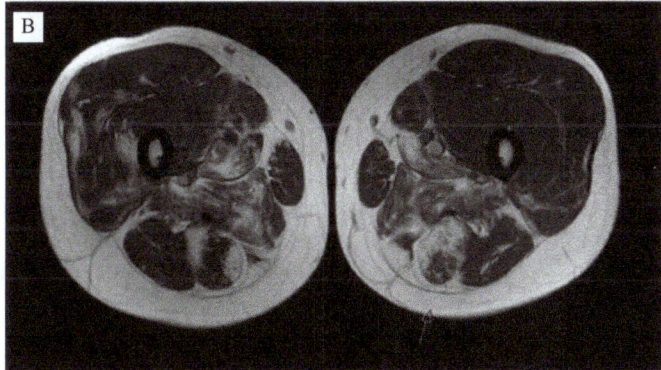

Figure 51.1 (A,B) Increased signal on a T2 STIR sequence indicating oedema (A) and fatty replacement of muscle tissue on a T1-weigted scan (B) affecting proximal anterior and posterior muscles of the upper legs in the described patient.

Follow-Up

As the attacks of weakness seriously impaired his social and professional life, we advised him to increase the potassium dose when noticing first weakness in order to more effectively abort attacks. However, he was reluctant to follow this advice because of fear of inducing hyperkalaemia. Acetazolamide is a carbonic anhydrase inhibitor, which probably has a positive effect on the frequency and severity of attacks, and possibly also on permanent weakness, but he declined to take this drug because of fear of side effects on cognition. He was also afraid of worsening of weakness by taking this medication, although we explained that this adverse effect was observed only occasionally, mainly in patients with a pathogenic variant in the *SCN4A* gene. Dichlorphenamide is probably more effective, with fewer side effects than acetazolamide, but this drug is unavailable in many countries. He was then started on eplerenone, an oral aldosterone antagonist increasing serum potassium levels, with fewer side effects (gynecomastia, impotence) than spironolactone, the effects of which have to be awaited. We also advised him to start moving gently at the start of an attack (swinging the arms, walking around), because this may diminish the attacks. We referred him to the department of rehabilitation medicine for advice on sporting activities and he was offered genetic counselling.

General Remarks and Suggested Reading

See **Case 50**.

Pompe Disease (Glycogen Storage Disease (GSD) Type II; α-Glucosidase Deficiency)

Clinical History

A 49-year-old man, who had always been very active, noted backache and pain in his neck starting four years ago. During this period, it became more difficult to rise from a chair and from his bed, to climb the stairs, or to carry heavy objects. Walking became a bit more difficult over time. He still went to the gym, but noticed that flexing his knees against resistance became more difficult. He slept well, could easily lie flat during the night, and did not experience myalgia, and there were no sensory disturbances. There were no symptoms of respiratory insufficiency. Family history was unremarkable.

Examination

He walked with hyperlordosis and a broad-based, waddling gait (Fig. 52.1). There were no contractures and the calves were not hypertrophic. Fasciculations were not found. There was no ptosis and also no abnormalities of the tongue. Neck extensors were slightly weak (MRC grade 5−). Shoulder girdle muscles (deltoid, infra- and supraspinatus) were weak (bilateral MRC 4). There was some muscular atrophy of hip abductors and adductors, and weakness of the hip flexors, abductors, and adductors and of the knee flexors (bilateral MRC 4). Knee and Achilles tendon reflexes were symmetrically reduced. When lying in supine position, he needed to use his arms to turn over to sitting position. Inspection of his back revealed clear atrophy of the lumbar paravertebral muscles. Forward flexing appeared normal, but with an attempt to get to a standing position, he made a swing with his upper body. Trendelenburg sign was (bilaterally) positive, and there was a positive Gowers sign (see **Videos 52.1 and 52.2**).

Diagnostic Considerations

Based on the symptoms and neurological examination, a clinical diagnosis of limb girdle weakness in combination with weakness of the lumbar

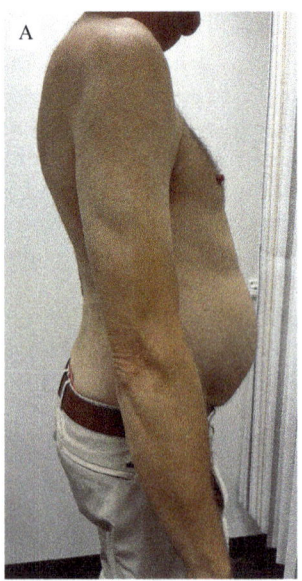
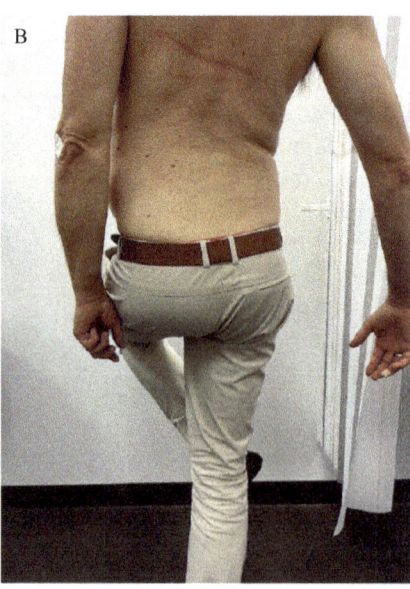

Figure 52.1 (A,B) Patient with hyperlordosis (A) and Trendelenburg sign due to weakness of hip abductors at the right side (B) in the described patient with late-onset Pompe disease.

paravertebral muscles was made. The duration of symptoms (several years) was considered more likely to be compatible with a genetic disorder than an acquired disease.

We considered adult Pompe disease, largely because of the combination of slowly progressive limb girdle weakness in combination with the obvious weakness of the lumbar paravertebral muscles. Other diagnostic considerations were AR limb girdle muscular dystrophy (LGMD), Becker muscular dystrophy (considered less likely because of the distribution of weakness, the absence of enlarged calves, and the relative low CK, see below), and spinal muscular atrophy (SMA) type 4.

Ancillary Investigations

Serum CK 494, TSH normal; pCO2: within normal range. Acid alpha-glucosidase (GAA) in leucocytes was deficient (3 nmol/mg; normal value > 40 nmol/mg).

Forced vital capacity (FVC) seated: 4.1 l (76%), supine 2.4 l (45%): postural drop 31pp), indicating diaphragmatic dysfunction. A muscle biopsy revealed myopathic changes with some vacuoles with PAS-positive staining. The diagnosis of late-onset Pompe disease (LOPD) was confirmed genetically by the finding of two pathogenic variants in the GAA gene: IVS1 / c.379-380delTG. Currently, genetic analysis after showing GAA deficiency in blood in leucocytes or dried blood spot is the preferred diagnostic sequence in patients suspected to have Pompe disease. A muscle biopsy as an intermediate diagnostic step can still be considered if there is initially substantial doubt about the clinical diagnosis, when genetic diagnostics is not readily available, or when there is some more urgency in the diagnostic process (to exclude, e.g., an inflammatory myopathy).

Follow-Up

The diagnosis of late-onset Pompe disease (LOPD) was suspected based on the medical history, predominant weakness of the hip muscles (waddling gait), the proximal lower leg muscles (especially the knee flexors), the lower paraspinal muscles (standing with hyperlordosis), and the weakness of the diaphragm (Figs. 52.1 and 52.2), and was confirmed genetically. We started treatment with enzyme replacement therapy (ERT) (alglucosidase alfa, intravenously once every 2 weeks). Over the years there initially was some relief of symptoms, especially muscle force of the extremities was slightly improved, and he felt more energetic. Pulmonary function initially remained stable. Over the following years, both muscle force and pulmonary function slightly decreased. Now, 11 years after start of ERT, the patient remains able to continue an active life style, including a lot of travel. He is still able to walk 7 km and to cycle (on an electric bike) for about 30 km, and he does not need noninvasive ventilation.

General Remarks

Pompe disease, glycogen storage disease type II (GSDII), is a rare autosomal recessive neuromuscular disease that is caused by deficiency of the enzyme acid alpha-glucosidase (GAA), also called acid maltase, which degrades lysosomal glycogen. Patients are compound heterozygotes. Different mutations in the *GAA* gene lead to different levels of residual GAA and glycogen accumulation. Pompe disease includes a large variation in both the age of onset and the severity of muscle weakness.

Infantile-onset Pompe disease (IOPD) becomes manifest before birth with diminished child movements, or before the age of six months (Fig. 52.3). Patients have two mutations with a severe pathogenic effect, and GAA activity is virtually absent. Ubiquitous glycogen storage leads to hepatomegaly, cardiomegaly, and macroglossia. Without GAA enzyme replacement therapy (ERT), most infants die of cardiorespiratory failure before their first birthday (Table 52.1).

Late-onset Pompe disease (LOPD) is the most frequent form. It is caused by two mutations, one with a severe pathogenic effect, and the other with a mild pathogenic effect. A similar genotype, however, may lead to variation between patients and within families. Some patients have a juvenile onset after the first year and before the age of 18 years. Far more frequently, the onset is after the age of 18 years. In LOPD, glycogen accumulation does only occur in skeletal muscle (the heart is not involved). Serum CK activity is elevated in almost all patients and may be as high as 10 × ULN. Fatigue and muscle soreness are common initial complaints. Most patients have a symmetric limb

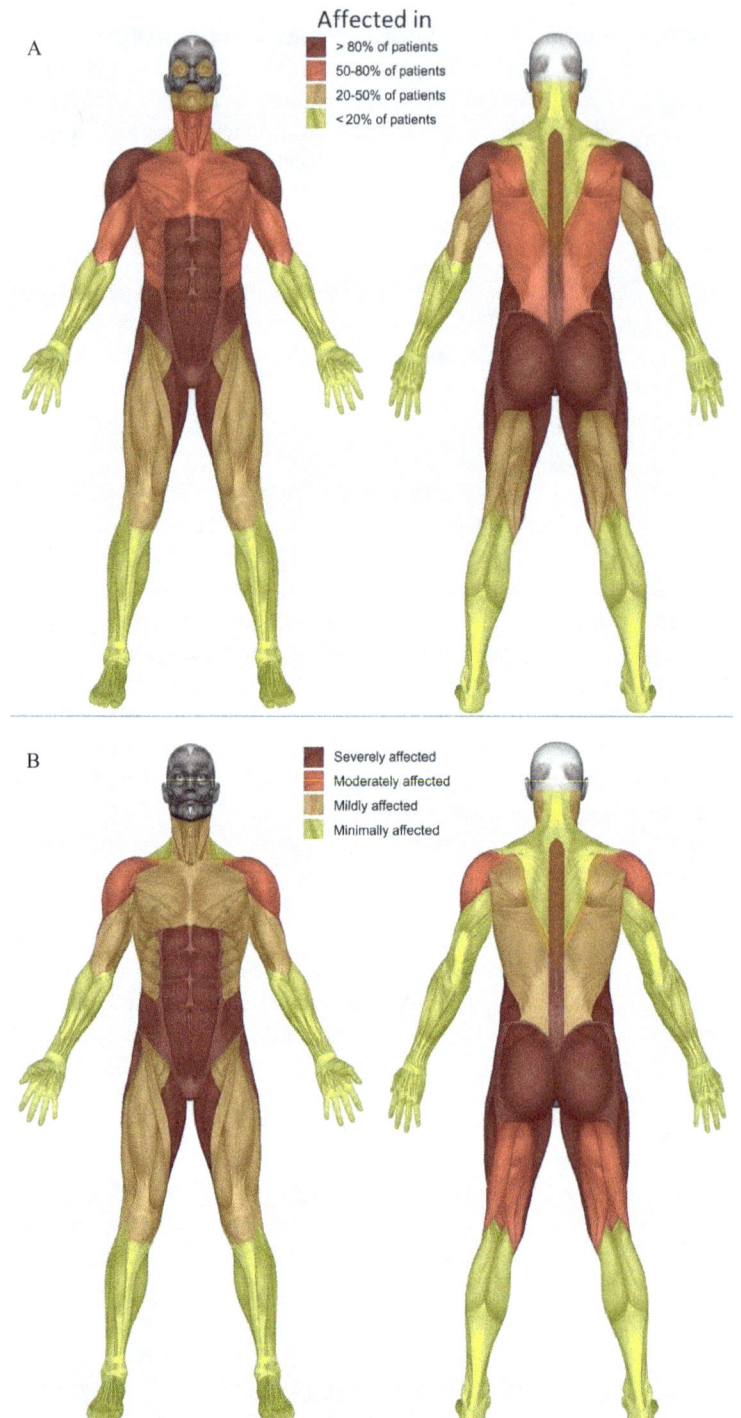

Figure 52.2 (A,B) Distribution (A) and severity (B) of muscle weakness in late-onset Pompe disease. From Van der Beek et al., *Orphanet Journal of Rare Diseases* 2012;7:88, with permission.

girdle type of weakness and a varying degree of axial weakness and respiratory insufficiency. Lumbar lordosis occurs in two-thirds of patients, asymmetric scapular winging in one-third, asymmetric ptosis and bulbar weakness in one-quarter. Respiratory insufficiency from weakness of the

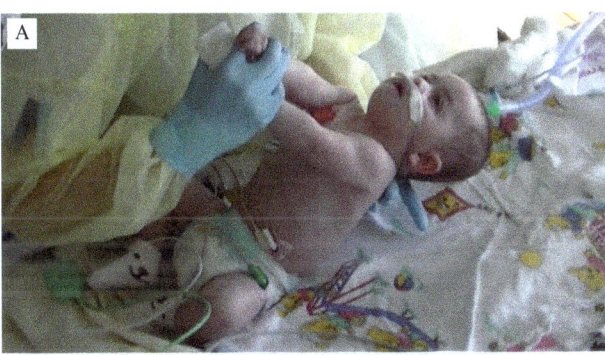
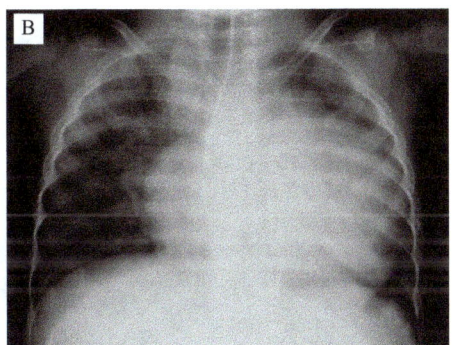
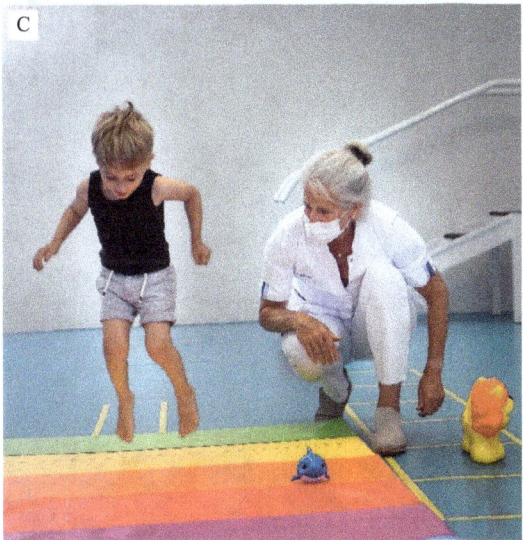

Figure 52.3 (A–C) Hypotonic six-month-old child with severe head lag (A) and hypertrophic cardiomyopathy (B) due to infantile-onset Pompe disease, at start of enzyme replacement therapy (ERT). Same patient, four years old, treated with ERT (C). From Reuser and Schoser, *Pompe Disease*, 3rd edition. Chapter 9: Enzyme replacement therapy in Pompe disease. UNI-MED Verlag AG, Bremen 2021, with permission.

Table 52.1 Main features of infantile-onset Pompe disease (IOPD) and late-onset Pompe disease (LOPD)

	Age at onset	Clinical features	Residual enzyme activity (% of normal)	Life expectancy without treatment	Effect of enzyme replacement therapy (ERT)
IOPD	< 1 yr	Severe hypotonia, progressive limb girdle and facial weakness, macroglossia, cardiomegaly, respiratory insufficiency	< 1%	< 1 yr	Rapid decrease of cardiac enlargement. Improved muscle strength and pulmonary function
LOPD	Childhood: 1–18 yr; adulthood: > 18 yr	Weakness of limb girdle and lumbar paraspinal muscles. Slowly progressive weakness of limb muscles. Diaphragm weakness.	3–25%	55 yr (range: 23–77)	Most patients have improved muscle strength; slight improvement or stabilization of lung function. Increased survival.

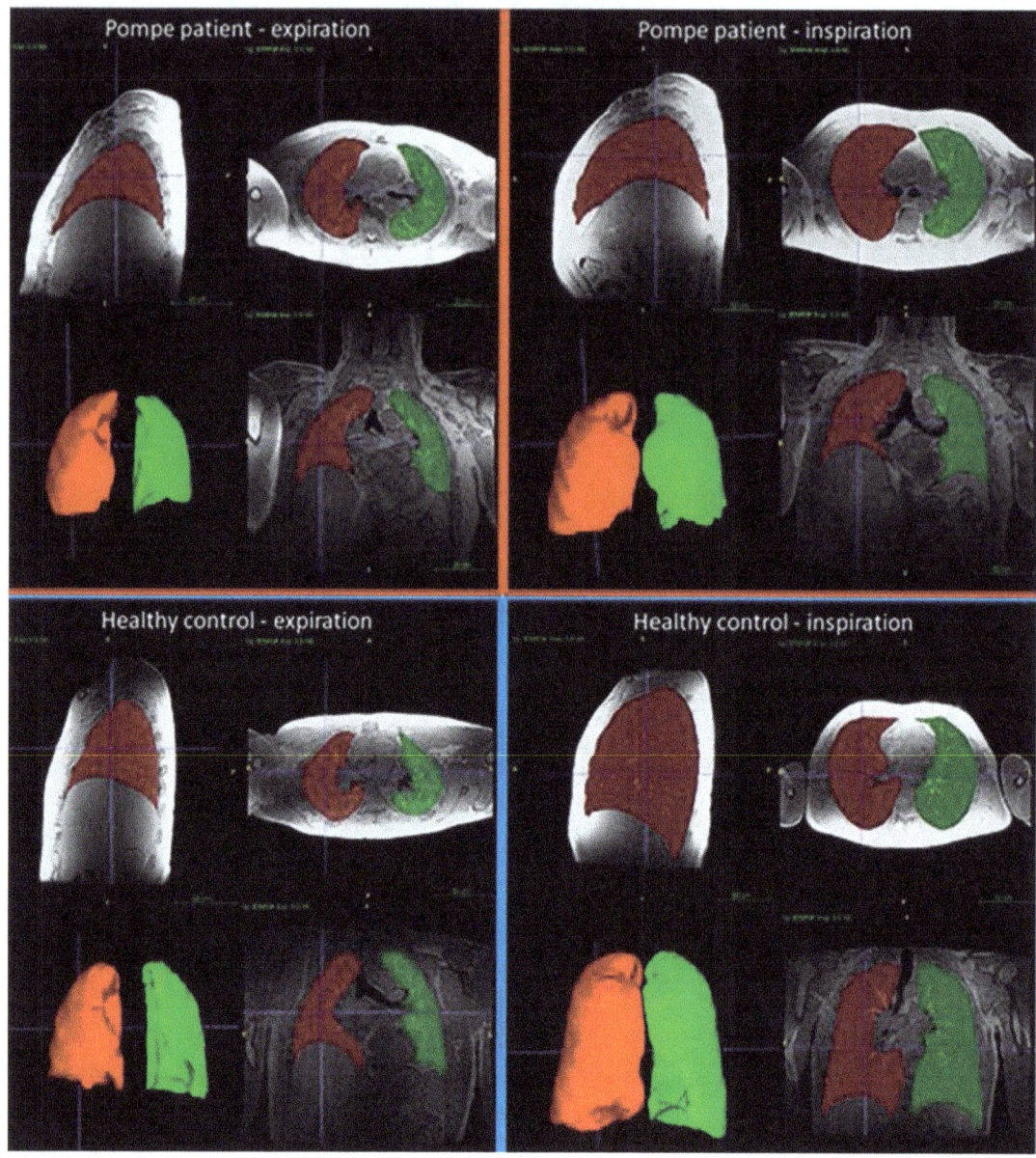

Figure 52.4 Inspiration and expiration in a patient with Pompe disease and in a healthy control. Severely decreased downward movement of the diaphragm in the patient with Pompe disease while anterior–posterior movement of the thorax is still possible. From Harlaar et al., MRI changes in diaphragmatic motion and curvature in Pompe disease over time. *Eur Radiol* 2022;32:8681–8686, with permission.

diaphragm can be disproportional compared with limb muscle weakness, and can be an early sign of disease (Fig. 52.4). A postural drop (> 20% reduction in FVC in lying compared with sitting position) is common. Complaints of respiratory insufficiency are feeling uncomfortable when lying flat, morning headaches, and daytime fatigue. The natural history of LOPD is characterized by slow but unrelenting progression of predominantly limb girdle weakness and pulmonary involvement. The decline in skeletal muscle strength and in respiratory function does not always occur at a similar pace. Respiratory function should be monitored at regular intervals (usually yearly) to ensure a timely start of noninvasive ventilation.

Treatment

Without ERT, patients with IOPD usually die before the age of one year. ERT with recombinant human enzyme in infants is effective in improving muscle strength and cardiac function, and the oldest IOPD patients that received ERT starting within a few weeks–months after birth are now over 20 years of age. A major problem, however, is that the infused enzyme does not cross the blood–brain barrier, and most of these surviving children eventually develop cerebral white matter abnormalities. Furthermore, surviving patients may develop ptosis, facial and distal weakness, and scoliosis.

In adults with LOPD Pompe disease, ERT is also effective, but after a few years, for reasons unknown, there may be some secondary decrease in muscle strength. New RCTs and follow-up studies have been conducted, and much research is being done to develop and assess a more effective variant of ERT, to develop treatment that inhibits the intracellular conversion from glucose to glycogen (substrate reduction therapy), and to further develop gene therapy for this disease. Over the next few years it is to be expected that gene therapy will be tested and, it is hoped, this will be effective and safe for use in patients with Pompe disease.

Suggested Reading

Bolano-Diaz C, Diaz-Manera J. Therapeutic options for the management of Pompe disease: current challenges and clinical evidence in therapeutics and clinical risk management. *Ther Clin Risk Manag* 2022;18:1099–1115. doi: 10.2147/TCRM.S334232. PMID: 36536827; PMCID: PMC9759116.

Diaz-Manera J, Kishnani PS, Kushlaf H, et al.; COMET Investigator Group. Safety and efficacy of avalglucosidase alfa versus alglucosidase alfa in patients with late-onset Pompe disease (COMET): a phase 3, randomised, multicentre trial. *Lancet Neurol* 2021;20(12):1012–1026. PMID: 34800399.

Dimachkie MM, Barohn RJ, Byrne B, et al.; NEO-EXT investigators. Long-term safety and efficacy of avalglucosidase alfa in patients with late-onset Pompe disease. *Neurology* 2022;99(5):e536–e548. doi: 10.1212/WNL.0000000000200746. Epub ahead of print. PMID: 35618441; PMCID: PMC9421599.

Harlaar L, Ciet P, van Tulder G, et al. Chest MRI to diagnose early diaphragmatic weakness in Pompe disease. *Orphanet J Rare Dis* 2021;16(1):21. doi: 10.1186/s13023-020-01627-x. PMID: 33413525; PMCID: PMC7789462.

Schoser B, Laforet P. Therapeutic thoroughfares for adults living with Pompe disease. *Curr Opin Neurol* 2022;35(5):645–650. doi: 10.1097/WCO.0000000000001092. Epub 2022 Aug 8. PMID: 35942661.

Schoser B, Roberts M, Byrne BJ, et al.; PROPEL Study Group. Safety and efficacy of cipaglucosidase alfa plus miglustat versus alglucosidase alfa plus placebo in late-onset Pompe disease (PROPEL): an international, randomised, double-blind, parallel-group, phase 3 trial. *Lancet Neurol* 2021;20(12):1027–1037. doi: 10.1016/S1474-4422(21)00331-8. Erratum in: Lancet Neurol 2023 Aug 9; PMID: 34800400.

van der Beek NA, de Vries JM, Hagemans ML, et al. Clinical features and predictors for disease natural progression in adults with Pompe disease: a nationwide prospective observational study. *Orphanet J Rare Dis* 2012;7:88. doi: 10.1186/1750-1172-7-88. PMID: 23147228; PMCID: PMC3551719.

van der Ploeg AT, Kruijshaar ME, Toscano A, et al.; European Pompe Consortium. European consensus for starting and stopping enzyme replacement therapy in adult patients with Pompe disease: a 10-year experience. *Eur J Neurol* 2017;24(6):768–e31. doi: 10.1111/ene.13285. Epub 2017 May 6. PMID: 28477382.

van der Ploeg AT, Reuser AJ. Pompe's disease. *Lancet* 2008;372(9646):1342–1353. doi: 10.1016/S0140-6736(08)61555-X. PMID: 18929906.

CASE 53: McArdle Disease (Glycogen Storage Disease (GSD) Type V); Myophosphorylase Deficiency, Rhabdomyolysis

Clinical History

A 40-year-old woman was referred because she complained about cramping and swelling of the hands and leg muscles for more than four years. The referring neurologist also found hyperCKaemia (> 10 × ULN). The symptoms bothered her when using her computer or when she was performing squats. She had never produced dark urine and she had never noticed muscle weakness. Previous disease history was inconspicuous except for goiter. The family history was negative for neuromuscular disorders.

Examination

The neurological examination was normal.

Diagnostic Considerations

The diagnosis of McArdle disease seemed likely based on the physical activity-induced cramps, rapidly diminishing at rest, the episode of rhabdomyolysis (i.e., physical activity-related cramping and muscle swelling associated with a CK > 10 × ULN), and the normal neurological examination.

Ancillary Investigations

Serum CK activity was markedly elevated (> 13,000 U/L, i.e., > 10 × ULN). The patient admitted to having done some exercises the day prior to the lab test. Repeat measurement after a few weeks showed activities of 3389 and 1550 U/L, respectively.

A nonischaemic forearm test was performed and showed only a minimal increase in serum lactate (from resting value of 0.4 to 0.7 mmol/L after forced contraction), whereas ammonia rose from 14 to 489 µmol/L. This result is highly suggestive of a disorder of muscle glycolysis of which McArdle disease is the most common. Ammonia production is enhanced in glycolytic disorders, due to an activation of the myokinase/myoadenylate deaminase pathway.

At the time, a muscle biopsy was the next diagnostic step. It was diagnostic for McArdle disease with subsarcolemmal vacuoles – visible on the H&E stain – that contained glycogen on the periodic acid-Schiff (PAS) stain (Fig. 53.1). Immunohistochemistry showed that myophosphorylase was absent in the muscle fibres. Biochemically, there was deficiency of the enzyme myophosphorylase (8 IU/L, normal > 12 to 560) in the muscle tissue. Subsequent sequencing of the

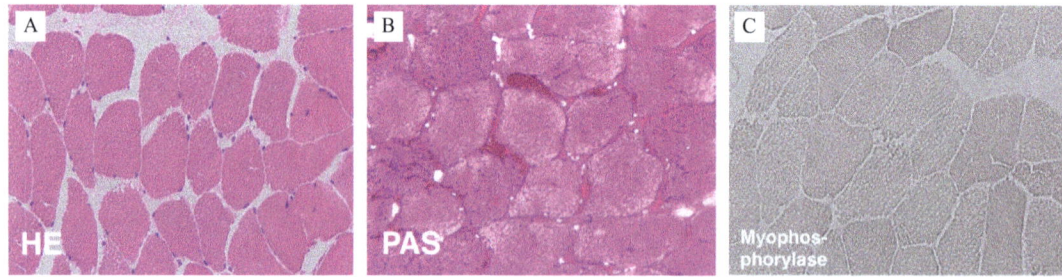

Figure 53.1 (A–C) A skeletal muscle biopsy shows small subsarcolemmal vacuoles on H&E staining (A), and a positive periodic acid-Schiff (PAS) reaction, also at the subsarcolemmal level (B). The intense staining disappears after digesting by diastase (not shown). Myophosphorylase staining showed no enzyme activity throughout the muscle fibres (C).

gene revealed that she was compound heterozygote for two missense variants in exons 4 and 12 of the *PYGM* (phosphorylase, glycogen, muscle) gene.

Follow-Up

We advised the patient to avoid strenuous physical activity. A carbohydrate-rich diet was prescribed. In subsequent years, no weakness developed.

General Remarks

McArdle disease (glycogen storage disease (GSD) type V) is a rare but the most frequent type of carbohydrate metabolic myopathies. The disease is autosomal recessively inherited and is caused by bi-allelic mutations of the *PYGM* gene, which encodes for the myophosphorylase protein, the muscle isoform of glycogen phosphorylase. In most affected patients, there is no detectable glycogen phosphorylase activity. Since the liver and heart isoforms are produced normally, McArdle disease is a pure myopathy.

Myophosphorylase is involved in converting glycogen into glucose-1-phosphate. This, in turn, is converted to glucose-6-phosphate, which enters glycolysis and subsequently the Krebs cycle and oxidative phosphorylation to generate ATP under aerobic conditions. In patients with McArdle disease, glycolysis is blocked upstream, but patients can still absorb glucose from the blood and convert it into glucose-6-phosphate, which then enters the downstream steps of glycolysis.

Onset can be in childhood but diagnosis is frequently delayed until after 30 years of age. Patients with McArdle disease suffer from physical activity-related symptoms (fatigue, muscle stiffness, myalgia, and weakness) when brief and intense isometric muscle contractions take place, such as lifting a heavy object or dynamic physical activity with a high intensity, like climbing stairs or running (Table 53.1). There is marked variation even within families. If physical activity is sustained, painful contractures occur. One should always ask whether the patient experiences a 'second wind' phenomenon which is almost pathognomonic and characterized by the sudden improvement of physical activity tolerance after 6–8 minutes of aerobic, dynamic physical activity (walking or cycling). It occurs in ~80% of the patients and is attributable to an improved delivery of extramuscular energy substrates, free fatty acids, and glucose to working muscles, which partially compensates for the impaired glycogen breakdown.

Rhabdomyolysis is encountered in more than half of the patients after intense muscle contractions. Proximal muscle weakness is usually mild and only found in patients > 40 years of age.

The diagnosis is based on the history and the inability of the patient to produce lactate during a nonischaemic forearm physical activity test, and genetic analysis. Resting CK (in between attacks of rhabdomyolysis) is markedly elevated. Currently, a muscle biopsy as a diagnostic step to show the lack of muscle glycogen phosphorylase activity can be omitted, but may be useful in case of uncertain genetic analysis. EMG does not have added value.

A Cochrane review showed that there was only low-quality evidence of improvement in physical activity performance with creatine, oral sucrose, ramipril, and a carbohydrate-rich diet. It is of utmost importance to educate the patient about the risks of rhabdomyolysis provoked by physical activity. Resistance training could be a useful adjunct to aerobic physical activity. However, implementation of the resistance training approach should be done under close supervision to avoid rhabdomyolysis. Patients suffering from McArdle disease are known to have difficulty increasing their muscle mass. As a consequence, with advancing age, muscle atrophy and weakness occur, especially involving the shoulder girdle and paraspinal muscles. Many patients learn, by experience or by instruction, to improve their exercise tolerance by exploiting the 'second wind' phenomenon.

Rhabdomyolysis (RML)

Based on a systematic review, rhabdomyolysis (RML) is defined as a clinical syndrome of acute muscle weakness, myalgia, and muscle swelling

Table 53.1 Main features of McArdle disease

- Onset can be in childhood, but diagnosis is frequently delayed > 30 years.
- Patients suffer from physical activity-related symptoms (fatigue, muscle stiffness, myalgia, and weakness) with brief and intense isometric muscle contractions.
- Marked – even intrafamilial – variability.
- 'Second wind' phenomenon is almost pathognomonic and occurs in ~80% of the patients.
- Rhabdomyolysis occurs in half of the patients.
- Fixed proximal muscle weakness is usually mild and found in patients > 40 years.

combined with a CK cut-off value of > 1000 IU/L or CK > 5 × ULN. Serum CK activity rises 2–12 hours after onset of muscle injury, peaks at 3–5 days after injury, and declines over the subsequent 6–10 days, unless a neuromuscular disease is underlying an RML episode, such as is the case in the McArdle patient described above. Myoglobinuria is only present in half of the cases and thus its absence does not rule out the diagnosis. The classic clinical triad of rhabdomyolysis includes muscle weakness, myalgia, and dark urine and is only present in 10–20%. RML may range in severity from an asymptomatic elevation of CK activity in blood to a potentially life-threatening syndrome associated with very high CK (> 15,000 U/L), and myoglobinuria resulting in acute kidney injury (AKI) due to combined ischaemic tubular injury (prerenal injury) and direct myoglobin toxicity (renal injury). The treshhold of CK causing AKI is unknown and so is its occurrence (13–50%).

Other complications of RML include the compartment syndrome, which may also be the cause of RML, disseminated intravascular coagulation, and cardiac arrhythmias.

Rhabdomyolysis has an extensive differential diagnosis (see Chapter 3, Box 3.23). Traumatic causes are more common in the developing countries, while anoxia/ischaemia and drug abuse are the most frequent causes in the Western world. Infections are largely responsible for RML in children, whereas drugs and trauma are the most common causes in adults (up to 80% of cases).

Neuromuscular causes include *RYR1*-related exertional rhabdomyolysis, disorders of glycogen metabolism (McArdle disease and others), disorders of long chain fatty oxidation (CPT2 (see **Case 54**), VLCAD), mitochondrial myopathies, and a group of miscellaneous hereditary myopathies. Among the latter, one can distinguish dystrophinopathy, limb girdle muscular dystrophy R2 (LGMDR2), LGMDR9, LGMDR12, and others. Next-generation sequencing (NGS) panels (combination of both sequencing and deletion/duplication copy number variant (CNV) analysis) are currently used to disclose the causative pathological gene variant.

There is no solid evidence about the timing of a work-up for neuromuscular causes. If there has been only one event and the patient has no history of muscle complaints (physical activity-related myalgia, cramps, muscle swelling or weakness) or if the CK normalizes after the RML episode, an extensive search for a neuromuscular cause often does not take place. However, recurrent rhabdomyolysis, a positive family history for attacks, or persistent hyperCKaemia warrant further investigations. If a muscle biopsy is part of the work-up, a word of caution about its timing: it should not be done immediately after the attack since this will show extensive muscle damage.

A substantial proportion of patients presenting with rhabdomyolysis in whom a hereditary myopathy is suspected remain currently genetically unsolved. Different genes may possibly be involved in an increased susceptibility for developing rhabdomyolysis.

RML treatment should be aimed at elimination of the toxic agent if possible and avoidance of cardiovascular (associated with electrolyte abnormalities) or renal complications. Pharmacological therapy of RML is based on volume replacement therapy in combination with diuretics under regular control of potassium, calcium, and phosphate levels. Considering the frequent occurrence of cardiac arrhythmias in RML, ECG monitoring is advisable. In case of myoglobinuric AKI, the basic principles of treatment are adequate nutrition, management of metabolic complications, and kidney replacement therapy if overt renal failure develops. Dialysis is indicated when uremic encephalopathy, deteriorating kidney function, uncontrolled hyperkalaemia, metabolic acidosis, and fluid overload occur.

Prevention of a rhabdomyolysis attack is difficult, since we currently do not know all of the risk factors. However, there are ways one can lower one's risk.

- Be aware that job or recreational activities involving exertion and/or heat exposure (e.g., military personnel) could increase the risk for rhabdomyolysis and try to avoid these risk factors if possible.
- Learn to recognize the signs and symptoms of heat-related illnesses and take steps to prevent getting overheated. Take frequent rest breaks and use cooling stations if available.
- Stay hydrated. Drink caffeine-free and low-sugar products. Avoid alcohol use when working in the heat.
- If one starts experiencing any rhabdomyolysis symptoms, stop the current activity right away, cool down, start drinking fluids, and go to a healthcare provider to get checked for rhabdomyolysis.

Suggested Reading

Godfrey R, Quinlivan R. Skeletal muscle disorders of glycogenolysis and glycolysis. *Nat Rev Neurol* 2016;12(7):393–402. doi: 10.1038/nrneurol.2016.75. Epub 2016 May 27. PMID: 27231184.

Kazemi-Esfarjani P, Skomorowska E, Jensen TD, Haller RG, Vissing J. A nonischemic forearm exercise test for McArdle disease. *Ann Neurol* 2002;52(2):153–159. doi: 10.1002/ana.10263. PMID: 12210784.

Kruijt N, van den Bersselaar LR, Kamsteeg EJ, et al. The etiology of rhabdomyolysis: an interaction between genetic susceptibility and external triggers. *Eur J Neurol* 2021;28(2):647–659. doi: 10.1111/ene.14553. Epub 2020 Oct 25. PMID: 32978841; PMCID: PMC7821272.

Martín MA, Lucia A, Arenas J, Andreu AL. Glycogen storage disease type V. 2006 Apr 19 [updated 2019 Jun 20]. In Adam MP, Mirzaa GM, Pagon RA, et al., editors. *GeneReviews®* [Internet]. Seattle, WA: University of Washington; 1993–2023. PMID: 20301518.

Nance JR, Mammen AL. Diagnostic evaluation of rhabdomyolysis. *Muscle Nerve* 2015;51(6):793–810. doi: 10.1002/mus.24606. Epub 2015 Mar 14. PMID: 25678154; PMCID: PMC4437836.

Scalco RS, Gardiner AR, Pitceathly RD, et al. Rhabdomyolysis: a genetic perspective. *Orphanet J Rare Dis* 2015;10:51. doi: 10.1186/s13023-015-0264-3. PMID: 25929793; PMCID: PMC4522153.

Stahl K, Rastelli E, Schoser B. A systematic review on the definition of rhabdomyolysis. *J Neurol* 2020;267(4):877–882. doi: 10.1007/s00415-019-09185-4. Epub 2019 Jan 7. PMID: 30617905.

Zutt R, van der Kooi AJ, Linthorst GE, Wanders RJ, de Visser M. Rhabdomyolysis: review of the literature. *Neuromuscul Disord* 2014;24(8):651–659. doi: 10.1016/j.nmd.2014.05.005. Epub 2014 May 21. PMID: 24946698. d

Carnitine Palmitoyltransferase-II (CPT2) Deficiency

Clinical History

A 39-year-old man was referred because of three attacks of severe myalgia accompanied by 'bloody urine'. There were no complaints about muscle weakness. There had been preceding exercise, but not excessively. Prior to one attack, he had suffered from a viral infection.

During childhood, at sports he had often noticed having muscle ache, once accompanied by 'red urine'. There was no 'second wind' phenomenon. After three days, the muscle complaints usually disappeared. At age 20 years he had suffered a similar attack during a soccer game and again at age 37 after playing volleyball. On that occasion, CK was determined and found to be approximately 800,000 IU/L, which led to admission to hospital for hydration and monitoring of his kidney function. His CK normalized rapidly. At that time, a muscle biopsy was performed that showed no accumulation of fat or glycogen and no mitochondrial abnormalities.

Medical history was otherwise unremarkable. Family history was negative for muscle disease.

Examination

The examination was found to be normal, no muscle weakness.

Diagnostic Considerations

The patient's history is characteristic of recurrent attacks of rhabdomyolysis (RML): exercise-elicited acute onset myalgia, sometimes accompanied by myoglobinuria and markedly elevated CK, rapidly normalizing.

The cause of recurrent RML is very likely a muscle disease (see Chapter 3, Box 3.23). A disorder of glycogen metabolism (e.g., McArdle disease, Case 53) is unlikely because of the normal CK in between the attacks and normal muscle biopsy. The same holds true for a mitochondrial disorder as the cause of RML. Becker muscular dystrophy and limb girdle muscular dystrophies (LGMDs, i.e., dysferlin-related LGMD (*DYSF*)(**Case 47**), anoctamin 5-related LGMD (*ANO5*), fukutin-related protein LGMD (*FKRP*) **Case 42**, and sarcoglycanopathies (*SGCA*, *SGCC*)) may be associated with RML, but can be ruled out because the patient did not have muscle weakness and had a normal CK between attacks. Other potential causes are disorders of fatty acid metabolism, including carnitine palmitoyltransferase-II deficiency (*CPT2*), very long-chain acetyl-CoA dehydrogenase deficiency (*ACADVL*), and multiple acyl-coenzyme A dehydrogenase deficiency (*ETFB*, *ETHDH*). In addition, RML can be *RYR1*-related (see **Case 56**), due to Brody disease (*SERCA1*), occur in TANGO2-syndrome, and can be caused by LPIN1 deficiency. TANGO2-syndrome is an autosomal recessively inherited disorder, characterized by metabolic encephalopathy and arrhythmias, in addition to RML. LPIN1 deficiency is autosomal recessively inherited and the second most common cause of severe, recurrent episodes of rhabdomyolysis in early childhood, which can result in serious morbidity and mortality.

Given the prevalence of CPT2 or very long-chain acyl-CoA dehydrogenase (VLCAD) deficiency as a cause of RML, and normal CK, diagnostic investigations were targeted at those enzymes.

Ancillary Investigations

Acylcarnitine profile analysis showed abnormalities indicative of CPT2 deficiency (i.e., accumulation of C16 and C18 carnitines). Subsequently gene analysis showed compound heterozygosity for two pathogenic variants in the *CPT2* gene (338c>T (S113L) and 370C>T (R124X)).

Follow-Up

After we had diagnosed the patient with CPT2 deficiency, we referred him to a dietitian who prescribed a high-carbohydrate and low-fat diet and further advised him to consume carbohydrates before exercise and to avoid night-time fasting longer than 12 hours. We stressed that he consult us immediately in case of symptoms of rhabdomyolysis. He has not experienced any serious attacks associated with myoglobinuria since.

General Remarks

Fatty Acid Oxidation Disorders (FAODs)

During periods of decreased carbohydrate intake, prolonged fasting, or increased energy demands, the body's glycogen stores fall short and energy needs of the heart, skeletal muscle, and liver are derived from the oxidation of fatty acids in healthy individuals. Short-chain and medium-chain fatty acids can enter the mitochondria directly, but long-chain fatty acids (LCFAs) must be transferred in via a shuttle involving three enzymes/transporters (CPT1, carnitine-acylcarnitine translocase (CACT), and CPT2) and carnitine (Fig. 54.1). Once inside the mitochondrial matrix, the breakdown of LCFAs (β-oxidation) progresses, resulting in the sequential cleavage of 2-carbon acetyl-coenzyme A (CoA) from the fatty acid chain and the transfer of electrons to the respiratory chain for adenosine triphosphate (ATP) production.

Fatty acid oxidation disorders (FAODs) are inborn errors of metabolism due to disruption of either mitochondrial β-oxidation or the fatty acid transport using the carnitine transport pathway. FAODs are characterized by exercise intolerance, muscle pain, and episodes of RML related to prolonged exercise, as well as other triggers such as fever, fasting, stress, drugs (such as sodium valproate and statins), and certain anaesthetic drugs. The most common FAODs resulting in rhabdomyolysis are CPT2 and VLCAD deficiency.

CPT2 Deficiency

There are three forms of CPT2 deficiency: lethal neonatal, severe infantile hepatocardiomuscular, and myopathic. The adult myopathic form of CPT2 deficiency is inherited in an autosomal recessive manner and has a variable onset (first to sixth decade). This form is characterized by recurrent attacks of myalgia accompanied by myoglobinuria and precipitated by prolonged exercise (especially after fasting), cold exposure, or stress. During attacks, there may be muscle weakness. Usually CK is normal between attacks.

High-performance liquid chromatography tandem mass spectrometry demonstrates increased levels of acylcarnitine levels C16 and C18:1, specifically with an overall increase of C12 to C18 acylcarnitines. The diagnosis is established by the identification of bi-allelic pathogenic variants in the *CPT2* gene. Muscle biopsy is usually normal and therefore not helpful if CPT2 deficiency is considered.

Recommendations are the following once the diagnosis has been established: a high-carbohydrate (70%), low-fat (<20%) diet, take

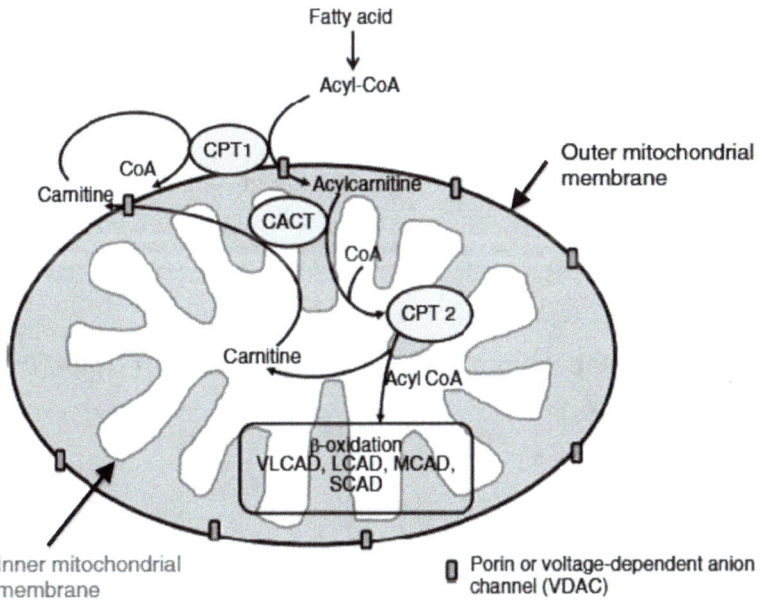

Figure 54.1 Diagram of the acylcarnitine shuttle and β-oxidation of fatty acids in mitochondria. From: Beger et al., Acylcarnitines as translational biomarkers of mitochondrial dysfunction. In *Mitochondrial Dysfunction Caused by Drugs and Environmental Toxicants*, edited by Will et al. 2018: pp. 383–393, John Wiley and Sons, Hoboken, New Jersey, USA, with permission.
CACT = carnitine/acylcarnitine translocase; CPT1 = carnitine palmitoyltransferase-I; CPT2 = carnitine palmitoyltransferase-II; LCAD = long-chain acyl-CoA dehydrogenase deficiency; MCAD = medium-chain acyl-CoA dehydrogenase deficiency; SCAD = short-chain acyl-CoA dehydrogenase deficiency; VLCAD = very long-chain acyl-CoA dehydrogenase deficiency.

carbohydrates before exercise, and avoid night time fasting longer than 12 hours.

Very Long-Chain Acyl-CoA Dehydrogenase (VLCAD) Deficiency

Very long-chain acyl-CoA dehydrogenase (VLCAD) is an enzyme associated with the inner mitochondrial membrane that plays an important role in the initial step of mitochondrial β-oxidation of long-chain fatty acids with a chain length of 14 to 20 carbons. There are several phenotypes, ranging from a severe neonatal/early childhood-onset form presenting with cardiomyopathy, hepatic disease, intermittent hypoglycaemia, and hypotonia with high mortality in infancy to a childhood- to adult-onset form presenting with exercise intolerance, muscle cramps, and RML. Identification of VLCAD deficiency is possible through newborn screening. Patients presenting with the adult-onset form may have symptoms between episodes of RML. Triggers for RML include fasting, prolonged aerobic exercise, emotional stress, shivering and cold, or other catabolic stress such as infections and fever and certain drugs such as sodium valproate and statins. Serum CK may be normal or raised between attacks. Muscle biopsy is unhelpful, and the most important first-line investigation is analysis of the blood acylcarnitine profile, which shows accumulation of long-chain acyl-carnitines usually with prominent acylcarnitine levels (C14:1). Diagnosis is confirmed by finding homozygous or compound heterozygous variants in the *ACADVL* gene, albeit gene panel testing may also be the first-tier diagnostic test.

Other FAODs manifesting with rhabdomyolysis include long-chain 3-hydroxy acyl-CoA dehydrogenase deficiency (LCHADD, *HADHB*), mitochondrial trifunctional protein deficiency (TFPD/MTP, *HADHA*, *HADHB*), and carnitine-acylcarnitine translocase (CACT) deficiency (*SLC25A20*); see also Chapter 3, Box 3.23.

Suggested Reading

Kruijt N, van den Bersselaar LR, Kamsteeg EJ, et al. The etiology of rhabdomyolysis: an interaction between genetic susceptibility and external triggers. *Eur J Neurol* 2021;28(2):647–659. doi: 10.1111/ene.14553. Epub 2020 Oct 25. PMID: 32978841; PMCID: PMC7821272.

Merritt JL 2nd, Norris M, Kanungo S. Fatty acid oxidation disorders. *Ann Transl Med* 2018;6(24):473. doi: 10.21037/atm.2018.10.57. PMID: 30740404; PMCID: PMC6331364.

Scalco RS, Gardiner AR, Pitceathly RD, et al. Rhabdomyolysis: a genetic perspective. *Orphanet J Rare Dis* 2015;10:51. doi: 10.1186/s13023-015-0264-3. PMID: 25929793; PMCID: PMC4522153.

Wieser T. Carnitine palmitoyltransferase II deficiency. 2004 Aug 27 [updated 2019 Jan 3]. In Adam MP, Mirzaa GM, Pagon RA, et al., editors. *GeneReviews*® [Internet]. Seattle, WA: University of Washington; 1993–2023. PMID: 20301431.

Mitochondrial Myopathies: Chronic Progressive External Ophthalmoplegia (CPEO)

Clinical History

A 52-year-old woman visited the neurologist because of drooping eyelids, which had not changed much over the past 10 years. She felt socially disabled because of the constant need to tilt her head upwards. Old photographs showed slight drooping from her mid-teens onwards. At one point she had experienced transient double vision. Speaking, swallowing, and limb muscle strength were reportedly normal. The family history was negative.

Examination

There was symmetric ptosis partly covering the pupils when looking straight ahead, which did not increase when looking upwards or laterally. Eye movements were impaired in all directions (external ophthalmoplegia); there was no diplopia.

Diagnostic Considerations

A mitochondrial disease was a likely explanation. In patients with this typical mitochondrial presentation of chronic progressive external ophthalmoplegia (CPEO), it is justified to refrain from performing a skeletal muscle biopsy and to start the diagnostic process with analyses of a mitochondrial gene panel. Arguments against myasthenia gravis (MG) were the slow and steady progression, symmetry, absence of evident diplopia, absence of worsening of ptosis, and diplopia on looking upwards or sideways. However, as myasthenia gravis is a treatable disease, it should be properly excluded. Arguments against myotonic dystrophy were the absence of clinical myotonia, absence of other weakness or signs of this disease, and a negative family history. Arguments against oculopharyngeal muscular dystrophy were the age at onset and absence of dysphagia at age 52, and the negative family history. A congenital myopathy and congenital myasthenia were considered possible alternative diagnoses.

Ancillary Investigations

Electrophysiological tests (repetitive nerve stimulation and single-fibre EMG) for neuromuscular transmission disorder were negative. Subsequently, DNA analysis on leukocytes revealed compound heterozygosity for two pathogenic variants in the *POLG* gene, which explains the clinical phenotype. Cardiac evaluation with Holter and echocardiography was normal.

Follow-Up

She declined eyelid crutches and surgery, despite the perceived disability. Ten years after presentation, she reported no change of symptoms.

General Remarks

Primary Mitochondrial Disorders (PMDs)

Primary mitochondrial disorders (PMDs) are caused by variants in the nuclear DNA (nDNA) or in the mitochondrial DNA (mtDNA) affecting oxidative phosphorylation. Disorders of fatty acid oxidation, which take place within the mitochondrion, and conditions that lead to secondary mitochondrial dysfunction (e.g., inclusion body myositis, immobilization, and ageing) are not counted among the PMDs. Over 1000 nuclear genes encode proteins that are now known to be needed for mitochondrial structure and for proteins involved in oxidative phosphorylation, including the electron transport (or respiratory) chain. Mutations in nuclear genes that are responsible for mtDNA maintenance cause mtDNA defects, often multiple deletions or depletion (reduction in the amount of mtDNA).

Primary mitochondrial disorders can present at any age and potentially affect any organ (Table 55.1). A PMD may involve one single organ only, but often there are multiple features that may cluster into overlapping central and/or neuromuscular system syndromes. The most common manifestation in infants is Leigh syndrome (developmental delay or retardation, hypotonia, respiratory dysfunction, epileptic seizures, lactate acidosis, poor feeding, death within one year in early-onset cases). PMDs predominantly involving the neuromuscular system are mostly found in adults and are listed in Table 55.2. Chronic progressive external ophthalmoplegia (CPEO) is the most prevalent neuromuscular manifestation of PMDs. Isolated limb weakness, myalgia, and exercise intolerance without any other feature of mitochondrial dysfunction are not features of PMD.

Because of the multisystem nature of many PMDs, a clinically suspected diagnosis can be supported by careful history taking, including the family history, and clinical examination. Various metabolic tests associated with mitochondrial dysfunction are advocated. High lactate and high lactate:pyruvate ratios in blood have low sensitivity and high specificity. Cerebral MRI abnormalities may be closely correlated to certain distinct PMDs, in particular in children. The final diagnosis rests upon genetic testing. In the case of pathogenic mtDNA changes, genetic testing is complicated by the phenomenon of heteroplasmy: each cell contains thousands of mtDNA copies, and the amount of mutated mtDNA relative to the amount of wild-type mtDNA differs between cells and between tissues. Heteroplasmy levels may be too low to be detected in leukocytes (but may be somewhat higher in urinary epithelial cells). Therefore, a diagnosis may require the genetic investigation of clinically involved tissue such as muscle, in which the proportion of mtDNA pathogenic variants exceeds a critical threshold. A muscle biopsy can also confirm mitochondrial dysfunction by showing ragged red fibres (H&E stain) and cytochrome c oxidase-negative fibres (COX-SDH stain) (Fig. 55.1). As a PMD may be transmitted autosomal dominantly, autosomal recessively, X-linked, maternally, or is not transmitted at all, a diagnosis at the molecular genetic level is paramount for adequate genetic counselling. At present, there is no drug treatment for PMDs, and also no robust evidence for the benefit of nutritional supplements or carnitine.

Table 55.1 Common clinical features of primary mitochondrial disorders

Neuromuscular	Central nervous system	Other
Ptosis, external ophthalmoplegia	Developmental, retardation	Lactate acidosis
Myopathy, CK mildly elevated	Cerebellar ataxia	Diabetes mellitus
Prolonged physical activity intolerance	Dystonia	Exocrine pancreatic dysfunction
Rhabdomyolysis	Stroke-like episodes	Cochlear sensorineural hearing loss
Peripheral neuropathy, sensory ataxia	Myoclonic epilepsy	Gastrointestinal dysmotility
Cardiomyopathy	Epileptic encephalopathy	Renal tubulopathy/failure
	Migraine	Nephrotic syndrome
	Retinitis pigmentosa	Sideroblastic anaemia
	Spasticity	Pregnancy loss
	Parkinsonism	Early menopause
	Optic neuropathy	

Table 55.2 Primary mitochondrial disorders (PMDs) with prominent neuromuscular features

PMD	Genes	Inheritance
Chronic progressive external ophthalmoplegia (CPEO)	*POLG* (*POLG1*), *POLG2*, *PEO1* (*TWNK*), *SLC25A4* (*ANT1*), *RRM2B*, *DNA2*, *OPA1*, *SPG7*, causing secondary mtDNA multiple deletions; single large-scale mtDNA deletion. Rarely a single nucleotide mtDNA variant, including m.3243A>G	AD or AR (*POLG*), AD (other nuclear genes), maternal, or sporadic, not transmitted (large single mutations)
Kearns–Sayre syndrome (KSS): onset < 20 years, CPEO, retinitis pigmentosa, ataxia, cardiac conduction block, elevated CSF protein	Single large-scale deletion of mtDNA	Sporadic, not transmitted
Sensory ataxic neuropathy, dysarthria, ophthalmoplegia (SANDO) Myoclonic epilepsy, myopathy, sensory ataxia (MEMSA)	*POLG*, *PEO1* (*TWNK*)	AR
CPEO, proximal weakness, respiratory insufficiency, neuropathy, dysphagia, rhabdomyolysis. Infantile, childhood-onset and adult-onset forms. Possibly treatable (nucleoside replacement therapy)	*TK2*	AR
Mitochondrial neurogastrointestinal encephalomyopathy (MNGIE), also CPEO, polyneuropathy	*TYMP*	AR
Mitochondrial myopathy, lactic acidosis, and sideroblastic anaemia (MLASA)	*YARS2*	AR
Mitochondrial encephalomyopathy with lactic acidosis and stroke-like episodes (MELAS)	m.3243A>G, *MT-TL1* (80%), amongst other mitochondrial genes	Maternal
Myoclonus epilepsy with ragged red fibres (MERRF)	m.8344A>G, m.8356T>C, m.8363G>A, and m.8361G>A. *MT-TK* (> 90%), among other mitochondrial genes	Maternal
Neuropathy, (episodic) ataxia and retinitis pigmentosa (NARP), various CNS abnormalities	m.8993T > G; m.8993T>C (*MT-ATP6*)	Maternal
Rhabdomyolysis, intolerance to prolonged exercise, with or without weakness	*MTCYB*, *MTCO1*, *MTCO2*, *MTCO3* *TK2*	Maternal AR
Reversible infantile respiratory chain deficiency (RIRCD) (reversible infantile cytochrome c oxidase deficiency myopathy): floppy infant, spontaneous recovery after age 6 months	Probably digenic: common homoplasmic m.14674T>C/G mt-tRNA^{Glu} mutation and heterozygous mutation in a nuclear gene, e.g., *TRMU*	Digenic inheritance

AD = autosomal dominant; AR = autosomal recessive; genes in italics

Chronic Progressive External Ophthalmoplegia

In adolescence and adulthood, CPEO (bilateral ptosis and external ophthalmoplegia, Fig. 55.2) can occur isolated and can be mild, but there can additionally be proximal limb weakness ('CPEO plus'), and CPEO can also be part of a more complex syndrome, such as the Kearns–Sayre syndrome (KSS) and sensory ataxia neuropathy dysarthria and ophthalmoplegia (SANDO), see Table 55.2.

On genetic testing, most patients have a single or multiple mtDNA deletions. Only in a minority of cases, a nuclear gene panel can identify a responsible mutation. By far the most frequent involved nuclear gene is the DNA polymerase subunit gamma (*POLG*). *POLG* mutations

Case 55 Chronic Progressive External Ophthalmoplegia (CPEO)

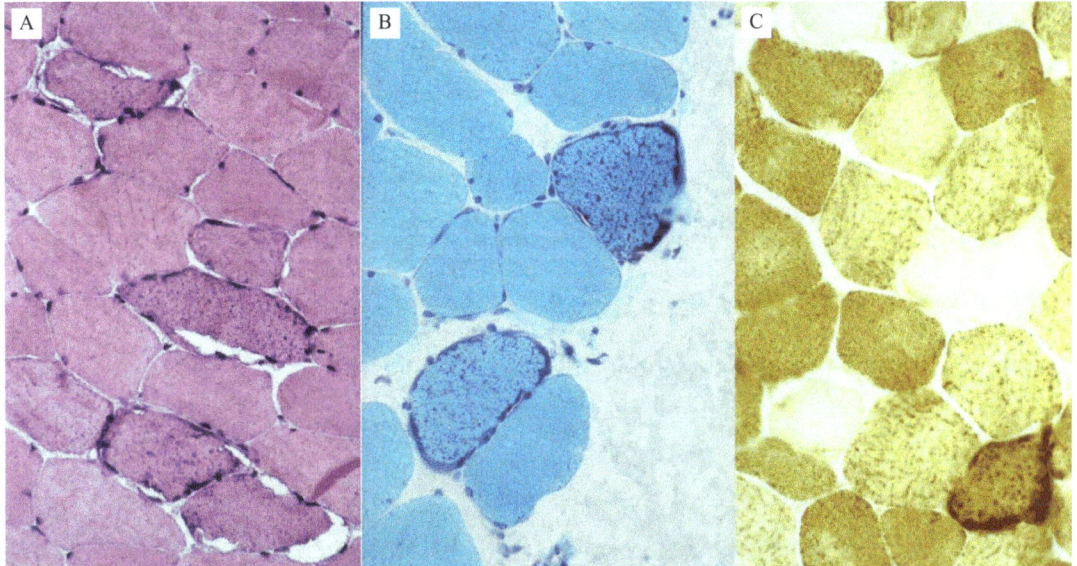

Figure 55.1 (A–C) 'Ragged-red' and 'ragged-blue' muscle fibres on H&E (A) and modified Gomori trichrome stain (B), caused by abnormal subsarcolemmal accumulation of mitochondria. Negative staining for the mitochondrial enzyme cytochrome oxidase (C).

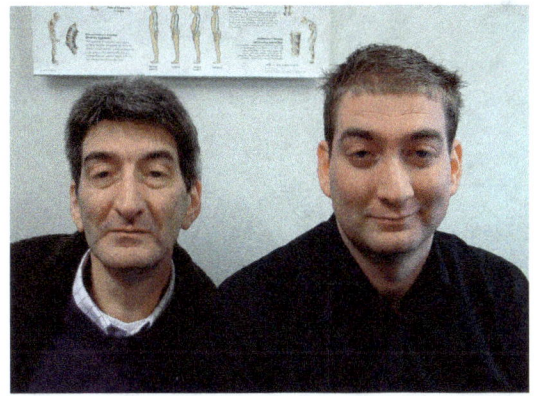

Figure 55.2 Father and son with symmetric ptosis and a progressive external ophthalmoplegia due to a pathogenetic variant in the nuclear *TWNK* PEO1 gene.

in particular can result in extremely heterogeneous phenotypes, especially in infancy and childhood. They can cause Alpers syndrome (psychomotor retardation, epilepsy, and liver failure) or Alpers-like syndromes with proximal myopathy or hypotonia. Sodium valproate given for seizure control can trigger liver failure in patients with a *POLG* mitochondrial disease. Other *POLG*-related features are proximal myopathy, large-fibre sensory neuropathy, dysarthria, parkinsonism, cerebellar ataxia, myoclonus, various forms of epilepsy, diabetes mellitus, and early menopause.

Management of CPEO includes advice on the symptomatic treatment of ptosis leading to functional blindness and social handicap. Ptosis may be alleviated by prosthetic inserts placed inside spectacles to raise the eyelids, albeit they can cause discomfort if not properly fitted. Most patients prefer surgical correction. In isolated CPEO, patients should be screened for cardiac conduction and rhythm disturbances, diabetes mellitus, and hearing loss. Genetic advice in case of a *POLG* or other nuclear gene mutation follows the Mendelian rules. In the case of an mtDNA defect, it is more difficult to provide accurate genetic counselling.

Suggested Reading

Chinnery PF. Primary mitochondrial disorders overview. 2000 Jun 8 [updated 2021 Jul 29]. In Adam MP, Mirzaa GM, Pagon RA, et al., editors. *GeneReviews®* [Internet]. Seattle, WA: University of Washington; 1993–2023. PMID: 20301403.

Hathazi D, Griffin H, Jennings MJ, et al. Metabolic shift underlies recovery in reversible infantile respiratory chain deficiency. *EMBO J* 2020;39(23): e105364. doi: 10.15252/embj.2020105364. Epub 2020 Oct 31. PMID: 33128823; PMCID: PMC7705457.

Heighton JN, Brady LI, Sadikovic B, Bulman DE, Tarnopolsky MA. Genotypes of chronic progressive external ophthalmoplegia in a large adult-onset cohort. *Mitochondrion* 2019;49:227–231. doi:

10.1016/j.mito.2019.09.002. Epub 2019 Sep 12. PMID: 31521625.

McClelland C, Manousakis G, Lee MS. Progressive external ophthalmoplegia. *Curr Neurol Neurosci Rep* 2016;16(6):53. doi: 10.1007/s11910-016-0652-7. PMID: 27072953.

Orsucci D, Caldarazzo Ienco E, Rossi A, Siciliano G, Mancuso M. Mitochondrial syndromes revisited. *J Clin Med* 2021;10(6):1249. doi: 10.3390/jcm10061249. PMID: 33802970; PMCID: PMC8002645.

Parikh S, Karaa A, Goldstein A, et al. Diagnosis of 'possible' mitochondrial disease: an existential crisis. *J Med Genet* 2019;56(3):123–130. doi: 10.1136/jmedgenet-2018-105800. Epub 2019 Jan 25. PMID: 30683676.

Quadir A, Pontifex CS, Lee Robertson H, Labos C, Pfeffer G. Systematic review and meta-analysis of cardiac involvement in mitochondrial myopathy. *Neurol Genet* 2019;5(4):e339. doi: 10.1212/NXG.0000000000000339. PMID: 31403078; PMCID: PMC6659349.

Schon KR, Ratnaike T, van den Ameele J, Horvath R, Chinnery PF. Mitochondrial diseases: a diagnostic revolution. *Trends Genet* 2020;36(9):702–717. doi: 10.1016/j.tig.2020.06.009. Epub 2020 Jul 13. PMID: 32674947.

CASE 56 Ryanodine Receptor 1 (RYR1)-Related Disorders

Clinical History

A five-month-old girl was referred with hypotonia and muscle weakness from birth onwards. She was born after an unremarkable pregnancy during a planned home birth at 40 weeks' gestational age as the second child from healthy, unrelated parents. In the first days after her birth, they noted a paucity in movements and a low muscle tone. Breastfeeding failed, as she was unable to suck sufficiently. Bottle feeding with an adapted nipple also was a problem, and she often coughed or threw up after drinking. At the age of three months, a percutaneous endoscopic gastrostomy (PEG) probe had been placed to ensure caloric intake. Swallowing had gradually improved in the past month and now she managed to swallow small quantities of purified fruit and vegetables.

Examination

The girl was interactive and alert, and made a variety of sounds. There was a haemangioma on the forehead (Fig. 56.1). She had normal eye movements and no ptosis. However, facial expression was slightly reduced and she had a high arched palate. There was wheezing on each inhalation with retraction of the intercostal muscles, but normal extension of the belly (i.e., no paradoxical breathing pattern). Although she was able to raise the arms and legs against gravity, there was an axial hypotonia with a prominent head lag upon arm traction, and only little head balance when kept supported in a sitting position. Lying on the belly, she was able to lift her head only briefly. Tendon reflexes were very low or absent.

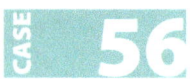

Figure 56.1 Frontal haemangioma in *RYR1*-related congenital myopathy.

Diagnostic Considerations

Congenital hypotonia was considered (i.e., a floppy infant has a broad differential diagnosis (Chapter 3, Box 3.20)). Central nervous system involvement is

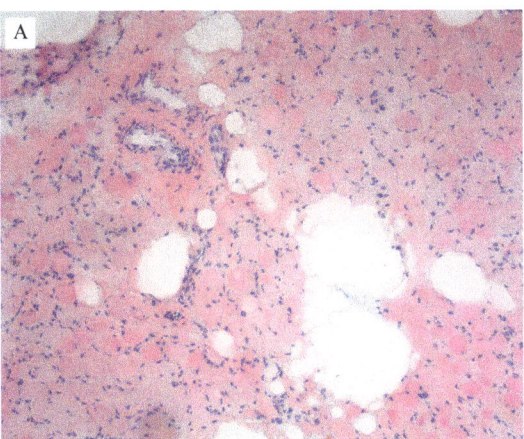 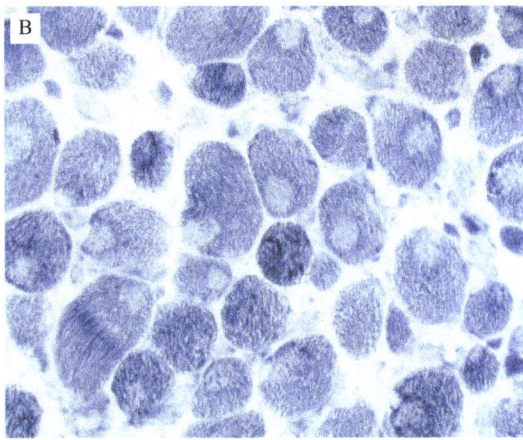

Figure 56.2 (A,B) Increased variation in fibre size, with rounded fibres, peri- and endomysial fibrosis, and fatty infiltration on H&E stain (A). Central cores on the NADH stain (B).

more common than neuromuscular diseases as a cause of floppiness. Both can present with feeding difficulties. To discriminate hypotonia from muscle weakness is challenging, especially in very young children. However, reduced tendon reflexes in the present case point towards a neuromuscular condition. The facial weakness, a high arched palate, frontal haemangioma, and gradual improvement with time are consistent with a congenital myopathy rather than a motor neuron disorder.

Ancillary Investigations

CK was normal (150 U/L). A muscle biopsy taken from the quadriceps femoris revealed an increased variation in fibre size, rounded fibres, increased peri- and endomysial fibrosis, and fatty infiltration as well as central cores in the NADH staining (Fig. 56.2A,B).

DNA sequencing revealed a *de novo* variant in the *RYR1* gene (c.14740 A>G, p.Arg4914Gly).

Follow-Up

Motor development improved and she achieved sufficient oral intake. She developed hip dysplasia with subsequent surgical treatment. She suffered from repeated respiratory infections requiring prophylactic antibiotic treatment in the first year. She reached independent walking at the age of three, but uses a wheelchair for longer distances.

General Remarks

The *RYR1* gene encodes for the type 1 ryanodine receptor, a calcium^{2+} release channel located in the sarcoplasmatic reticulum of skeletal muscles that is essential for excitation–contraction coupling and calcium homeostasis. Variations relate to a spectrum of clinical phenotypes including various congenital myopathies, malignant hyperthermia syndrome (MHS), King–Denborough syndrome (including skeletal abnormalities and dysmorphic features), rhabdomyolysis-myalgia syndrome (**Case 66**), or, more rarely, atypical periodic paralysis, adult-onset myopathy, and bleeding abnormalities. This has led to the concept of a spectrum of *RYR1*-related disorders of which neuromuscular phenotypes are a major part.

Congenital myopathies can be classified according to the main histological findings in a muscle biopsy. Historically, *RYR1* mutations have been linked to central core disease, as presented in this case. These cores represent local areas with disrupted myofibrils and absent mitochondria and may also develop over time. Central cores, however, are not unique to *RYR1*-related myopathy, but can also occur in, for example, *ACTA1* mutations. On the other hand, muscle histology in *RYR1* congenital myopathy may also show multiminicores, congenital fibre type disproportion, internalized or centralised nuclei, or nemaline rods with or without cores. Predominant fibrosis and fatty replacement may resemble a muscular dystrophy. As each of these histological phenotypes can be caused by multiple genes, it is clear that the relation between histology and genotype is complex in congenital myopathies. Due to the widespread availability of next-generation sequencing, genetic testing would currently be the most likely first step in case of a clinical diagnosis of a congenital

Part II Neuromuscular Cases: Myopathies

Table 56.1 Features of *RYR1*-related disease

- *RYR1* mutations are the most frequent cause of congenital myopathies.
- Congenital myopathies are historically defined according to the histopathology: central core disease (CCD), multiminicore disease, centronuclear myopathy, congenital fibre type disproportion.
- In *RYR1*-related disease, the typical core histopathology may be absent in a muscle biopsy.
- *RYR1*-related myopathy typically has an early onset with proximal or generalized weakness, and little progression.
- Adult patient may present with axial weakness or distal weakness.
- *RYR1* variations are the most frequent cause of exertional rhabdomyolysis and malignant hyperthermia.
- Unlike core diseases associated with some other genes, *RYR1*-related disease is not complicated by cardiac involvement.
- *RYR1* is a relatively large gene and therefore genetic testing may easily result in finding a variant of unknown significance (VUS). As the clinical phenotypes are heterogeneous, the histopathology may be helpful in reverse phenotyping.

myopathy, reserving the biopsy for unsolved or more complex cases.

RYR1-related myopathies can be caused by autosomal dominant (AD) or autosomal recessive (AR) transmitted variants resulting in gain-of-function and loss-of-function of the ryanodine receptor. There is a wide spectrum of severity ranging from severe weakness in the neonatal period to only muscle cramps and pain or mild disability in adulthood (Table 56.1; Fig. 56.3). Generally, the most severe end of the spectrum is related to AR variations. However, both in AD and AR disease young children may have progressive respiratory and feeding difficulties, and be nonambulant. Presentation can be with polyhydramnios and reduced fetal movements. Neonates show generalized hypotonia and facial weakness, often with ophthalmoparesis and ptosis. Respiratory insufficiency can require permanent support, and children may have limited life expectancy. In AD central core disease, proximal weakness is more prominent in the legs with frequent hip

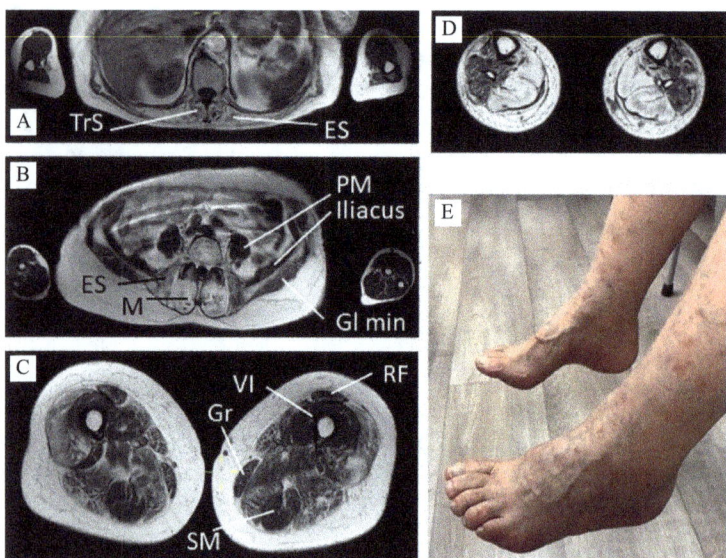

Figure 56.3 (A–E) A 76-year-old woman with autosomal dominantly inherited central core disease due to a heterozygous pathogenic variant in the *RYR1* gene (c.14438A>G). She had never been able to run and suffered from frequent falls as a child because of equinus foot deformities. At age 40 years, clinical examination because of an incidentally found hyperCKaemia (365) showed very mild weakness of proximal leg muscles and foot dorsal flexors and a rigid lumbar back. A muscle biopsy showed type 1 fibre predominance and core-like structures. She at present has some difficulty using the stairs. Whole-body muscle MRI shows fatty replacement of the paraspinal muscles at all levels (thoracic transversospinal (TrS), and erector spinae (ES) muscles (A) and lumbar multifidus (M) and erector spinae muscles (B)), and all calf muscles (D). Proximal leg muscles and anterior lower leg muscles are also affected, with relative sparing of the rectus femoris (RF), vastus intermedius (VI), gracilis (Gr), and semimembranosus (SM) muscles (C). Sparing of the psoas major (PM), iliacus, and gluteal (Gl min) muscles (B). Note that the bilateral pes cavus is not accompanied by distal atrophy or hammer toes, which are seen if hollow feet are of neurogenic origin (E).

dysplasia, but gradually improves with time. Ocular movements are more frequently preserved, and facial weakness may be minimal. Cardiomyopathy is not part of the *RYR1*-related myopathy spectrum. The adult onset phenotype in *RYR1* myopathies has been reported as variable including axial weakness with bent spine, slowly progressive proximal weakness, and rare cases of calf predominant weakness and distal weakness with jaw contractures. Characteristic histopathological features (i.e., cores or minicores) are found in about half of the cases; otherwise, fibre type disproportion or nonspecific myopathic changes are observed.

Exertional rhabdomyolysis (ERM) with malignant hyperthermia susceptibility (MHS) and ERMS without MHS have both been linked to *RYR1* variations, both AD and AR. Patients can be without muscle weakness or even show muscle hypertrophy (**Case 66**). The European Malignant Hyperthermia (MH) Group lists diagnostic MH mutations in the *RYR1* gene. Much more rarely, MHS is caused by a mutation in the *CACNA1S* or *STAC3* gene. In case of diagnostic uncertainty, increased susceptibility to MH can be tested using an in vitro contracture test with halothane and caffeine on a muscle biopsy. Exertional myalgia and rhabdomyolysis can be triggered by excessive exercise, heat, viral infection, alcohol, or drugs such as statins. In between episodes, patients may have mild, mostly aspecific muscle biopsy abnormalities and mildly elevated CK. MHS, either as part of an *RYR1*-related myopathy or as an isolated syndrome, is a potentially life-threatening susceptibility to the use of volatile anaesthetics, such as sevoflurane or desflurane, and depolarizing muscle relaxants, such as succinylcholine (see section on Anaesthetic Management in Chapter 8). An intramuscular excess of calcium leads to sustained muscle contraction and hypermetabolic state, resulting in heat production, combined respiratory and metabolic acidosis, and ultimately rhabdomyolysis with hyperkalaemia and myoglobinuria. MHS can thus result in arrhythmias, disseminated intravascular coagulation, and multiorgan failure with a significant mortality. Treatment is by withdrawal of the causative agent and intravenous dosing of dantrolene at 2.5 mg/kg. Dantrolene is an antagonist of the ryanodine receptor, and dosing may need to be repeated until symptoms subside. Further treatment consists of correction of electrolyte disturbances and acidosis, cooling, and ensuring sufficient urine output. taken from the quadriceps muscle.

Suggested Reading

Claeys KG. Congenital myopathies: an update. *Dev Med Child Neurol* 2020;62(3):297–302. doi: 10.1111/dmcn.14365. Epub 2019 Oct 2. PMID: 31578728.

Dosi C, Rubegni A, Baldacci J, et al. Using cluster analysis to overcome the limits of traditional phenotype-genotype correlations: the example of *RYR1*-related myopathies. *Genes (Basel)* 2023;14(2):298. doi: 10.3390/genes14020298. PMID: 36833224; PMCID: PMC9956305.

Kruijt N, den Bersselaar LV, Snoeck M, et al. RYR1-related rhabdomyolysis: a spectrum of hypermetabolic states due to ryanodine receptor dysfunction. *Curr Pharm Des* 2022;28(1):2–14. doi: 10.2174/1381612827666210804095300. PMID: 34348614.

Lawal TA, Todd JJ, Witherspoon JW, et al. Ryanodine receptor 1-related disorders: an historical perspective and proposal for a unified nomenclature. *Skelet Muscle* 2020;10(1):32. doi: 10.1186/s13395-020-00243-4. PMID: 33190635; PMCID: PMC7667763.

O'Connor TN, van den Bersselaar LR, Chen YS, et al; RYR1 Myopathy Consortium.RYR-1-Related Diseases International Research Workshop: From Mechanisms To Treatments Pittsburgh, PA, U.S.A., 21-22 July 2022. *J Neuromuscul Dis* 2023;10(1):135–154. doi: 10.3233/JND-221609. PMID: 36404556; PMCID: PMC10023165.

Papadimas GK, Xirou S, Kararizou E, Papadopoulos C. Update on congenital myopathies in adulthood. *Int J Mol Sci* 2020;21(10):3694. doi: 10.3390/ijms21103694. PMID: 32456280; PMCID: PMC7279481.

Sarkozy A, Sa M, Ridout D, et al. Long-term natural history of pediatric dominant and recessive *RYR1*-related myopathy. *Neurology* 2023;101(15): e1495–e1508. doi: 10.1212/WNL.0000000000207723. Epub 2023 Aug 29. PMID: 37643885.

Snoeck M, van Engelen BG, Küsters B, et al. RYR1-related myopathies: a wide spectrum of phenotypes throughout life. *Eur J Neurol* 2015;22(7):1094–1112. doi: 10.1111/ene.12713. Epub 2015 May 11. PMID: 25960145.

Case 57 Congenital Myopathies: X-Linked Myotubular Myopathy

Clinical History

A boy was born at 33 weeks' gestational age via caesarean delivery because of a transverse position and difficulties in obtaining an adequate cardiotocography. Pregnancy had been complicated by fetal growth restriction with an abdominal circumference at p10, and polyhydramnios. His mother had noticed a reduction in fetal movements the day before delivery. Immediately after birth, he was hypotonic, pale, bradycardic, and without spontaneous breathing. Resuscitation was started with bag and mask ventilation and thoracic compressions. Heart rate and oxygen levels quickly normalized. However, breathing remained insufficient. Arterial CO_2 levels rose to 14.0 kPa (ref 4.7–6.4) and he was intubated. He was the first child of unrelated parents. His mother had been diagnosed with obesity and gestational diabetes. The maternal grandmother had a sister whose daughter had a son who had died two days after birth more than 20 years earlier.

Examination

The child was ventilated via a nasal tube and did not trigger support from the ventilator. He showed severe hypotonia without antigravity movements. There was facial weakness and a high arched palate, and he did not make any sounds or attempts to swallow. There was no cough reflex. Extraocular movements were limited in all directions. Tendon reflexes were absent. Fingers and toes were strikingly long (Fig. 57.1). Testicles were nonpalpable.

Diagnostic Considerations

Neonatal hypotonia (i.e., the floppy infant) poses a diagnostic challenge to differentiate between central and peripheral neurological conditions. Neonatal asphyxia is common and should be considered in newborns requiring immediate resuscitation. However, ancillary investigations such as the cerebral ultrasound and cerebral function monitoring were normal. Polyhydramnios is generally associated with reduced swallowing and fetal akinesia and/or muscle weakness, although it could have been caused by increased fetal urination as part of the gestational diabetes in the present case. In the first days of life, respiratory insufficiency did not improve. Together with the high arched palate, facial weakness, and absent tendon reflexes, congenital myopathy or myasthenia became the most likely clinical diagnosis. This was supported by the family history and confirmed by histology and DNA. Whether or not to perform a muscle biopsy before DNA analysis can be

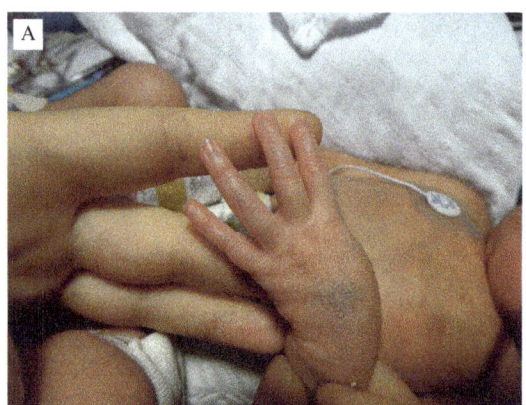
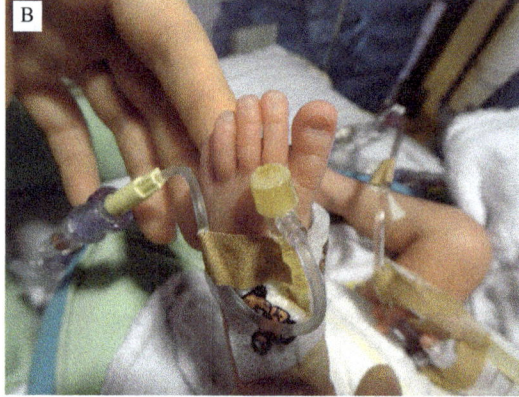

Figure 57.1 (A,B) Long fingers (A) and toes (B) (arachnodactyly) as part of the X-linked myotubular myopathy phenotype.

debated and is dependent on the turnaround time of the genetic laboratory. In the present case, DNA results were expected after two weeks. As it was considered very likely that a muscle biopsy would provide an aetiological diagnosis instantaneously, this was the preferred option for the medical team and the parents.

Ancillary Investigations

Serum CK was normal. Ultrasound revealed an undescended testis on the left side; the right testis could not be visualized. Cerebral ultrasound was normal. Cerebral function monitoring revealed a continuous normal voltage pattern for 48 hours. Information on the deceased relative revealed that the child had been diagnosed with myotubular myopathy based on a muscle biopsy that had shown centralized nuclei. In the patient, it was decided to also take a muscle biopsy from the left quadriceps femoris muscle while waiting for the DNA results. H&E staining showed some variation in fibre size and centralized myonuclei in almost all the fibres (Fig. 57.2). DNA analysis revealed a frameshift mutation in the *MTM1* gene located on the X chromosome (c.969dup; p.Val324Serfs*fs).

Follow-Up

The diagnosis and poor prognosis were discussed extensively with the parents and the medical team including a medical ethics consultant and a social worker. In a shared decision process that took place over several days, there was agreement that prolonged respiratory support and thus continuation of treatment was not in the child's best interest. Planned extubation took place under sedation with midazolam and morphine on day 6, after which the child died quietly. The parents were referred to the clinical geneticist for counselling and genealogy.

General Remarks

X-linked myotubular myopathy is a severe neuromuscular condition affecting approximately 1 in 50,000 male births. Presentation is with polyhydramnios and often reduced movements in utero. At birth, there is a myopathic phenotype with dolichocephaly, facial weakness, high arched palate, often ophthalmoparesis, and severe respiratory insufficiency. Most-severely affected patients show no breathing effort or limb movement at birth and often die within the first months of life. Survivors often require permanent respiratory support via tracheostomy and are wheelchair dependent. Comorbidity is significant including scoliosis, frequent respiratory infections, gastrointestinal symptoms, and an increased occurrence of learning difficulties. At the milder end of the spectrum are occasional patients who achieve independent walking and live into adulthood. Weakness is then relatively stable, although with significant disease burden. Associated features include arachnodactyly, cryptorchidism (undescended testicle(s)), and hepatobiliary disease (Table 57.1).

Similar to many other X-linked neuromuscular conditions, female carriers are most often not affected, but can be symptomatic as well, varying

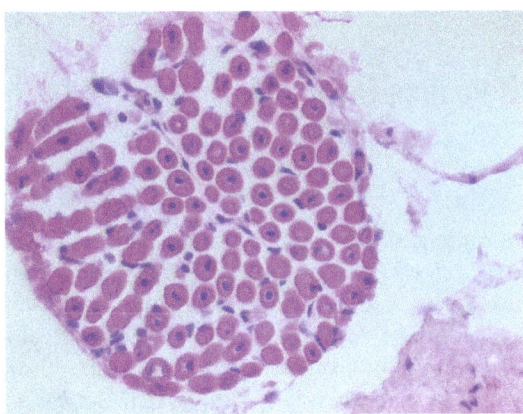

Figure 57.2 Centralized nuclei on an H&E stain of a muscle biopsy in a neonate with *MTM1* myopathy.

Table 57.1 Findings suggestive of an X-linked myotubular myopathy

- Severe weakness in a male infant at birth
- Distribution of weakness comparable with that of a congenital myopathy, i.e., facial weakness, high arched palate, and respiratory insufficiency
- Dolichocephaly (elongation of the head)
- Arachnodactyly (long fingers and toes)
- Cryptorchism (undescended testicle(s))
- Hepatobiliary disease, including enlarged liver, gallstones, and peliosis hepatis
- Laboratory testing: increased serum transaminases and gamma-glutamyl-transferase
- Muscle biopsy: centralized nuclei

from exercise intolerance to a myopathic phenotype with generalized muscle weakness, even to the same extent as that of male neonates.

The disease is caused by variations in the *MTM1* gene on Xq28, which encodes for a 3-phosphoinositide phosphatase called myotubularin. Variations lead to a complete or partial loss of function of a protein that normally deactivates phosphoinositides like phosphoinositol-3-phosphate by removing phosphate. Myotubularin is thought to regulate endosomal trafficking and is involved in the development and maintenance of muscle cells. Histopathological classification is that of a centronuclear myopathy, a multigenetic group of myopathies in which most nuclei are located centrally in the myofibres (see Fig. 57.2).

Therapeutic strategies are being developed targeting various aspects of the pathophysiology. These include enzyme replacement, modulation of dynamin-2 via antisense oligonucleotides or tamoxifen, and adeno-associated virus (AAV) vector-mediated gene transfer. A clinical trial using AAV8 showed an improvement in motor function and a reduction in respiratory support, but unfortunately was complicated by cases with fatal liver failure due to the underlying liver involvement in X-linked myotubular myopathy. Therefore, the trial had to be prematurely stopped. The use of an antisense oligonucleotide for dynamin-2 was also stopped because of increases in liver enzymes and a reduction of platelets already at low doses.

Suggested Reading

Amburgey K, Tsuchiya E, de Chastonay S, et al. A natural history study of X-linked myotubular myopathy. *Neurology* 2017;89(13):1355–1364. doi: 10.1212/WNL.0000000000004415. Epub 2017 Aug 25. PMID: 28842446; PMCID: PMC5649758.

Annoussamy M, Lilien C, Gidaro T, et al. X-linked myotubular myopathy: a prospective international natural history study. *Neurology* 2019;92(16):e1852–e1867. doi: 10.1212/WNL.0000000000007319. Epub 2019 Mar 22. PMID: 30902907; PMCID: PMC6550499.

Biancalana V, Scheidecker S, Miguet M, et al. Affected female carriers of MTM1 mutations display a wide spectrum of clinical and pathological involvement: delineating diagnostic clues. *Acta Neuropathol* 2017;134(6):889–904. doi: 10.1007/s00401-017-1748-0. Epub 2017 Jul 6. PMID: 28685322.

D'Amico A, Longo A, Fattori F, et al. Hepatobiliary disease in XLMTM: a common comorbidity with potential impact on treatment strategies. *Orphanet J Rare Dis* 2021;16(1):425. doi: 10.1186/s13023-021-02055-1. Erratum in: Orphanet J Rare Dis 2022;17(1):18. PMID: 34641930; PMCID: PMC851335.

Graham RJ, Muntoni F, Hughes I, et al. Mortality and respiratory support in X-linked myotubular myopathy: a RECENSUS retrospective analysis. *Arch Dis Child* 2020;105(4):332–338. doi: 10.1136/archdischild-2019-317910. Epub 2019 Sep 4. PMID: 31484632; PMCID: PMC7054136.

Shieh PB, Kuntz NL, Dowling JJ, et al. Safety and efficacy of gene replacement therapy for X-linked myotubular myopathy (ASPIRO): a multinational, open-label, dose-escalation trial. *Lancet Neurology* 2023; 22 (12):1125–1139.

Congenital Myopathies: Nemaline Myopathy

Clinical History

After a normal pregnancy without hydramnios, delivery of a healthy-looking girl was uneventful. At four months of age, she had had a respiratory infection and was noted to have a weak cough. At eight months of age she was just able to keep her head in an upright position but was not able to sit unsupported. Her mother admitted that she had not been very active since birth, but there was no progressive muscle weakness and no swallowing difficulty. She was referred to a paediatric neurologist because of a suspected neuromuscular disorder. The parents were healthy and there was no consanguinity.

Examination at Age Eight Months

She was found to have generalized wasting and muscle weakness of arms and legs, proximal more than distal. There were spontaneous antigravity movements of the arms and legs, but when pulling the body at the shoulders, there was a head lag. On horizontal suspension, she was able to lift her head only to the level of the spinal column. She achieved a sitting position when supported at the shoulders and showed poor head balance. She was able to roll over, but not able to bear her weight on her legs. There were normal eye movements and no ptosis, but bilaterally there was facial weakness and she had a high arched palate. The tongue was not enlarged and there was no organomegaly. She was able to swallow mashed food. Tendon reflexes were absent. Breathing was normal, but she had a weak cough. Joints were hypermobile; there were no contractures and no fasciculations.

Diagnostic Considerations

She showed signs of floppiness and delayed motor milestones. The floppy infant syndrome is mostly of central origin (Chapter 3, Box 3.20). Given the apparent muscle weakness including that of the face and absent tendon reflexes, a central origin of hypotonia was highly unlikely in this patient. Spinal muscular atrophy may manifest with hypotonia and proximal weakness and tongue fasciculations, but no facial weakness. Infantile-onset Pompe disease (IOPD) should be considered, albeit IOPD is associated with hepatomegaly, cardiomegaly, an enlarged tongue, and fast progression of muscle weakness. Congenital myasthenic syndrome can present shortly after birth. Characteristic features include hypotonia, feeding difficulties, facial weakness, ptosis, and respiratory problems. All these diseases were thought to be unlikely, and therefore, a congenital myopathy or muscular dystrophy was considered.

Ancillary Investigations

Serum CK activity was normal, making a congenital muscular dystrophy unlikely. A muscle biopsy performed at age eight months showed 'rods', which are characteristic of a nemaline myopathy (Fig. 58.1). Nemaline bodies are small, spindle-shaped rods or short, thread-like structures primarily distributed in the sarcoplasm. Rods are often observed in continuation with the Z-disk and are considered to be derived from Z-lines, as they have a similar structure and express similar proteins.

DNA analysis was performed, and she was found to have a compound heterozygote variant of the nebulin gene (*NEB*): a splice site mutation in intron 36 inherited from her mother and a frameshift mutation in exon 138 from her father.

Follow-Up

Motor development was delayed, but gradually she was able to sit and slide on her buttocks. Since age 3 she was able to stand with support and over the years managed to walk short distances. She used a wheelchair first for outdoor transportation and became wheelchair dependent at age 15, and a year later she underwent surgery because of progressive scoliosis. She went to high school and found herself a job, working from home. Since age 19 she complained about shortness of breath on exertion and she was found to have a forced vital capacity (FVC) of 40% of expected. From age 23 years FVC was decreasing, pCO2 was increasing to the upper limit of normal, and night-time ventilation was discussed. However, she had to be admitted to the hospital because of a pneumonia, developed restlessness at night, became 'psychotic', and was found in bed with an apnoea and cardiac arrest. Unfortunately, cardiopulmonary resuscitation was not effective and she died at age 23.

General Remarks

A floppy infant has hypotonia at birth or in early infancy. Hypotonia is a common symptom

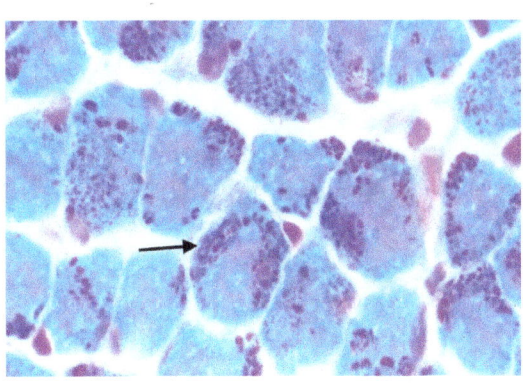

Figure 58.1 Modified Gomori trichrome stain showing rods (arrow), which are found in nearly all muscle fibres.

associated with disorders of brain, spinal cord, nerve, the neuromuscular junction, and muscle (Chapter 3, Box 3.20). Parents commonly complain to physicians that their baby is not very active. When these babies pass through infancy, parents notice the delay in the motor milestones.

Nemaline myopathy is defined by nemaline rods or nemaline bodies that stain red with the modified Gomori trichrome technique. Sometimes only a few fibres with rods are present in a muscle biopsy, or rods are only observed on electron microscopic examination of the muscle tissue. There may be additional pathological features such as cores, caps, and fibre type disproportion, which overlap with other congenital myopathies. Histopathological features have a major role not only in guiding molecular analysis, but also in suspected congenital myopathies. Next-generation sequencing (NGS) gene panels are rapidly replacing the muscle biopsy in daily clinical practice. However, a recent study showed that muscle biopsy may still play a role if the genetic analysis turns out negative, which was the case in 50% of patients in whom a histological diagnosis of congenital myopathy had been established, or when NGS yields a difficult-to-interpret result.

Nemaline myopathy is one of the most common congenital myopathies, ranging in severity from severe forms, developing in utero, associated with early fatal outcome to milder forms with onset in childhood, sometimes presenting as late as in adulthood (Table 58.1). It is a genetically and clinically heterogeneous group of disorders, characterized by usually nonprogressive or slowly progressive generalized (proximal more than distal) muscle weakness. In the typical form, there is also weakness of the neck flexors and the face (Fig. 58.2A). Milder forms may present later in childhood with delayed motor milestones or other signs of muscle weakness. Patients presenting in adulthood with muscle weakness or respiratory failure may, on examination, be found to have a myopathic facies, high arched palate, and other signs of early muscle weakness, which are clues that the disorder was, in fact, congenital. In adults with rod myopathy, a severe autoimmune sporadic late-onset nemaline myopathy (SLONM), which is potentially treatable, is much more likely than hereditary nemaline myopathy.

There is not only a wide spectrum of clinical phenotypes; variations in many (> 12) genes are known. Nemaline myopathies may have an autosomal dominant or recessive inheritance or may appear *de novo*. Dependent on the gene variation, there may be associated features,

Table 58.1 Main features of nemaline myopathy

- One of the most common congenital myopathies
- Pathologically characterized by nemaline rods or nemaline bodies
- Usually congenital onset, but age of onset may vary: from prenatal (in utero) to adulthood. Severity also very variable.
- Nonprogressive or slowly progressive generalized weakness (proximal > distal), including the face
- > 12 known genes. Most frequent genes *ACTA1*, *NEB*
- Autosomal recessive or autosomal dominant inheritance
- CK normal or mildly elevated
- Cardiac involvement rare

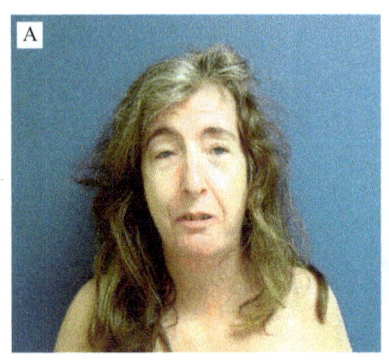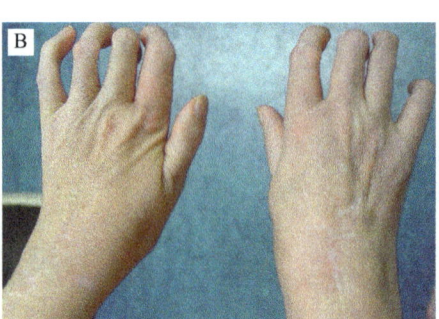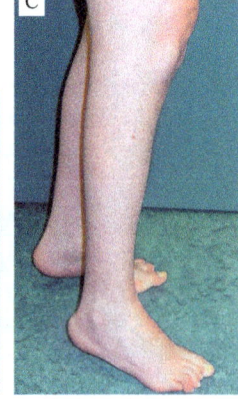

Figure 58.2 (A–C) Patient with nemaline myopathy caused by a *TPM2* mutation. Myopathic face (A); arthrogryposis of hands (B) and ankles (C).

such as arthrogryposis (Fig. 58.2B,C) and external ophthalmoplegia. The commonest causes are mutations in the genes encoding skeletal muscle α-actin (*ACTA1*) and nebulin (*NEB*).

Currently, there is no curative treatment, so management should have a multidisciplinary approach, targeted at maintaining muscle strength, mobility, and independence in the activities of daily living. Regular monitoring of respiratory function and addressing orthopaedic problems are paramount. In retrospect, the described patient should have been treated more aggressively and probably offered noninvasive ventilation as soon as she complained about shortness of breath.

Cardiac monitoring is dependent on genetic findings. Cardiac involvement is rare and has been reported in a few patients with variants in *ACTA1* or *MYPN* or with a contiguous deletion of *TNNT1* and *TNNI3*.

Suggested Reading

Ahmed MI, Iqbal M, Hussain N. A structured approach to the assessment of a floppy neonate. *J Pediatr Neurosci* 2016;11(1):2–6. doi: 10.4103/1817-1745.181250. PMID: 27195025; PMCID: PMC4862282.

Laitila J, Wallgren-Pettersson C. Recent advances in nemaline myopathy. *Neuromuscul Disord* 2021;31 (10):955–967. doi: 10.1016/j.nmd.2021.07.012. Epub 2021 Jul 24. PMID: 34561123.

Nicolau S, Milone M. Sporadic Late-Onset Nemaline Myopathy: Current Landscape. Curr Neurol Neurosci Rep. 2023 Nov;23(11):777–784. doi: 10.1007/s11910-023-01311-0. Epub 2023 Oct 19. PMID: 37856049.

Veneruso M, Fiorillo C, Broda P, et al. The role of muscle biopsy in diagnostic process of infant hypotonia: from clinical classification to the genetic outcome. *Front Neurol* 2021;12:735488. doi: 10.3389/fneur.2021.735488. PMID: 34675869; PMCID: PMC8523832.

Juvenile Dermatomyositis (JDM)

Clinical History

A 12-year-old boy had a three-year history of exercise-induced pain in his limbs; in particular, the shoulders, elbows, and knees were affected. For six months he had also experienced loss of strength. He noted difficulty with walking and cycling and was hardly able to climb stairs. He developed toe walking and complained about an itchy skin rash with focal depigmentation at his neck and trunk, diagnosed as eczema. He did not complain about swallowing difficulty, yet he became cachexic because his nutritional intake was lagging, and he suffered from mood swings.

Previous history was unremarkable. His parents were healthy, as was his older brother.

Examination

He was examined by a dermatologist who found a V-sign purplish rash on the anterior chest accompanied by scaling (Fig. 59.1A). In the abdominal region, the rash showed lichenification. There was an erythematous macular rash on the palms. There were no facial skin abnormalities, or Gottron papules at the knuckles of the fingers.

Neurological examination revealed bilateral scapular winging (Fig. 59.1B) and atrophy and contractures in shoulders, elbows, and ankles (Fig. 59.1C). Because of the latter, he walked on tiptoes. There was weakness MRC grade 2 of the neck flexors and the deltoid muscles, and weakness MRC 4 of the biceps and triceps brachii muscles. Gowers sign was positive and standing on one leg caused a positive Trendelenburg sign. He had a waddling gait. There was MRC 4+ weakness of the quadriceps femoris muscles and hamstrings. Distal muscles of arms and legs showed normal strength. Otherwise, there were no abnormalities (normal sensation and reflexes).

Diagnostic Considerations

There was subacute onset and progressive pain of the joints, followed by development of skin

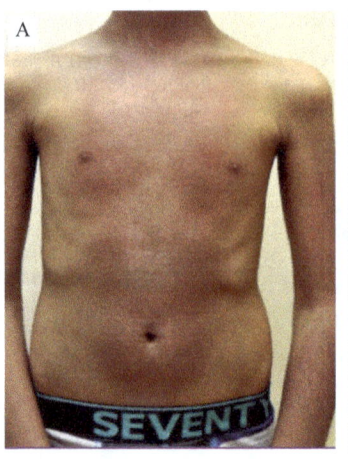 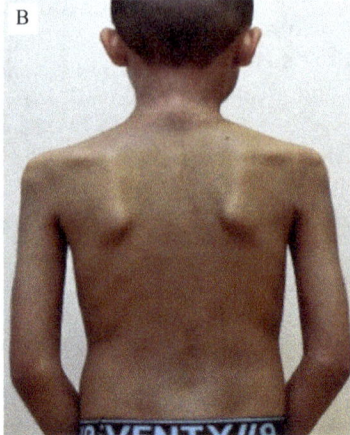 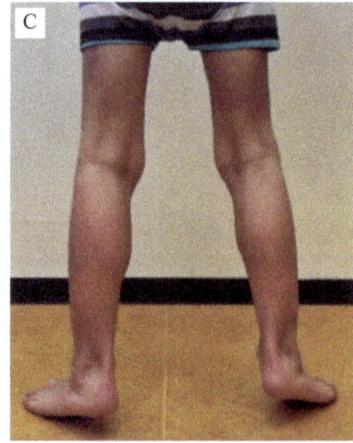

Figure 59.1 (A–C) Skin rash on trunk (A); scapular winging, shoulder girdle atrophy, and elbow contractures (B); upper leg atrophy and Achilles tendon contractures (C).

abnormalities and progressive moderate to severe proximal muscle weakness of his limbs accompanied by contractures. The skin abnormalities and contractures were not characteristic of but still consistent with a long-lasting dermatomyositis. The most likely diagnosis was juvenile dermatomyositis (JDM). However, since there were some 'atypical' features, he was subjected to ancillary investigations: muscle MRI, muscle biopsy, and assessment of myositis-specific antibodies (MSAs).

Ancillary Investigations

Serum CK activity was 497 U/L (ULN 143 U/L). Immunoblot for MSAs and myositis-associated antibodies (MAAs) showed weakly positive Mi-2beta and PM-Scl autoantibodies. T2-weighted FATSAT MRI revealed hyperintensities of multiple leg muscles. Muscle biopsy revealed perifascicular atrophy (Fig. 59.2) and microtubular inclusions on EM.

Follow-Up

The clinically suspected diagnosis of dermatomyositis was confirmed by MRI and, above all, by the muscle biopsy. Perifascicular atrophy is highly characteristic of dermatomyositis with a longer duration. The MSAs were weakly positive and thus cannot be considered to be of any significance. He was treated with pulse methylprednisolone and intravenous immunoglobulins (IVIg), followed by oral methotrexate and prednisolone. Skin lesions and contractures disappeared and muscle strength normalized in a period of two years, and thereafter the medication could be tapered and eventually stopped.

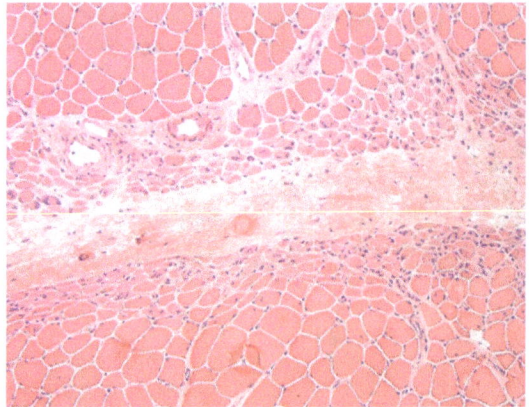

Figure 59.2 Muscle biopsy from the quadriceps femoris. H&E stain shows prominent perifascicular atrophy.

General Remarks

Juvenile dermatomyositis (JDM) is the most common idiopathic inflammatory myopathy of childhood, yet a rare disease with a characteristic rash and symmetric limb girdle muscle weakness evolving over weeks–months. It is primarily classified as a vasculopathy, albeit the microvascular damage is not limited to the skin and muscle and may also include the vasculature of the gastrointestinal tract. A dysregulated interferon (IFN) pathway plays an important role in the pathogenesis of dermatomyositis.

Girls are more often affected than boys. The mean age at JDM diagnosis is around seven years with about 25–30% being younger than five years at onset. The mean time between the onset of the first symptoms and confirming the diagnosis is six months, ranging from five weeks to two years.

As in adult DM, skin abnormalities include pathognomonic features, that is, Gottron papules (violaceous plaques with subtle scaling) and Gottron sign (erythematous macules or patches) over the metacarpophalangeal, interphalangeal, and distal interphalangeal joints, or – less frequently – over the extensor surfaces of elbows and knees, and a heliotrope rash (purplish) with oedema on the upper eyelids. Painful periungual erythema with telangiectasia, cuticular hypertrophy, facial oedema, shawl sign (erythema over the neck and upper back), and V sign (erythema over the upper chest) may also occur.

Muscle weakness is usually symmetric and proximal, with legs more affected than arms.

As in adults, children can have skin abnormalities without muscle weakness (clinically amyopathic JDM). Calcinosis is the intracellular deposition of insoluble calcium salts in the skin, subcutaneous tissue, fascia, tendons, and muscles. Calcinosis occurs due to injury and affects approximately 40% of JDM patients and can lead to skin ulcers, recurrent infection, and joint contractures. Contractures occur more frequently in JDM as compared with adult DM. The commonest sites are ankles, elbows, and knees. Swallowing difficulty, including silent aspiration, is under-recognized and not always predicted by generalized muscle weakness. Therefore, it is recommended to subject children with nasal speech or coughing during swallowing to speech and language therapy assessment and instrumental assessments according to local experience.

Ancillary Investigations

Blood tests include serum creatine kinase activity ($10 \times$ ULN in ~60%), MSAs, and MAAs. The most common type of MSA in JDM is anti-TIF1-γ and associated with a more prolonged and severe disease course. In contrast, in adults, TIG1-γ is associated with the occurence of a malignancy. Anti-NXP-2 is the second most frequent MSA and is associated with calcinosis, especially in children diagnosed below the age of five years who manifest with more severe muscle disease and gastrointestinal bleeding, resulting in a worse disease outcome with a lower functional status. The next most common MSA in children is melanoma differentiation MDA-5, especially in Japanese children. Usually, the clinical features include an amyopathic disease course, interstitial lung disease (ILD), and digital ulcers. Identification of ILD is facilitated by a biomarker called Krebs von den Lungen-6 (KL-6) and is associated with increased IL-18 and ferritin. If ILD is suspected, high-resolution computerized tomography (CT) or ultrasound as well as pulmonary function testing, in children older than six years, should be performed.

There may also be MAAs identifying overlap syndromes, such as those associated with antibodies to ribonuclear proteins. Children positive for MAA usually have a more chronic and relapsing disease course and have an increased frequency of calcinosis. Anti-Ro-52 is associated with ILD in children with JDM.

MRI is a helpful aid to support diagnosis in children with JDM showing muscle oedema, fascial or perimuscular oedema in the thighs, which can also be observed in a proportion of patients with chronic disease. Oedema is most frequently found in proximal muscles, legs more than arms, but also in distal and axial muscles. Replacement of muscle by fat has a pattern similar to that of oedema. Calcinosis in the muscle or subcutaneous tissue and lipodystrophy may also be found on MRI. Ultrasound studies have been performed only on small JDM cohorts demonstrating increased echogenicity of the tibialis anterior muscle more than biceps or forearm flexors. There is also a decrease in the muscle thickness, as a measure of muscle atrophy, in proximal muscles, such as biceps and quadriceps, in JDM patients with disease activity.

Muscle biopsy is not done on a routine basis but can be performed in case of atypical presentation. It is a matter of preference whether this is done via a needle or open biopsy. The histological picture resembles that found in adults – profound upregulation of MHC I expression on muscle fibres, increased expression of integrins and complement and membrane attack complex deposition on capillaries and perimysial large vessels, a type 1 IFN signature (measured by the myxovirus resistance protein A (MxA) stain), and cell infiltrates consisting mostly of mature plasmacytoid dendritic cells, CD3+ T cells, macrophages, and B cells. Perifascicular atrophy is found more often in children.

Lung involvement (interstitial lung disease (ILD)) is present in only 8% of patients, and often asymptomatic, but assessment is recommended since ILD is a significant cause of morbidity and mortality. All children should have assessment of lung involvement at time of diagnosis by pulmonary function tests, including carbon monoxide (CO) diffusion capacity. Further testing is necessary in those with an abnormal restrictive pattern. High-resolution CT is a noninvasive and sensitive test for detecting ILD in JDM, but radiation risk associated with repeated CT scan must be considered.

There are promising biomarkers that may aid the clinician in prognostication. Measurement of two IFN-related biomarkers (galactin-9 and CXCL10) outperform CK in distinguishing between active disease and remission.

Management

With early treatment, 30–50% of patients reach remission within two to three years of disease onset with few complications and a low mortality rate (< 4%). However, polycyclic or persistently active disease has been described in 41–60% of cases.

According to consensus-based recommendations, corticosteroids are the mainstay of JDM medical therapy. It is now customary to start with high-dose intravenous methylprednisolone for two months (followed by prednisone), combined with methotrexate (MTX) subcutaneously. One should advise sun protection and sufficient intake of calcium and vitamin D. Rituximab may be useful in refractory cases. Based on the IFN-type 1 involvement in the pathogenesis, treatment with JAK-inhibitors is evolving, and case series show promising results. IVIg may also be a useful adjunct for resistant disease. A challenge in the treatment of JDM is calcifications. As yet there are no evidence-based recommendations. Some treatments can be considered, such as colchicine, diltiazem, bisphosphonates, minocycline, or biologicals (TNF-α inhibitors or rituximab).

Treatment of JDM should include a safe and appropriate exercise programme, monitored by a physiotherapist.

Juvenile Immune-Mediated Necrotizing Myopathy (IMNM)

Juvenile immune-mediated necrotizing myopathy (IMNM) – associated with anti-SRP or anti-HMGCR antibodies – also occurs, but is very rare (~3% in juvenile IIM). There are no reports of anti-HMGCR-positive juvenile IMNM patients with prior use of statins. Girls are more often involved than boys. The average age at onset is ~9 years, but the youngest case was 10 months old. Most commonly, there is 1–3 months onset, but a more insidious onset (> 6 months) does also occur, which may hamper the distinction from genetic limb girdle muscle dystrophies.

Muscle weakness can be severe, involving the proximal muscles, but neck flexors and bulbar muscles may also be affected, in particular in anti-SRP-positive juvenile IMNM. As in adults, there can be DM-like and antisynthetase syndrome-like skin features.

Serum CK is usually markedly elevated (up to 1000 × ULN). Muscle biopsy is compatible with the histopathological features in adults.

Suggested Reading

Bellutti Enders F, Bader-Meunier B, Baildam E, et al. Consensus-based recommendations for the management of juvenile dermatomyositis. *Ann Rheum Dis* 2017;76(2):329–340. doi: 10.1136/annrheumdis-2016-209247. Epub 2016 Aug 11. PMID: 27515057; PMCID: PMC5284351.

Liang WC, Uruha A, Suzuki S, et al. Pediatric necrotizing myopathy associated with anti-3-hydroxy-3-methylglutaryl-coenzyme A reductase antibodies. *Rheumatology (Oxford)* 2017;56(2):287–293. doi: 10.1093/rheumatology/kew386. Epub 2016 Nov 6. PMID: 27818386; PMCID: PMC5410926.

Pachman LM, Nolan BE, DeRanieri D, Khojah AM. Juvenile dermatomyositis: new clues to diagnosis and therapy. *Curr Treatm Opt Rheumatol* 2021;7(1):39–62. doi: 10.1007/s40674-020-00168-5. Epub 2021 Feb 6. PMID: 34354904; PMCID: PMC8336914.

Wang CH, Liang WC. Pediatric immune-mediated necrotizing myopathy. *Front Neurol* 2023;14:1123380. doi: 10.3389/fneur.2023.1123380. PMID: 37021281; PMCID: PMC10067916.

CASE 60 Dermatomyositis (DM)

Clinical History
A 38-year-old woman was referred to a dermatologist because of a rash in the face. She had been feeling low in energy for several months and in the past two months her arms and legs felt weak accompanied by myalgia. The rash had expanded to the extensor surfaces of hands and knees, upper chest, and neck. Serum CK was 4313 U/L (20 × ULN), and she was referred to the outpatient department for neuromuscular disorders with a presumed diagnosis of dermatomyositis.

Examination
Body weight was 103 kg (BMI 34.7). The skin of the upper eyelids showed a subtle heliotrope rash and oedema, a rash in the face, positive V- and shawl signs, Gottron papules, and erythema on the extensor surfaces of upper arms, elbows, and knees (Fig. 60.1). Physical examination was otherwise normal. There was symmetric weakness MRC grade 4+ of the deltoid and iliopsoas muscles.

Diagnostic Considerations
The pathognomonic skin abnormalities together with symmetric limb girdle weakness leaves dermatomyositis as the only possible diagnosis. The subacute disease course and elevated CK are in line with this diagnosis.

Ancillary Investigations
A whole-body muscle MRI was performed (Fig. 60.2), but it was considered unnecessary to proceed with a muscle biopsy because the diagnosis was clear clinically. Antinuclear antibody (ANA) test was positive. Line blot showed positive anti-SS-B antibody. Myositis blot showed anti-Mi2 strongly positive. HRCT scan thorax showed no interstitial lung disease (ILD). Whole-body FDG-PET/CT, mammography, and a faecal occult blood test revealed no signs of a malignancy and were planned to be repeated yearly for three years after disease onset.

Follow-Up
Prednisone was started at a dose of 60 mg daily, which was lower than the recommended starting dose of 1 mg/kg body weight, because she was obese and the weakness not severe. No second-line drug was added. Two months later, at a prednisone dose of 50 mg, all muscles showed normal strength and the skin abnormalities were much improved and quickly resolved altogether. CK activity was normalized. Functioning in daily life was completely normal. Body weight had increased by 14 kg. Prednisone was slowly tapered and discontinued seven months later. Four months after that, there was a slight flare-up of the skin abnormalities over the hands, the face,

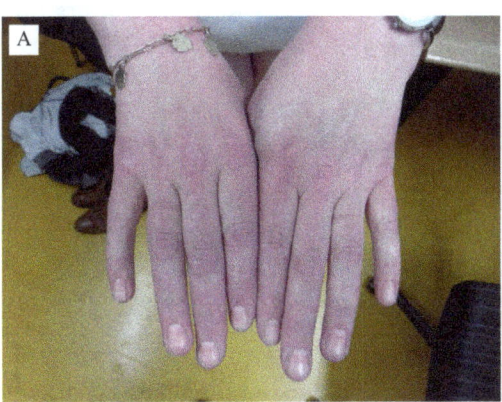
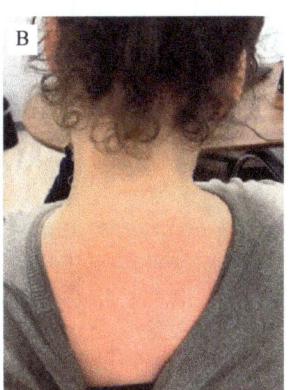
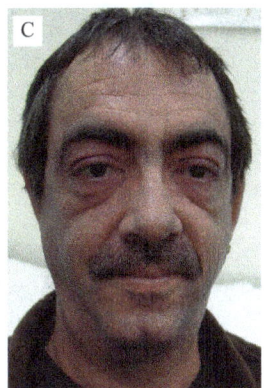

Figure 60.1 (A–C) Gottron papules (A) and shawl sign (B) in the described patient. Facial and heliotropic rash in another patient with dermatomyositis (C).

Part II Neuromuscular Cases: Myopathies

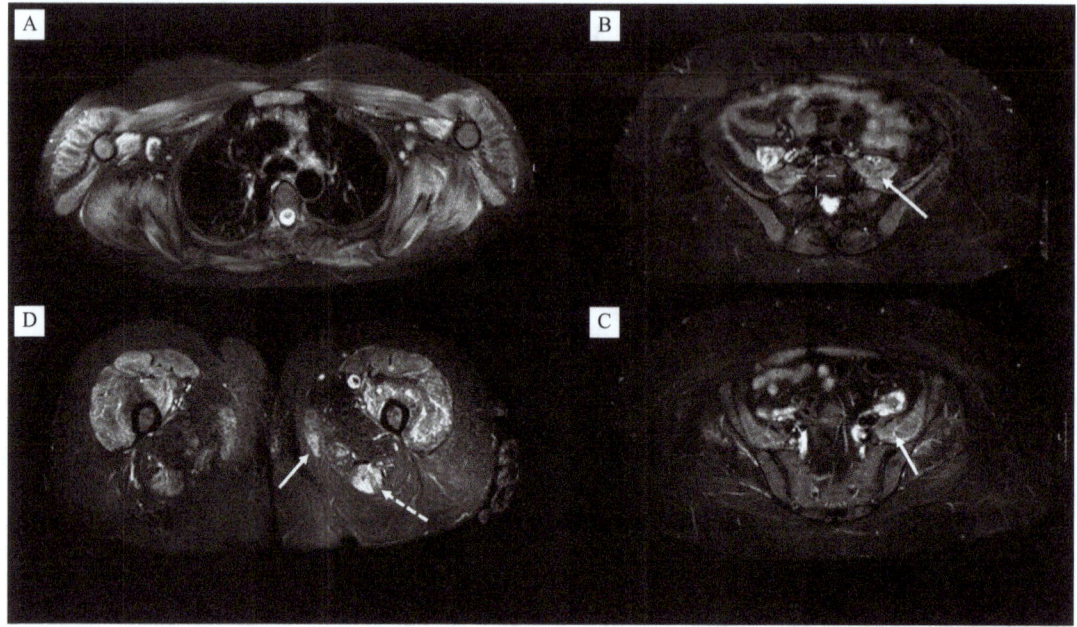

Figure 60.2 (A–D) T2-STIR (fat-suppressed) MRI in the described patient. High-intensity abnormality indicates symmetric oedema in shoulder girdle muscles (A), psoas (B), iliacus (C), and quadriceps muscles, gracilis (solid arrow), and semitendinosus muscles (dashed arrow), D).

neck, and upper chest, without myalgia or muscle weakness. CK activity was still normal (85 U/L). Topical treatments were not successful. Two months later, there was slight weakness (MRC 4 +) of the deltoid muscle, and the iliopsoas, hip abductors, and hamstring muscles, and CK activity had risen to 1399 U/L. Oral dexamethasone pulses were started at 40 mg daily on four consecutive days, once every four weeks, and azathioprine 50 mg tid was added. After two courses of dexamethasone, muscle strength had nearly normalized, the skin abnormalities had almost disappeared. CK was 750 U/L. There was no further weight gain, but the dexamethasone caused notable sleeping disturbances and agitation on the days she took the medication. Dexamethasone dose was lowered to 28 mg daily on four consecutive days. After the third course, CK was 150 and she felt almost completely well, without weakness but with a slight rash in the face on examination. The next courses were shortened from four to two days, and the dose was reduced to 8 mg daily, which was well tolerated. She felt completely well and the rash had disappeared. Nine months after onset of the relapse, CK was 38 U/L. It was planned to further taper the dexamethasone and to continue the azathioprine.

General Remarks

Idiopathic Inflammatory Myopathies, Myositis

The idiopathic inflammatory myopathies (IIMs), or myositis, have for a long time been divided into dermatomyositis, polymyositis, and inclusion body myositis (IBM). However, IBM is different from the other IIMs, sharing only the presence of an inflammatory infiltrate in a muscle biopsy, and not the clinical features (see **Case 62**). Polymyositis has become a disputed entity, and doctors from different disciplines confusingly used this term for different conditions. Currently, the following subtypes of myositis are recognized: besides IBM dermatomyositis (DM), anti-synthetase syndrome (ASyS), overlap or nonspecific myositis (OM), and immune-mediated necrotizing myopathy (IMNM). Several attempts have been made recently to formulate criteria for diagnosis and classification. Table 60.1 lists the myositis subtypes and their major distinctive features. In children, juvenile dermatomyositis (JDM, **Case 59**) is the least rare form of myositis, but the other types occur also. Autoimmune myositis further also includes sarcoid myopathy, eosinophilic fasciitis,

Table 60.1 Main features of dermatomyositis (DM), anti-synthetase syndrome (ASyS), overlap myositis, immune-mediated necrotizing myopathy (IMNM), and inclusion body myositis (IBM)

	Distinctive clinical features, associated conditions	Muscle biopsy (see Fig. 60.3)	Myositis-specific autoantibodies (MSAs)
DM	Skin abnormalities, (see Table 60.2). Interstitial lung disease, cardiac involvement. Haematological malignancies and solid tumours	Perimysial and perivascular inflammation, consisting of macrophages, B cells, and CD4 T cells; perifascicular atrophy; expression of IFN-1 regulated proteins (MHC-1, MxA) (Fig. 60.4) on muscle fibres; MAC deposition on capillaries	DM-specific autoantibodies (DMSAs) directed at TIF-1-γ, NXP-2, Mi-2, MDA-5, SAE (Table 60.3)
ASyS	Nonerosive arthritis, interstitial lung disease, Raynaud phenomenon, mechanic's hands, DM-like skin changes	Perimysial and perivascular inflammation, mostly CD68+ cells; perifascicular atrophy, necrotic, and regenerating fibres; damaged perimysium MxA negative	Anti-synthetase (anti-aminoacyl-tRNA synthetase (ARS)) antibodies directed at: Jo-1, OJ, PL-7, KS, EJ, PL-12, Zo, Ha, SC, JS
Overlap myositis	As part of a connective tissue diseases, e.g., scleroderma, M Sjogren, MCTD, SLE, RA, either concomitant, before, or after onset of myositis	Perivascular perimysial inflammation, scattered necrosis ('nonspecific')	Myositis-associated antibodies (MAAs), directed at SSA-52, SSA-60, SS-B, Sm, nRNP/Sm, AMA-M2, centromere-B, dsDNA, histones, nucleosomes, PCNA, PM-Scl, ribosomal-P, Scl-70, U1-RPN, Ku
IMNM (Case 61)	Severe disease, high CK. Increased risk of cancer in HMGCR-positive IMNM	Necrotic muscle fibres; minimal inflammatory infiltrate; MHC1 and MAC expression on sarcolemma of non-necrotic muscle fibres	Anti-HMGCR Anti-SRP
IBM (Case 62)	Age at onset > 40 yr. Weakness more distal than other IIMs (deep finger flexors). Asymmetric. Treatment-resistant.	CD8+ T cells surrounding and invading non-necrotic muscle fibres, grouped atrophy, ~60% rimmed vacuoles, COX-negative fibres	Anti-cN1A

focal myositis, and immune-checkpoint inhibitors-induced myasthenia-myositis (**Case 33**).

The clinical hallmark in DM, ASyS, OM, and IMNM is symmetric muscle weakness with a limb girdle distribution, often associated with myalgia. Onset is subacute in most cases, and progression is over weeks to months. The differential diagnosis of subacute proximal weakness is limited and can be found in Chapter 3, Box 3.7. The differential diagnosis of myalgia can be found in Chapter 3, Box 3.17.

Dysphagia, neck flexor weakness, and head drop may occur early in the disease. Systemic involvement includes skin abnormalities, ILD, and sometimes cardiac manifestations (myocarditis and arrhythmias). In ASyS, ILD and arthritis may precede myositis. Serum CK activity is often markedly increased, up to 50 × ULN, but may be normal, in particular in DM. Muscle MRI shows oedema in the T2 sequence with fat suppression (Fig. 60.2). This may corroborate a clinical suspicion of myositis and can also be useful in selecting the optimal location for the muscle biopsy.

A muscle biopsy is often needed for making the diagnosis and for excluding sarcoid myopathy and amyloid myopathy, which may also present with subacute limb girdle weakness. However, a muscle biopsy may be omitted if the diagnosis is clear clinically, for instance in the presence of characteristic DM skin abnormalities (Table 60.2), clinical features of ASyS and the presence of anti-Jo1 antibody, or in the presence of a connective tissue disease. The muscle biopsy should be taken from a clinically affected muscle (i.e., weak, myalgic, or showing oedema on MRI) which is not weaker than MRC grade 4, especially in more long-

Table 60.2 Most characteristic skin abnormalities in dermatomyositis, typically present in Mi-2 positive patients, but also in other DM types (and also present in 25% of ASyS patients)

- Gottron papules (violaceous plaques with subtle scaling) and Gottron signs (erythematous macules or patches) over the metacarpophalangeal, interphalangeal, and distal interphalangeal joints (Fig. 60.1A), or extensor surfaces of elbows and knees.
- Heliotrope rash, (purplish, pruritic, erythematous rash with oedema on the upper eyelids) (Fig. 60.1C)
- Nail fold changes (periungual erythema and telangiectasia, haemorrhagic nail fold infarcts)
- Shawl sign (erythema over the neck and upper back (Fig. 60.1B)), V sign (erythema over the upper chest), holster sign (poikiloderma of the hips and lateral thighs)
- In patients with a dark skin, dyschromia (skin discolouration or patches of uneven colour) is more pronounced than erythema as compared with patients with a lighter skin tone, and calcinosis in adult patients with a dark skin tone is more frequent

Table 60.3 Dermatomyositis-specific autoantibodies (DMSAs) in adult and juvenile dermatomyositis

DMSAs	Typical clinical features
Anti-Mi-2	Classical DM skin changes (see Table 60.2), more severe weakness and higher CK than in Mi-2 negative DM. Good prognosis.
Anti-MDA-5	Severe skin abnormalities, including mechanic hands and palmar skin ulceration, CADM, ILD, more frequent in Asians. Usually little muscle weakness. Arthritis in JDM. Cancer in adults.
Anti-NXP-2	Severe weakness, peripheral oedema, contractures, little skin involvement, calcinosis in children, cancer in adults. Most frequent MSA in JDM
Anti-TIF-1-γ	Severe, photosensitive cutaneous disease with palmar involvement, may be hypomyopathic, cancer in adults.
Anti-SAE	Skin changes possibly more pronounced than muscle involvement, diffuse erythema, fever, weight loss. Cancer in adults.

standing disease, and does not show fatty or fibrous replacement of muscle on MRI (or CT). A lateral vastus muscle is usually a good choice. About half the patients have a myositis-specific antibody (MSA). The role of MSAs and myositis-associated antibodies (MAAs) in the pathophysiology of myositis is not yet fully understood. These antibodies are associated with different comorbidities, for instance ILD or cancer, and different clinical and histopathological features.

Treatment of Myositis

Treatment of first choice is corticosteroids by expert consensus. Prednisone 1 mg/kg/day is given for four to six weeks, followed by very slow tapering to avoid a relapse. The first doses of corticosteroids may be given intravenously (methylprednisolone). From the start, co-medication with azathioprine or methotrexate can be given as prednisone-sparing drug. Oral dexamethasone pulses (40 mg daily on four consecutive days, once every four weeks) can also be effective and does not cause a moon face or weigh gain. Underdosing of corticosteroids or tapering too fast, often out of fear of afverse effects, is a frequent cause of treatment failure in the early phases of the disease. If the treatment has been adequate but the effect is insufficient, other drugs (e.g., mycophenolate mofetil, rituximab, IVIg monthly – preferably

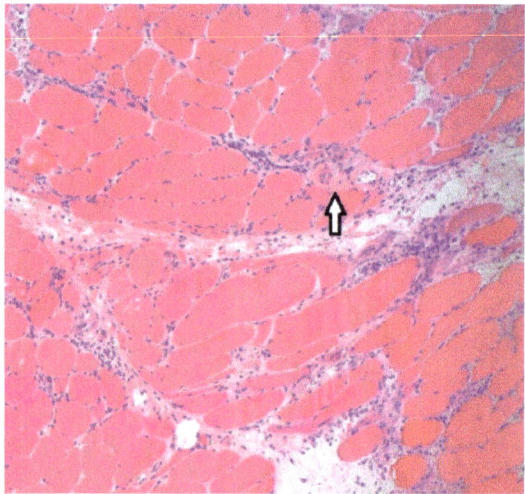

Figure 60.3 Mononuclear cell infiltrate around perimysial blood vessels (arrow) and 'overflow' from the perimysium. Courtesy Dr. Wim van Hecke.

at home) can be added. Low-dose subcutaneously administered Ig can also be considered, but its efficacy has not been proven in RCTs. Exercise therapy can improve endurance and myalgia.

In general, patients respond in weeks with an increase of muscle strength, always preceded by a decline in CK. In patients with severe weakness, it

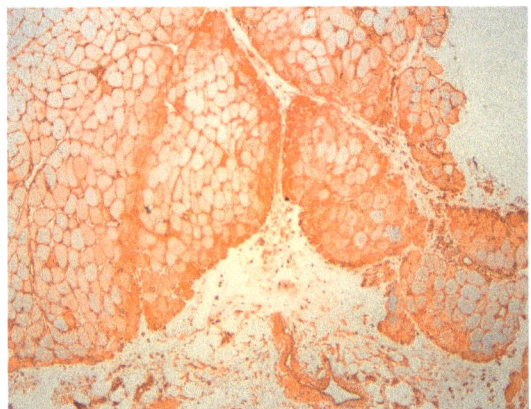

Figure 60.4 Perifascicular myxovirus resistance protein A (MxA)-positive stain in a patient with dermatomyositis. Courtesy Prof. Eleonora Aronica.

may take months before an increase of muscle strength can be noted. About 20–40% of patients achieve long-term (near) normal strength without medication. The majority, however, show a chronic persistent disease course or a polycyclic disease course with recurrent relapses (always preceded by an increase in CK). Mortality is increased, foremost attributable to cancer, and thus mainly in DM.

Dermatomyositis (DM)

The classic skin abnormalities in DM are listed in Table 60.2. In patients with a dark skin tone, the skin changes differ from the classic signs, typically showing dyschromia rather than erythema, which may lead to diagnostic delay. The type of skin abnormality and other clinical features differ according to the involved dermatomyositis-specific autoantibody (DMSA) (Table 60.3). Muscle involvement in DM may be mild or even absent (clinically amyopathic dermatomyositis, CADM), and CK activity may be normal.

Several classification criteria for DM have been formulated. In a 2018 ENMC workshop (Mammen et al., 2020), it was concluded that a DM classification (including CADM) can be made if the following features are present (either 1 and 2 or 1 and 3):

1. At least one of the following: Gottron papules, Gottron sign, heliotrope rash
2. Either a or b:
   a. Two of the three following: proximal muscle weakness, elevated muscle enzymes, suggestive muscle biopsy findings (see Table 60.1).
   b. Perifascicular atrophy and/or perifascicular MxA overexpression with rare or absent perifascicular necrosis in a muscle biopsy.
3. DM-specific MSA (Table 60.3)

Interstitial lung disease occurs in 15–20% of patients. DM is associated with a broad range of malignancies (in 10–15%) Following a recent guideline, screening for cancer should be basic or enhanced, done at the time of diagnosis only or yearly for three years, depending on risk factors such as the presence of certain MSAs. As in the other myositis subtypes, the pathogenesis of DM is yet unknown. Recent insights point to a pathogenetic role for pathways mediated by type I interferon, most likely interferon-β. The development of new treatments is currently directed at these presumed pathogenetic mechanisms, for example Janus kinase (JAK) inhibitors, which block the type 1 interferon pathway. B cell depletion by rituximab has not shown efficacy in a RCT, but has found to be sometimes useful in clinical practice. CAR T therapy targeting B cells (by engineering the patient's own T cells outside the body) causes deeper B cell depletion and might proove to be more effective. Skin abnormalities may be treated topically, but respond better to systemic immune suppression.

Suggested Reading

Bhai SF, Dimachkie MM, de Visser M. Is it really myositis? Mimics and pitfalls. *Best Pract Res Clin Rheumatol* 2022;36(2):101764. doi: 10.1016/j.berh.2022.101764. Epub 2022 Jun 23. PMID: 35752578.

Ezeofor AJ, O'Connell KA, Cobos GA, et al. Distinctive cutaneous features of dermatomyositis in Black adults: a case series. *JAAD Case Rep* 2023;37:106–109. doi: 10.1016/j.jdcr.2023.05.019. PMID: 37396484; PMCID: PMC10314225.

Gandiga PC, Ghetie D, Anderson E, Aggrawal R. Intravenous immunoglobulin in idiopathic inflammatory myopathies: a practical guide for clinical use. *Curr Rheumatol Rep* 2023;25(8):152–168. doi: 10.1007/s11926-023-01105-w. Epub 2023 Jun 1. PMID: 37261663

Goswami RP, Haldar SN, Chatterjee M, et al. Efficacy and safety of intravenous and subcutaneous immunoglobulin therapy in idiopathic inflammatory myopathy: a systematic review and meta-analysis. *Autoimmun Rev* 2022;21(2):102997. doi: 10.1016/j.autrev.2021.102997. Epub 2021 Nov 17. PMID: 34800685.

La Rocca G, Ferro F, Baldini C, et al. Targeting intracellular pathways in idiopathic inflammatory myopathies: a narrative review. *Front Med (Lausanne)* 2023;10:1158768. doi: 10.3389/fmed.2023.1158768. PMID: 36993798; PMCID: PMC10040547.

Lundberg IE, de Visser M, Werth VP. Classification of myositis. *Nat Rev Rheumatol* 2018;14(5):269–278. doi: 10.1038/nrrheum.2018.41. Epub 2018 Apr 12. PMID: 29651121.

Mammen AL, Allenbach Y, Stenzel W, Benveniste O ; ENMC 239th Workshop Study Group. 239th ENMC International Workshop: classification of dermatomyositis, Amsterdam, the Netherlands, 14-16 December 2018. *Neuromuscul Disord* 2020;30(1):70–92. doi: 10.1016/j.nmd.2019.10.005. Epub 2019 Oct 25. PMID: 31791867.

Oldroyd AGS, Callen JP, Chinoy H, et al.; International Myositis Assessment and Clinical Studies Group Cancer Screening Expert Group; Aggarwal R. International Guideline for Idiopathic Inflammatory Myopathy-Associated Cancer Screening: an International Myositis Assessment and Clinical Studies Group (IMACS) initiative. *Nat Rev Rheumatol* 2023;19(12):805–817. doi: 10.1038/s41584-023-01045-w. Epub ahead of print. PMID: 37945774.

Tanboon J, Nishino I. Update on dermatomyositis. *Curr Opin Neurol* 2022;35(5):611–621. doi: 10.1097/WCO.0000000000001091. Epub 2022 Aug 4. PMID: 35942671.

CASE 61 Immune-Mediated Necrotizing Myopathy (IMNM)

Clinical History

At the age of 44 years, this now 57-year-old woman noticed myalgia and difficulty walking, progressing over weeks. Two weeks after the first complaints, lifting the arms became troublesome too. CK activity was found to be > 10,000 U/L. TSH was normal. A diagnosis of myositis was made, and prednisone was started at a dose of 60 mg daily (body weight 80 kg). CK decreased, but the complaints worsened. Six weeks after disease onset, she was presented at our hospital. She was otherwise healthy, apart from well-controlled Graves disease with orbitopathy at the age of 31 years.

Examination

The following weakness was found (in MRC grades): deltoid muscles 4–/3, supraspinatus 4/3, pectoralis major 4/3, latissimus dorsi 3/4–, biceps brachii 5/4+, triceps brachii 5/4+, finger extensors 4+/4, iliopsoas 2+/2+, hamstrings 4/4, hip adductors and abductors 4–/4. She could not get from supine to sitting position or get up from a chair without support. The gait was waddling with hyperlordosis. There was no ocular, facial, or neck weakness. She had no problems swallowing. There was no dyspnoea. There were no skin abnormalities.

Diagnostic Considerations

Symmetric limb girdle weakness can have its origin in the anterior horn cell, nerves, neuromuscular junction, and muscles. Given a CK elevation of > 10 ×, however, a myopathy was the only plausible cause. In the absence of febrile illness, and no use of any toxins, the subacute disease onset pointed to an autoimmune pathogenesis. Since there were no dermatomyositis skin changes, an immune-mediated necrotizing myopathy (IMNM) was the most likely type of myositis. The fulminant disease course and high CK were in line with this diagnosis. In amyloid myopathy, CK is normal or mildly elevated. However, acute sarcoidosis myopathy with markedly elevated CK has been reported. A muscle biopsy and myositis blot were ordered.

Ancillary Investigations

Serum CK was 3837 U/L (under treatment with prednisone). TSH, T3, and T4 were normal. Antinuclear antibody (ANA) test was weakly positive. A muscle biopsy taken from the lateral vastus muscle at disease onset (after a CT scan had shown no fatty replacement of muscle tissue) showed abundant scattered necrosis and regeneration, and no mononuclear cell infiltrates or granulomatous abnormalities (Fig. 61.1). High-resolution

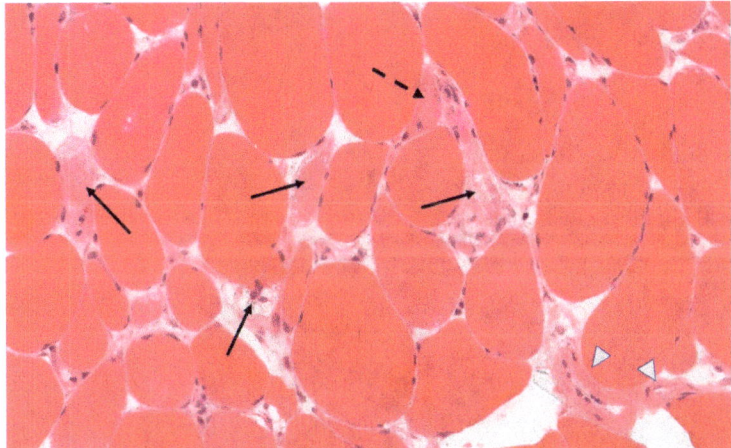

Figure 61.1 Biopsy taken from the lateral vastus muscle of the described patient at presentation. There are numerous necrotic fibres (arrows), and regenerating fibres (dashed arrow). Many atrophic fibres. No perivascular mononuclear cell infiltrate in perimysium or endomysium (white arrow heads). H&E stain. Courtesy Dr Wim van Hecke.

CT thorax did not show interstitial lung disease (ILD). Troponin in blood was normal. Screening for cancer was negative. Years after disease onset, the line blot showed positive anti-SSA antibodies, but the consulted rheumatologist could not find any clinical signs of Sjogren disease. The myositis blot showed positive anti-SRP antibodies.

Follow-Up

A diagnosis of immune-mediated necrotizing myopathy (IMNM) was made. The prednisone dose was increased to 80 mg daily and methotrexate was added in increasing doses up to 25 mg weekly. Four weeks after the prednisone dose had been increased, walking was no longer possible, weakness on examination had become more severe, and CK had increased to 5176 U/L. She was then treated with intravenous immunoglobulins (IVIg) 2 g/kg body weight in five days. During the following six to seven months, first CK levels decreased, followed by a slow increase of muscle strength, with weakness now found only in the deltoid and iliopsoas muscles, MRC grade 4 and 4–, respectively). However, it was not possible to lower the prednisone dose under 80/50 mg on alternate days. She was treated for hypertension and diabetes, and her body weight had increased to 92 kg. Therefore, she was treated with a second course of IVIg 2 g/kg, followed by 4-weekly infusions of 0.5 g/kg at home. Prednisone could be tapered to 40/15 mg, and weakness was now restricted to the iliopsoas muscles (MRC 4). CK levels remained around 400–600.

During the following years, she could function reasonably normally, albeit hampered by fatigue and overweight. She reported a strong effect of IVIg, with noticeable weakening of muscle strength just before every next dose. When CK levels slowly rose to around 1000, methotrexate was replaced by mycophenolate mofetil 2 × 1500 mg, which did not lower CK levels. Several attempts were made to taper the prednisone, eventually to 15 mg daily.

Twelve years after disease onset, gaining venous access became troublesome, and IVIg was replaced by subcutaneous Ig. Several months later, she reported a serious deterioration, and on examination there was severe weakness (MRC grade 0–2 of the iliopsoas muscles, severe weakness of shoulder girdle and other hip girdle muscles). Walking was hardly possible, with pronounced waddling gait and hyperlordosis. She could not climb the stairs, and she could not get up from a chair without support of the arms or get out of bed without her daughter's help. CK was 4294. Thereupon, she was admitted for treatment with rituximab and re-instalment of 4-weekly IVIg, in an increased dose of 2 g/kg in four days. Prednisone was increased to 30 mg daily and the mycophenolate mofetil was continued. Six months later, she feels much better: she can now climb the stairs and get out of bed on her own. Several muscles have improved by one

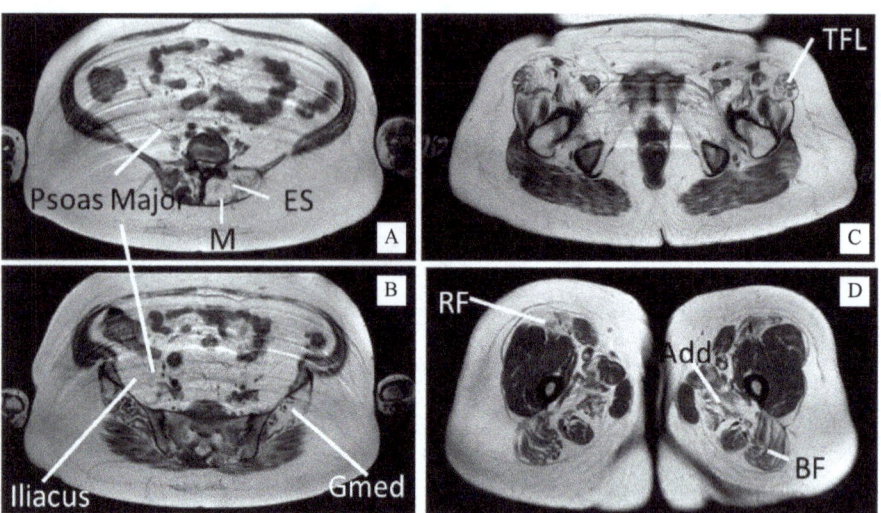

Figure 61.2 (A–D) Described patient: MRI 10 years after disease onset (T1). Pelvic girdle muscles, from rostral to caudal, and thigh levels: The psoas major and iliacus muscles have been completely replaced by fat. The paraspinal muscles (multifidus and erector spinae), gluteus medius (Gmed) and tensor fascia lata (TFL) muscles are also severely affected, left more than right. In the most proximal part of the thigh there is fatty replacement of the rectus femoris (RF), biceps femoris (BF), gluteus maximus (Gmax), and adductor (Add) muscles. T2 STIR images show oedema in anterior and posterior thigh muscles (not shown).

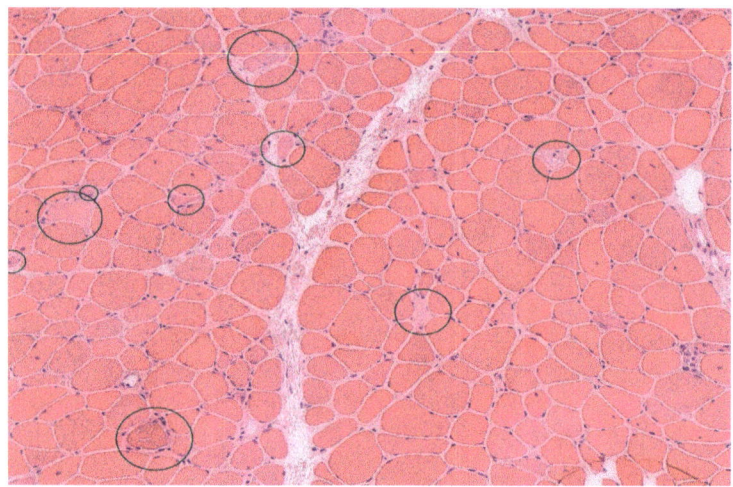

Figure 61.3 A 63-year-old man who had used a statin for 5 years presented with a 15-month history of proximal myalgia and weakness. On examination, weakness of the iliopsoas muscles (MRC 4) and deltoid muscles (MRC 4+), and a positive Gowers sign. CK 2500. Anti-HMGCR antibodies positive. The muscle biopsy (H&E) shows necrotic fibres (some encircled), increased variation in the size of the muscle fibres, no inflammatory cells in perimysium or endomysium, no increase in endomysial fibrosis, no abnormalities in other routine stains. The abnormalities are less prominent than in the described patient (see Fig. 69.1 61.1). Courtesy Prof. Eleonora Aronica and Dr Wim van Hecke

MRC grade. CK is 846 U/L. A whole-body muscle MRI four years earlier had shown muscle oedema and fatty degeneration of several muscles (Fig. 61.2).

We note that nowadays, given the rapidly progressive and severe weakness, we would have treated her with high-dose IVIg monthly together with corticosteroids from the start, and rituximab would also have been considered at an earlier phase during the disease course. A more aggressive strategy might have prevented irreversible damage.

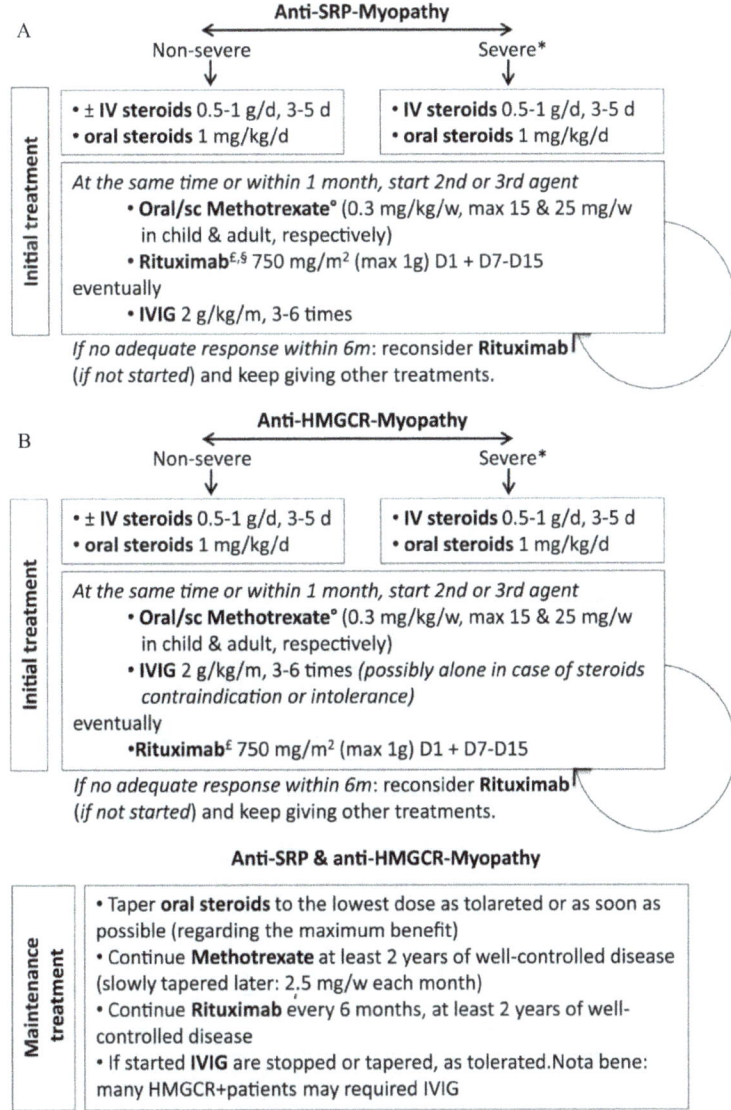

Figure 61.4 (A,B) Consensus recommendations on the initial treatment of IMNM. (A) Anti-SRP-myopathy. (B) Anti-HMGCR myopathy. From: Allenbach et al., *Neuromuscul Disord* 2018;28:87–99, with permission.

d = day; IVIG = intravenous immunoglobulins; m = month; sc = subcutaneous.
* walking difficulties and/or dysphagia; ° azathioprine or mycophenolate mofetil in case of methotrexate intolerance; £ rigorous data from the literature are however missing; § along with methotrexate, especially in severe cases.

General Remarks

Immune-mediated necrotizing myopathy (IMNM) is one of the myositis subtypes (see Case 60). It is diagnosed based on a subacute-onset, progressive, symmetric limb girdle weakness, (very) high CK, and a muscle biopsy showing scattered necrosis and regeneration with no or only minimal mononuclear cell infiltrates, (Fig. 61.1 and Fig. 61.3). Careful history taking showing progression in weeks–months in most cases differentiate IMNM from inherited diseases such as Pompe disease and limb girdle muscular dystrophies (LGMDs), but in particular in children the distinction from LGMD based on the disease course can be less clear. The differential diagnoses of subacute symmetric weakness and of myalgia are listed in Chapter 3, Boxes 3.7 and 3.17, respectively. Rhabdomyolysis (progression of myalgia, weakness and strong CK elevation in days) should not be mistaken for IMNM.

Weakness in IMNM, particularly anti-SRP IMNM (see below), is generally more severe, and CK is more increased than in the other myositis types. The iliopsoas muscles are the earliest and most severely affected. Deltoid muscles and hip abductors also become weak early. Weakness of neck muscles and dysphagia occur frequently. In IMNM, extra-muscular disease is much less frequent than in dermatomyositis, anti-synthetase syndrome and overlap myositis, but myocarditis may occur in SRP-positive patients.

IMNM is associated with anti-3-hydroxy-3-methylglutaryl-coenzyme A reductase (HMGCR) antibodies or anti-SRP antibodies in up to 61% and 16% of patients, respectively. These myositis-specific antibodies (MSAs) are regarded as highly specific for IMNM, and a muscle biopsy may be omitted in seropositive patients if the clinical presentation is typical. The enzyme HMGCR catalyses the synthesis of cholesterol and is inhibited by statins. About two-thirds of HMGCR-positive IMNM patients have been exposed to statins. HMGCR-positive IMNM should be distinguished from toxic statin-induced myopathy, a very rare adverse effect of statins that also manifest with proximal weakness and increased CK. Toxic statin-induced myopathy, but not IMNM, resolves in months after discontinuation of the medication. The group of sero-negative patients is not yet fully characterized.

Patients with seronegative IMNM and anti-HMGCR IMNM are considered at increased risk of cancer. Currently, it is recommended to screen all patients with IMNM yearly for at least three years after diagnosis.

IMNM is a severe disease. Treatment is often difficult, and should usually be aggressive from the start. In the absence of evidence from RCTs, recommendations are currently based on expert opinion and include corticosteroids, second-line drugs, IVIg, and rituximab (Fig. 61.4). Treatment usually is long term, and despite a favourable response, patients are often eventually left with considerable muscle damage and disabilities (**Video 61.1**). At present, there are no biomarkers for disease activity that could guide the therapeutic strategy, apart from CK activity.

Suggested Reading

Allenbach Y, Benveniste O, Stenzel W, Boyer O. Immune-mediated necrotizing myopathy: clinical features and pathogenesis. *Nat Rev Rheumatol* 2020;16(12):689–701. doi: 10.1038/s41584-020-00515-9. Epub 2020 Oct 22. PMID: 33093664.

Allenbach Y, Mammen AL, Benveniste O, Stenzel W ; Immune-Mediated Necrotizing Myopathies Working Group. 224th ENMC International Workshop: clinico-sero-pathological classification of immune-mediated necrotizing myopathies Zandvoort, the Netherlands, 14-16 October 2016. *Neuromuscul Disord* 2018;28(1):87–99. doi: 10.1016/j.nmd.2017.09.016. Epub 2017 Oct 23. PMID: 29221629.

Lim J, Rietveld A, De Bleecker JL, et al. Seronegative patients form a distinctive subgroup of immune-mediated necrotizing myopathy. *Neurol Neuroimmunol Neuroinflamm* 2018;6(1):e513. doi: 10.1212/NXI.0000000000000513. PMID: 30345336; PMCID: PMC6192692.

CASE 62 Inclusion Body Myositis (IBM)

Clinical History

A 64-year-old man suffered from progressive swallowing difficulty, in particular of solid food. There was a feeling of food getting stuck. He needed to take small bites and coughed while he was eating. Choking occurred frequently, and sometimes food came out his nose. He lost 7 kg over the past year. Gradually, drinking also became difficult. His GP first referred him to an ENT specialist and subsequently to a gastroenterologist who referred him to a neuromuscular centre. He was treated with Botox injections in the cricopharyngeal muscle, and this ameliorated his swallowing problems for about a year. He did not complain about limb weakness, diplopia, drooping eyelids, slurring of speech, shortness of breath, or muscle twitching. Family history was unremarkable.

Clinical Examination

There were no other abnormalities at neurological examination, in particular no ptosis, external ophthalmoplegia, dysarthria, or limb girdle muscle weakness. Myotatic reflexes were normal.

Diagnostic Considerations

Late-onset swallowing difficulty can have an extensive differential diagnosis: motor neuron disease (in particular, amyotrophic lateral sclerosis (ALS)), myasthenia gravis, oculopharyngeal muscular dystrophy, bulbospinal muscular atrophy, mitochondrial myopathy, and inclusion body myositis (IBM). ALS was very unlikely given the one-year history of dysphagia without other clinical features.

Ancillary Investigations

Videofluoroscopy (VF) was done by the gastroenterologist and showed hypertrophy of the m. cricopharyngeus, stasis of contract, and reflux from the stomach to the oesophagus. Antibodies against acetylcholine receptors and muscle-specific kinase were negative. At that time, an EMG or serum CK estimation did not seem to be appropriate.

Follow-Up

Given the negative family history, the absence of 'myasthenia' antibodies, and the absence of other pathological neurological signs and symptoms, no diagnosis could be made and a 'wait-and-see' approach was taken.

In the course of a year, the patient started to complain about fatigue in the legs ('feels like I have run the marathon'). Objective muscle weakness was not found. Thereupon, a CK test and MRI of the skeletal muscles were performed, which were normal. Subsequently, a quadriceps muscle biopsy was performed. This revealed a picture consistent with IBM: mononuclear cells surrounding and sometimes invading non-necrotic muscle fibres (Fig. 62.1A), and numerous SDH-COX-positive muscle fibres (Fig.62.1B) as an indication of mitochondrial involvement, which is often found in IBM. No rimmed vacuoles were observed (Fig. 62.1C).

Anti-cN1A IgG autoantibodies were absent.

Based on the history of progressive dysphagia, symptoms of thigh muscle weakness and the histopathology the diagnosis of inclusion body myositis (IBM) was established.

General Remarks

Inclusion body myositis (IBM) is the most common late-onset acquired myopathy. IBM is an autoimmune T cell-mediated disease and has a degenerative component manifesting with myofibre protein aggregates, which are present in < 1% of myofibres in patients with IBM.

See Table 62.1 for the main features of IBM. The age at onset is usually beyond 40 years with a mean age of symptom onset ranging from 61 to 68 years. The duration of symptoms is usually more than 12 months at presentation. In 35% of IBM patients, falls are the first manifestation. Decreased dexterity and swallowing difficulty may also be presenting symptoms. Patients presenting with dysphagia usually have a longer time to diagnosis as compared with patients with a more generalized presentation. Sometimes a drop foot or inability to walk on tiptoes may also be early manifestations.

Table 62.1 Main features of inclusion body myositis (IBM)

- Most frequent late-onset acquired myopathy
- Characteristic distribution of muscle weakness: deep finger flexors (often asymmetric), knee extensors, dysphagia
- Age at onset > 45 years; ≥ 12-month history of progressive weakness
- Diagnosis based on finger flexor and quadriceps weakness and an endomysial mononuclear cell infiltrate surrounding non-necrotic muscle fibres
- CK normal or mildly-moderately elevated up to 15 × ULN
- Supportive diagnostic features: anti cN1A autoantibodies, typical muscle MRI appearance (upper legs), or typical muscle ultrasound pattern (finger flexors)
- Slowly progressive
- Refractory to immunosuppressants or intravenous immunoglobulin

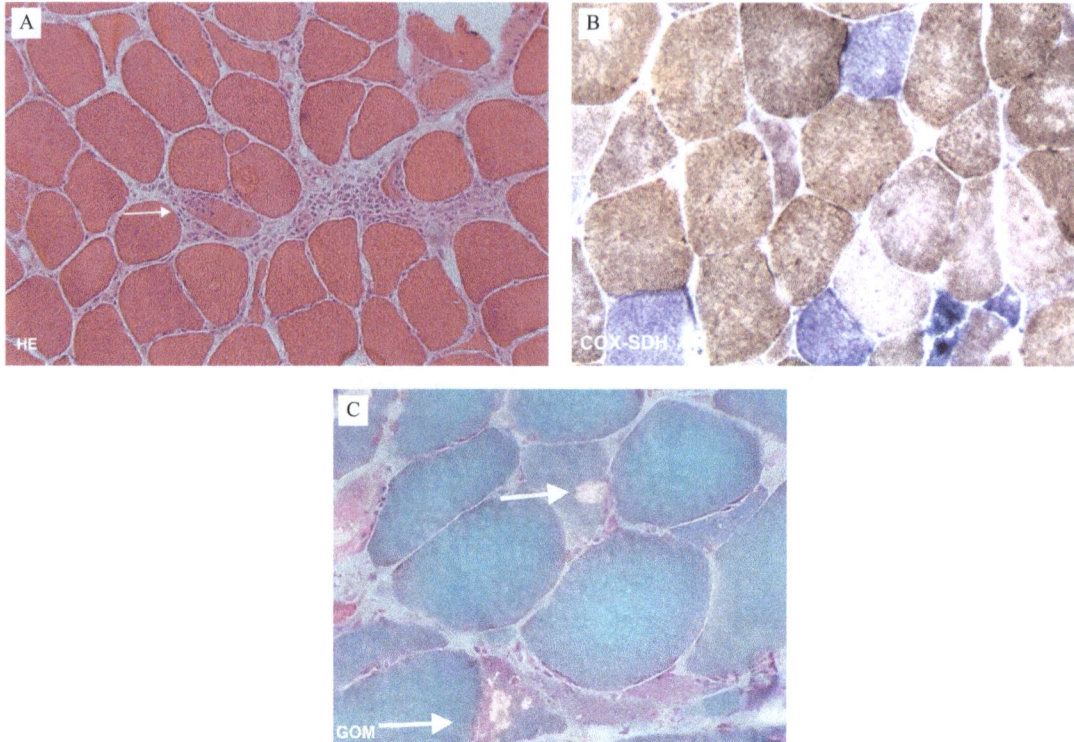

Figure 62.1 (A–C)Endomysial cell infiltrates composed of lymphocytes invading a non-necrotic muscle fibre (A, arrow), shown on H&E; COX-SDH stain showing blue (COX-negative, SDH-positive) muscle fibres, indicating mitochondrial abnormalities (B); and rimmed vacuoles (arrows) in a muscle biopsy of another patient with IBM (C, modified Gomori trichrome stain, GOM).

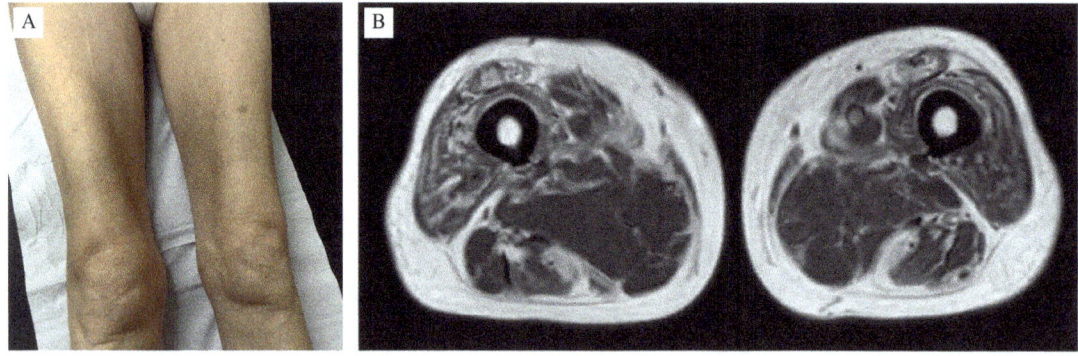

Figure 62.2 (A,B)Severely atrophic thigh muscles of a patient with IBM who presented with leg muscle weakness (A). MRI shows that hardly any quadriceps muscle tissue is left in contrast to the hamstrings and adductors, which seem to be well preserved (B).

There is a characteristic distribution of muscle weakness including quadriceps muscles (Fig. 62.2), deep finger flexors (which flex the distal phalanges, Fig. 62.3), oesophageal muscles, and facial muscles (Fig. 62.4, **Video 62.1**). Muscle weakness of the hands is often asymmetric and slowly progressive. Usually there is no muscle pain.

Dysphagia often goes unnoticed, in particular if not specifically asked for. Solid food gets stuck in the throat, requiring a drink of water. Meals can take a long time to consume, which may be socially disabling. Radiological studies including a VF swallowing study, fibreoptic endoscopic evaluation of swallowing, or real-time MRI may reveal

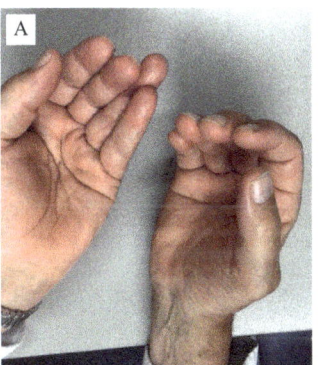
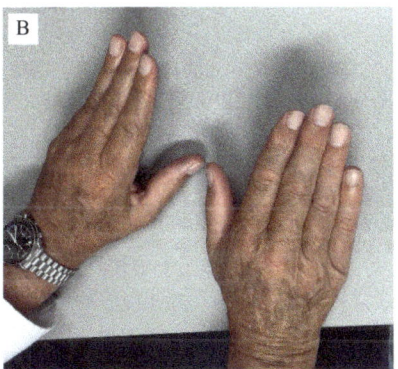

Figure 62.3 (A,B) Deep finger flexors are weak, left more than right in an IBM patient (A); the finger extensors have normal strength (B).

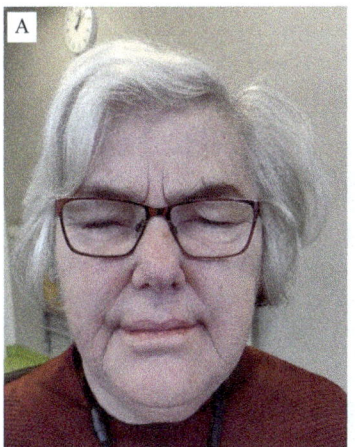
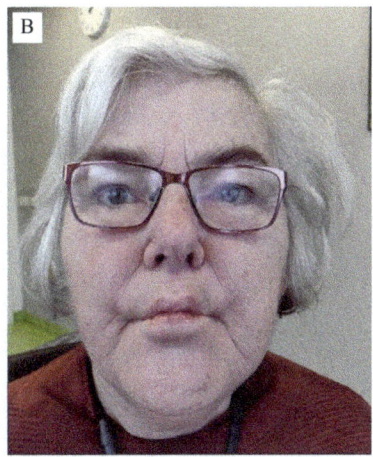

Figure 62.4 (A,B) A 72-year-old woman, severely affected with IBM after a disease duration of 20 years. She attempts to forcefully close the eyes, but her eyelashes remain visible, right more than left (A). Pouting the lips is also weak (B).

pharyngeal and suprahyoid muscle weakness. VF and MRI demonstrate a cricopharyngeal propulsion ('bar') in the region of the upper oesophageal sphincter during swallowing, which may be interpreted as functional achalasia.

Diagnosis

A diagnosis of IBM should be strongly considered in patients > 45 years, presenting with slowly progressive, proximal weakness of the legs, and/or often asymmetric weakness of the deep finger flexors over a period of more than one year. As mentioned above, there may be other, more uncommon manifestations (e.g., dysphagia, foot drop). A muscle biopsy is mandatory to show the presence of endomysial cytotoxic T cell infiltration surrounding non-necrotic fibres (with or without invasion). Supportive features are the following: rimmed vacuoles or protein aggregates (e.g., p62, TDP43), mitochondrial abnormalities (more than age-related). Also supportive of the diagnosis is a typical pattern of the thigh muscles on MRI (see Fig. 62.2B) or a typical pattern on ultrasound of the forearm, and the presence of elevated cN1A antibodies which have a sensitivity of 33–76% and a specificity of 80–96%. However, the antibodies can also be found in other myositis subtypes such as antisynthetase syndrome, immune-mediated necrotizing myopathy, and dermatomyositis. Seropositivity does not correlate with any prognostic factors or survival.

Serum CK activity is not very helpful as a diagnostic tool. CK is usually mildly to moderately elevated (<15x ULN).

IBM is a clinical mimic of ALS and multifocal motor neuropathy, in particular if there is asymmetric distal muscle weakness of the arms at onset. An EMG is not useful to differentiate IBM from other idiopathic inflammatory myopathies. However, in experienced hands, it is an important tool to distinguish IBM from diseases with a neurogenic cause.

Treatment

IBM is therapy-resistant. All immunosuppressants administered to patients with other idiopathic inflammatory myopathies have unfortunately failed in IBM. IBM is a disabling disorder. Patients become wheelchair dependent approximately 10–15 years after onset of the disease. Dysphagia, which develops in two-thirds of the patients, also progresses and may be associated with malnutrition, dehydration, and aspiration pneumonia, which may be the cause of death. Respiratory insufficiency caused by diaphragmatic weakness may occur at advanced stages. Overall, life expectancy is slightly shorter in IBM patients compared with the general population.

In patients with severe dysphagia in whom dietary measures are insufficient, botulinum toxin A, injected in the cricopharyngeus muscle, cricopharyngeus myotomy, or dilation or percutaneous endoscopic gastrostomy can be considered. Supportive strategies aim at improving quality of life, and a palliative care approach alongside the regular treatment seems appropriate, especially when swallowing difficulty occurs and when the patients lose the ability to walk and perform daily activities.

Suggested Reading

Cox FM, Titulaer MJ, Sont JK, et al. A 12-year follow-up in sporadic inclusion body myositis: an end stage with major disabilities. *Brain* 2011;134:3167–3175.

Greenberg SA. Inclusion body myositis: clinical features and pathogenesis. *Nat Rev Rheumatol* 2019;15(5):257–272.

Lilleker JB, Naddaf E, Saris CGJ, Schmidt J, de Visser M, Weihl CC; 272nd ENMC workshop participants. 272nd ENMC international workshop: 10 Years of progress - revision of the ENMC 2013 diagnostic criteria for inclusion body myositis and clinical trial readiness. 16-18 June 2023, Hoofddorp, The Netherlands. Neuromuscul Disord. 2024 Apr;37:36-51. doi: 10.1016/j.nmd.2024.03.001. Epub 2024 Mar 7. PMID: 38522330.

Shelly S, Mielke MM, Mandrekar J, et al. Epidemiology and natural history of inclusion body myositis: a 40-year population-based study. *Neurology* 2021;96(21):e2653–e2661.

Endocrine Myopathy: Hypothyroid Myopathy; Hyperthyroid Myopathy

Clinical History

A 41-year-old male was referred with a six-month history of progressive, exercise-related muscle pains, cramps, and muscle weakness. He also was found to have hyperCKaemia. His past medical history was unremarkable, and the family history was negative for neuromuscular disorders.

Examination

He had slight wasting and MRC grade 4 weakness of his shoulder girdle muscles. In addition, he had increased lumbar lordosis, firm calves, and a positive Gowers phenomenon. Sensation and reflexes were normal.

Diagnostic Considerations

The progressive muscle weakness with a limb girdle distribution and markedly elevated serum CK could be consistent with necrotizing immune-mediated myopathy, but muscular dystrophy (FSHD, BMD) and Pompe disease, despite the seemingly subacute onset and progression over months, were also considered.

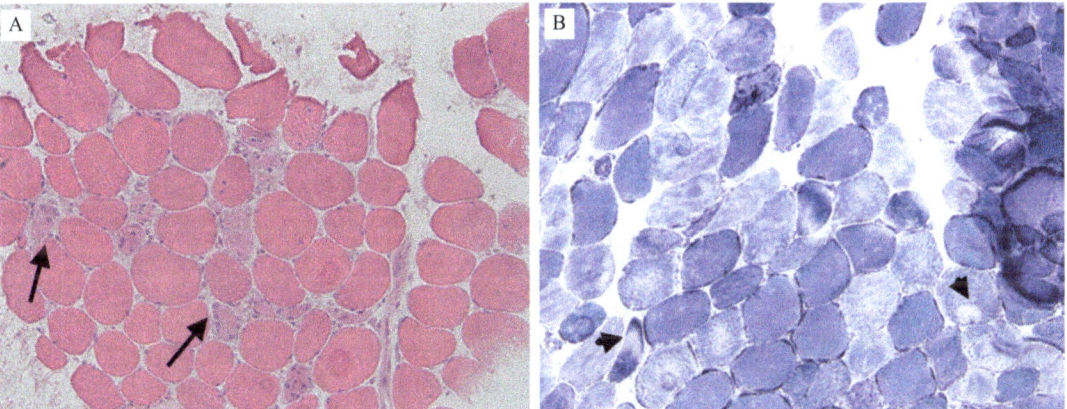

Figure 63.1 (A,B) A biopsy from the quadriceps femoris muscle shows marked variation in the size of the muscle fibres, necrotic and regenerating fibres (H&E stain, arrows) (A), and areas of decreased oxidative enzyme activity in numerous muscle fibres (NADH-TR stain, black arrow heads) (B).

Ancillary Investigations

Serum CK activity was 2530 IU/L (N < 130). Acid alpha-glucosidase activity in leucocytes was normal. Myositis-specific antibodies were negative.

A biopsy from the quadriceps femoris muscle showed marked variation in the size of the muscle fibres, foci of necrotic and regenerating fibres, areas of decreased oxidative enzyme activity in numerous muscle fibres (Fig. 63.1), and subsarcolemmal accumulations of glycogen. Immunohistochemical analysis, including dystrophin, sarcoglycan, and dystroglycan stains, was normal. DNA analysis for variations in the dystrophin gene (BMD) and in chromosome 4q35 (FSHD) was negative. At that time, next-generation sequencing was not yet available.

During the work-up, however, the patient's condition progressively deteriorated. Muscle weakness increased. He developed nasal dysarthria, and sleep-apnoea syndrome. The work-up of the latter includes analysis of the thyroid function, and subsequently a markedly increased TSH (185 mE/L, normal 0.4–4) was found. Free T4 was considerably decreased (< 2 mE/L, N 10–23), and anti-thyroid peroxidase antibodies were present.

These findings led to a diagnosis of autoimmune thyroiditis manifesting with hypothyroidism and myopathy.

Follow-Up

With treatment for hypothyroidism, he had complete recovery. All symptoms and signs subsided.

General Remarks

The endocrinological history of hypothyroidism includes tiredness, dry skin, cold intolerance, coarse voice, increase in weight, swelling of the tongue, and periorbital puffiness. Hashimoto thyroiditis is the most prevalent autoimmune disease worldwide and the most common cause of hypothyroidism. It is a T cell-mediated disease characterized by elevated levels of serum antithyroidperoxidase (anti-TPO) antibodies. Prior to hypothyroidism, there may be a few months of hyperthyroidism.

A prospective cohort study of newly diagnosed patients with thyroid dysfunction in a general hospital study in the Netherlands showed that complaints suggestive of muscle dysfunction were present in 79% of patients with untreated primary hypothyroidism (Duyff et al., 2000). Muscle complaints included weakness (54%), and fatigability, muscle pain, stiffness, or cramps (42%). In a few patients, these muscle complaints were the presenting symptom. Distal sensory symptoms occurred in 29%. On neurological examination, proximal muscle weakness was found in 30–40%. Neck flexor, deltoid, and iliopsoas muscles were predominantly affected, and weakness was usually mild. About 30% of patients had – usually bilateral – carpal tunnel syndrome. Mild, predominant sensory axonal neuropathy was observed in approximately 40%. One-third of patients had myopathic EMG abnormalities with short-duration motor unit action potentials. Serum CK is often elevated, and sometimes strikingly high. Muscle biopsy may present nonspecific findings (e.g., necrotic fibres and cell infiltrates, and 'core'-like structures), as was also the case in our patient.

Diagnostic delay ranged between two months and seven years (mean one year).

During treatment, muscle complaints resolved in 79% of the patients with an average time of seven months. Some patients remained symptomatic after one year of treatment. A significant correlation between the level of weakness and the biochemical severity of hypothyroidism in hypothyroid patients was not found. Only in a few cases was myxoedema or rhabdomyolysis observed.

The main message of this case vignette is that all patients who present with an elevated CK should undergo routine testing of serum thyroid stimulating hormone. Hypothyroidism may go unrecognized if there is no clear history of thyroid dysfunction.

In the above-mentioned cohort study, two-thirds of the patients with hyperthyroidism had complaints of weakness and fatigability, and muscle pain. Cramps occurred in 10%. The mean subjective duration of these symptoms was significantly shorter in hyperthyroid than in hypothyroid patients. Mild symmetric proximal leg muscle weakness was found in 62% of the patients with hyperthyroidism. However, EMG, CK, and muscle histology were normal. Because of the significant correlation between the severity of hyperthyroidism and clinical muscle weakness, a functional muscle disorder due to metabolic dysfunction is a more likely explanation than a structural myopathy.

Symmetric sensory polyneuropathy was found in 19%. Generalized hyperreflexia and tremor were frequently observed.

Thyrotoxic periodic paralysis is a complication of hyperthyroidism among individuals of Asian descent, characterized by sudden onset of hypokalaemia and muscle paralysis (see Case 50, Table 50.1).

Both Hashimoto thyroiditis and Graves disease may be associated with myasthenia gravis. Graves disease is an autoimmune disease characterized by hyperthyroidism, diffuse goitre, ophthalmopathy, and in rare cases, dermopathy. Thyroid-associated ophthalmopathy is an ocular condition that is the most common extrathyroidal manifestation of Graves disease. Diplopia can occur due to inflammation of the extra-ocular muscles.

Suggested Reading

Duyff RF, Van den Bosch J, Laman DM, van Loon BJ, Linssen WH. Neuromuscular findings in thyroid dysfunction: a prospective clinical and electrodiagnostic study. *J Neurol Neurosurg Psychiatry* 2000;68(6):750–755. doi: 10.1136/jnnp.68.6.750. PMID: 10811699; PMCID: PMC1736982.

Klein I, Ojamaa K. Thyroid (neuro)myopathy. *Lancet* 2000;356(9230):614. doi: 10.1016/s0140-6736(00)02601-5. PMID: 10968432.

Jordan B, Uer O, Buchholz T, Spens A, Zierz S. Physical fatigability and muscle pain in patients with Hashimoto thyroiditis. *J Neurol* 2021;268(7):2441–2449. doi: 10.1007/s00415-020-10394-5. Epub 2021 Jan 28. PMID: 33507372; PMCID: PMC8217009.

Drug-Induced Myopathies: Hydroxychloroquine Myopathy

Clinical History

A 55-year-old woman was referred because of increasing complaints about her legs for a few years. She had a continuous 'heavy feeling' in her legs and buttocks. There was no difficulty with walking or climbing stairs, but cycling was increasingly difficult. She had a dry mouth, which impaired swallowing.

The medical history included chronic discoid lupus erythematosus of her face and immune dysregulation for which she was treated with both prednisone for about 10 years (dosage 5 mg bid), hydroxychloroquine, also for about 10 years (dosage 200 mg bid), and intravenous immunoglobulins (IVIg). Other medications included alendronic acid, calcium carbonate/calciferol, cotrimoxazole, esomeprazole, labetalol, and salicylic acid.

Examination
There was a rash of the upper part of her torso. Otherwise, there were no abnormalities and, in particular, no leg weakness.

Diagnostic Considerations
A steroid myopathy was considered a possible explanation because of chronic prednisone use. An overlap myositis was considered, and also dermatomyositis, albeit the skin changes were restricted to the upper part of the torso. Chloroquine myopathy was also a diagnostic consideration.

Ancillary Investigations
Serum CK was elevated (600 IU/L; normal < 217). Muscle MRI of the legs showed no abnormalities, in particular no hyperintensity as sign of inflammation. A biopsy of the quadriceps muscle showed predominance of type 2 fibres, but no type 2 fibre atrophy. There were degenerating fibres and fibres with vacuoles. No inflammatory changes were found. Acid phosphatase was markedly positive, in particular in the fibres with vacuoles (Fig. 64.1A,B).

Follow-Up
Based on the histopathological findings in the muscle biopsy, a diagnosis of hydroxychloroquine myopathy was established. Hydroxychloroquine was discontinued and CK normalized in two months. Muscle symptoms persisted.

General Remarks
Many drugs and toxins have been reported to carry a risk of causing a myopathy. Pathogenetic mechanisms, clinical presentation, and laboratory and pathological abnormalities differ; see Doughty and Amato (2019) for a comprehensive overview. Some of these drugs are prescribed frequently and are discussed below (Table 64.1): (hydroxy)chloroquine, statins, immune checkpoints inhibitors, and steroids. Myotoxic effects of alcohol are here described too. Deficiencies are not a major cause of myopathies, but hypovitaminosis D is often considered as a cause of muscle weakness in clinical practice.

(Hydroxy)chloroquine
Chloroquine (CQ) and hydroxychloroquine (HCQ) are frequently prescribed in connective tissue diseases (CTDs) because of their immunomodulatory effect. Besides liver, kidney, and retina toxicity, skeletal and cardiac myopathy is a well-documented adverse effect. Case reports have also suggested that CQ/HCQ can unmask or worsen myasthenia gravis and cause a peripheral neuropathy.

CQ and HCQ have an effect on lysosomal function and membrane stability and CQ/HCQ myopathy is pathologically characterized by autophagic vacuoles or rimmed vacuoles, with an increase in the activity of the lysosomal enzyme acid phosphatase. These abnormalities, however, can be very subtle. Ultra-structural abnormalities (myeloid or curvilinear bodies) can be found more frequently. Clinically, there is proximal weakness. Myalgia is not a prominent feature. The duration of medication use before symptom onset is variable (between 6 months to > 10 years). Most studies have reported symptoms at doses of 200–400 mg/day. Swallowing muscles, respiratory muscles, and axial muscles (mainly neck flexors) may be affected, in particular after long exposure. Dysphagia and respiratory

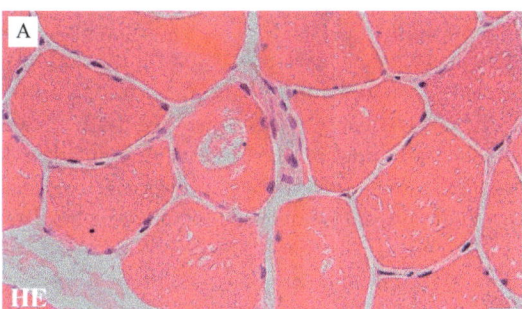
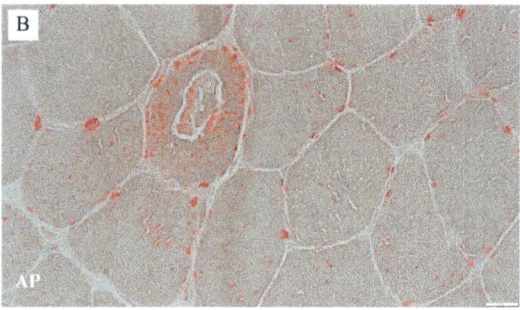

Figure 64.1 The H&E stain shows a muscle fibre with a large vacuole and muscle fibres with small vacuoles (A). Acid phosphatase (AP) is markedly elevated in the vacuolized fibre and in a punctate fashion in the other fibres (B). Courtesy Professor Eleonora Aronica.

Table 64.1 Features of selected drugs, toxins, and deficiencies that may cause myopathy

Drug/toxin deficiency	Weakness	Pain	CK	EMG	Muscle biopsy
(Hydroxy) chloroquine	Onset in proximal limb muscles, heart	No pain	Mildly elevated	Spontaneous muscle fibre activity	Vacuoles, increased acid phosphatase reactivity, ultra-structural abnormalities
Immune checkpoint inhibitors	Limb girdle muscles	Myalgia	Markedly elevated	Spontaneous muscle fibre activity	Inflammatory or necrotizing features
Statins	Proximal limb muscles	Myalgia, cramps	Elevated	Spontaneous muscle fibre activity	Necrosis and regeneration
Steroids	Atrophy and proximal weakness legs > arms	No pain	Normal	Normal	Type 2 fibre atrophy
Chronic alcohol abuse	Atrophy and proximal weakness legs > arms	No	Normal or mildly elevated	Normal	Type 2 fibre atrophy, oxidative changes
Vitamin D deficiency	Proximal weakness	Myalgia, bone pain	Normal	Insertional activity↑, small polyphasic muscle action potentials	Type 2 fibre atrophy

insufficiency may go unnoticed and need to be screened for. Cardiac screening is also strongly recommended since dilated cardiomyopathy and prolonged QT interval that predispose to lethal cardiac arrhythmias can occur. CK ranges from normal to moderately (< 10 ×) elevated. A muscle biopsy can be helpful for the distinction with an overlap myositis. The diagnosis is often delayed by months to years. Once diagnosed and the drug discontinued, the patients improve, but there may be residual weakness in those who were severely affected.

A vacuolar myopathy with increased acid phosphatase reactivity can also be caused by colchicine. This myopathy is featured by subacute symmetrical weakness and markedly elevated CK within weeks after start of the medication.

Statins

Hyperlipidaemia is a major risk factor for cardiovascular morbidity and mortality. Statins are the first-choice treatment. They lower cholesterol synthesis by blocking the enzyme HMGCoA-reductase (HMGCR). Statins can adversely affect muscle fibres, as shown by an elevation of serum CK activity (statin-associated myotoxicity (SAMT)). Almost always, CK elevation is mild (< 4 × ULN) and asymptomatic. It is advised to stop the medication for four to six weeks if CK is > 4 × ULN and start again at a lower dose, in combination with ezetimibe if needed, after CK has normalized.

Rarely, hyperCKaemia, usually > 10 × ULN, is accompanied by myalgia and/or muscle weakness (estimated incidence 9 per 10,000 person-years). Risk factors are, among other, high-dose statin, Chinese ethnicity, older age, female sex, low BMI, various drugs (e.g., fibrates, cyclosporine), and genetic factors. Onset of myopathy is within six months after initiation of the medication in one-third of patients, but it can also begin after years. Myalgia and cramps are more prominent than is weakness. A muscle biopsy shows necrosis and regeneration, but is not needed for making the diagnosis. The diagnosis is confirmed by resolution of hyperCKaemia and complains within three months after discontinuation of the medication. It is advised to restart the statin in a lower dose, or switch to another type of cholesterol-lowering drug, and add another type of lipid-lowering drug if needed. Extremely rarely, toxic statin myopathy takes the more severe, acute form of rhabdomyolysis.

Myalgia without CK elevation is reported by up to 25% of patients, and has been shown in randomized placebo-controlled trials to rest upon a nocebo effect in at least half of them. Misattribution probably occurs too. Statin-related myalgia (statin-associated muscle symptoms (SAMS)) is symmetric, located in proximal muscles and the calves, and develops within one to two months. In contrast, musculoskeletal discomfort of another cause is more diffuse and can develop later. In patients in which the complaint is not due to the statin, cessation of the medication should be avoided.

Apart from a direct myotoxic effect on muscle, the use of a statin is in extremely rare cases complicated by an immune-mediated necrotizing myopathy (HMGCR-IMNM, statin-associated autoimmune myopathy (SAAM), **Case 44**), hypothesized to be causally related to the formation of antibodies directed at HMGCR. Symmetric, proximal weakness can be severe and CK is often markedly elevated. HMGCR-IMNM does not resolve after cessation of the statin and needs to be treated by immunosuppressive and immunomodulatory medication. HMGCR-IMNM also occurs without prior use of a statin, both in children and adults.

Immune Checkpoints Inhibitors (see also Case 33)

Neuromuscular adverse effects occur in over 1% of patients using an immune checkpoints inhibitor (ICI). Over half the patients with an ICI-related myositis or necrotizing myopathy have a concurrent myasthenia gravis, myocarditis, or both.

Onset in these overlap manifestations is earlier (days–weeks), and prognosis is much worse than in isolated ICI-related myopathy. Mild, isolated ICI-related myopathy can be treated with prednisone while continuing the ICI treatment. In myositis-myasthenia-myocarditis overlap disease, ICI treatment should be discontinued and treatment with immune suppression and immune modulation should be prompt and aggressive.

Steroids

Corticosteroid-induced myopathy is characterized by insidious-onset, symmetric weakness and atrophy of pelvic more than shoulder girdle muscles without pain. Serum CK is normal, needle EMG is also normal, and a muscle biopsy shows atrophy of type 2 fibres, but various other abnormalities may be present. Evidence concerning duration of treatment or doses that increase the risk of myopathy, as well as studies on prevalence, is largely lacking. In cancer patients taking daily high-dose dexamethasone (which is 5 × as potent as prednisone), weakness can evolve after a few weeks of treatment, related to the cumulative dose. Muscle strength has been reported to improve after three to four weeks following the cessation of the medication. Impaired muscle function due to corticosteroid-induced myopathy should be differentiated from symptoms and signs of the underlying disease, such as immobilization, exercise intolerance, and general malaise, as well as from the impact of other adverse effects of corticosteroids, such as body weight gain. It is noted that immobilization may also show a type 2 muscle fibre atrophy in a muscle biopsy. In the treatment of myositis with prednisone, persisting weakness and even increasing weakness while CK activity is decreasing should not be mistaken for corticosteroid-induced myopathy. In these patients, improvement of muscle strength can lag behind the decrease of CK levels for months, and premature withdrawal of prednisone would be detrimental.

Alcohol

Binge-drinking can cause rhabdomyolysis. In almost half of chronic asymptomatic alcohol-addicted men, muscle strength and cardiac function are less than in age-matched controls. The toxic effect of chronic ethanol abuse on skeletal and cardiac muscle seems to be independent of the effects of nutritional deficiencies. In elderly persons after many years of very high ethanol intake (at least 10 drinks a day) it mainly manifests with limb girdle atrophy and weakness (typically mild) and normal or mildly elevated serum CK. A muscle biopsy shows predominant atrophy of type 2 fibres, but necrosis, regeneration, moth-eaten fibers, and oxidative changes may also be present. Cessation of alcohol consumption or lowering the daily ethanol intake reportedly results in improvement in strength in most patients within a year.

Vitamin D Deficiency

Rickets and osteomalacia in adults manifest with bone pain, symptoms and signs of pathological fractures, musculoskeletal pain, and proximal or diffuse muscle weakness. It is not clear whether the muscle symptoms are a direct effect of hypovitaminosis D or of the hypocalcaemia, secondary hyperparathyroidism, or hypophosphatemia that consecutively results from the vitamin D deficiency. Patients who present with proximal myalgia and weakness and severe vitamin D deficiency (< 20 nmol/L; < 8 ng/mL), which can occur in heavily veiled women with insufficient dietary calcium intake, may lack clinical symptoms and signs of bone disease, and show osteopenia only radiologically and by an increase of alkaline phosphatase. Weakness may be severe, leaving the patient wheelchair bound. In these patients, CK is normal, EMG shows increased insertional activity and small polyphasic muscle action potentials, and a muscle biopsy shows type 2 fibre atrophy. After supplementation with oral cholecalciferol (800 IU/day) and calcium supplements (1200 mg/day), weakness has been described to resolve within three months. A randomized placebo-controlled trial in post-menopausal women with moderate vitamin D deficiency (35–67 nmol/L; 14–27 ng/mL) showed no effect of supplementation with vitamin D_3 on timed up and go tests or falls. A randomized placebo-controlled trial in patients with diffuse musculoskeletal pain and moderate vitamin D deficiency (< 50 nmol/L; < 20 ng/mL) also showed no benefit.

Suggested Reading

Abudalou M, Mohamed AS, Vega EA, Al Sbihi A. Colchicine-induced rhabdomyolysis: a review of 83 cases. BMJ Case Rep. 2021 Jul 21;14(7):e241977. doi: 10.1136/bcr-2021-241977. PMID: 34290008; PMCID: PMC8296791.

Allenbach Y, Anquetil C, Manouchehri A et al. Immune checkpoint inhibitor-induced myositis, the earliest and most lethal complication among rheumatic and musculoskeletal toxicities. Autoimmun Rev. 2020 Aug;19(8):102586. doi: 10.1016/j.autrev.2020.102586. Epub 2020 Jun 11. PMID: 32535094.

Batchelor TT, Taylor LP, Thaler HT, Posner JB, DeAngelis LM. Steroid myopathy in cancer patients. *Neurology* 1997;48(5):1234–1238. doi: 10.1212/wnl.48.5.1234. PMID: 9153449.

Doughty CT, Amato AA. Toxic myopathies. *Continuum (Minneap Minn)* 2019;25(6):1712–1731. doi: 10.1212/CON.0000000000000806. PMID: 31794468.

Gunton JE, Girgis CM. Vitamin D and muscle. *Bone Rep* 2018;8:163–167. doi: 10.1016/j.bonr.2018.04.004. PMID: 29963601; PMCID: PMC6021354.

Mammen AL. Statin-associated myalgias and muscle injury-recognizing and managing both while still lowering the low-density lipoprotein. *Med Clin North Am* 2021;105(2):263–272. doi: 10.1016/j.mcna.2020.10.004. Epub 2020 Dec 24. PMID: 33589101.

Naddaf E, Paul P, AbouEzzeddine OF. Chloroquine and hydroxychloroquine myopathy: clinical spectrum and treatment outcomes. *Front Neurol* 2021;11:616075. doi: 10.3389/fneur.2020.616075. PMID: 33603707; PMCID: PMC7884308.

Penson PE, Bruckert E, Marais D, et al.; International Lipid Expert Panel (ILEP).Step-by-step diagnosis and management of the nocebo/drucebo effect in statin-associated muscle symptoms patients: a position paper from the International Lipid Expert Panel (ILEP). *J Cachexia Sarcopenia Muscle* 2022;13(3):1596–1622. doi: 10.1002/jcsm.12960. Epub 2022 Mar 10. PMID: 35969116; PMCID: PMC9178378.Bottom of Form

Simon L, Jolley SE, Molina PE. Alcoholic myopathy: pathophysiologic mechanisms and clinical implications. *Alcohol Res* 2017;38(2):207–217. PMID: 28988574; PMCID: PMC5513686.

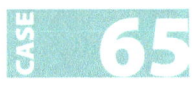

CASE 65 A- or Paucisymptomatic HyperCKaemia

Clinical History

A 44-year-old man was referred because of hyperCKaemia (elevated CK activity). CK ranged from 1300 to 2200 IU/L (normal < 171). Before referral some investigations were performed. TSH was normal. HyperCKaemia was initially considered to be related to the use of simvastatin, but four months after withdrawal of this drug, CK was still markedly elevated.

He did not complain about muscle weakness, muscle cramps, or myalgia. Previous history disclosed diabetes mellitus type 2, hypertension, and Asperger syndrome. Medication included metoprolol/hydrochlorothiazide, enalapril, and metformin. Family history was negative for neuromuscular disorders.

Examination

Hypertrophic calves and focal atrophy of the left thigh were noted, but there was no muscle weakness. Sensation was normal, reflexes could be normally elicited.

Diagnostic Considerations

Asymptomatic and paucisymptomatic hyperCKaemia has an extensive differential diagnosis (Chapter 3, Box 3.22). We submitted the patient to repeat history taking and he admitted that he had never been good at sports from childhood onwards. Running caused excruciating pain in the calves during childhood (without producing dark urine), and later he experienced stiffness of the muscles. However, he had been able to serve in the army.

Differential diagnosis in patients with calf hypertrophy and hyperCKaemia may include Becker muscular dystrophy, various forms of limb girdle muscular dystrophy, spinal muscular atrophy type 3, and Pompe disease.

Ancillary Investigations

CK ranged from 1300 to 2200 IU/L (normal < 171). TSH was normal

We first performed muscle imaging because this may be helpful in guiding the genetic work-up. MRI showed replacement of the adductor magnus, the long head of the biceps femoris and – to a lesser extent – the semimembranosus muscle on both sides, and the left vastus lateralis muscle by fat (Fig. 65.1). Since the patient's MRI of the thighs was compatible with Becker muscular dystrophy (BMD), DNA analysis of the dystrophin gene (multiplex ligation-dependent probe amplification (MPLA)) was performed. This disclosed an in-frame deletion of exons 2–7, consistent with a diagnosis of BMD. Subsequent cardiological examination did not reveal any abnormalities, but the patient was scheduled to undergo cardiological screening on a regular basis.

Follow-Up

Over the ensuing years, he mentioned mild functional limitations. He had to hold the railing when getting up the stairs and he was no longer able to run. On examination, he had a slight waddling gait and some atrophy of the pectoral major muscles. Cardiac screening was still normal.

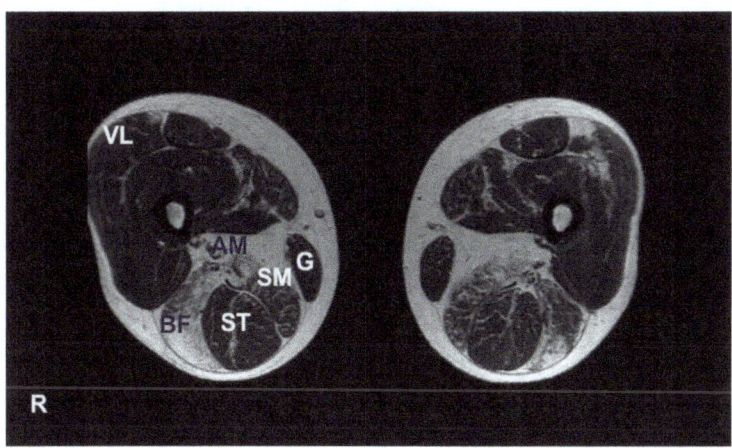

Figure 65.1 T1-weighted MR image shows preferential involvement of specific muscles. The adductor magnus (AM) is completely replaced by fat, as is the biceps femoris (BF); the semimembranosus (SM) is slightly involved, the vastus lateralis (VL) is slightly involved on the left. The gracilis (G) and semitendinosus (ST) muscles have a hypertrophic aspect.

General Remarks

Creatine kinase (CK) is an enzyme playing an important role in the energy metabolism of cells. It catalyses the reaction of creatine and adenosine triphosphate to create phosphocreatine and adenosine diphosphate. Three isoenzymes are involved: CK-MM, which is mainly present in skeletal muscle (93%), CK-MB in cardiac muscle (< 6%), and CK-BB, which is predominantly expressed in the brain (< 3%). The sum of these three isoenzymes quantifies the total serum CK (sCK) levels.

Increased CK activity indicates muscle damage with disruption of sarcolemmal integrity and may be caused by a variety of conditions (Chapter 3, Box 3.22). An exception is macro-CK. In macro-CK type 1 (not associated with disease), immunoglobulins bind to CK-BB, while in macro-CK type 2 (usually associated with significant disease) oligomeric mitochondrial CK is present.

The reference values of CK are still a matter of discussion. It is important to take into account that CK varies across gender and ethnicities. Men have a higher CK than women and Black people have a higher CK than non-Black individuals (see for definition of reference values Chapter 3, Box 3.22).

HyperCKaemia may be the initial sign of a neuromuscular disorder already known in the family, such as BMD or Duchenne muscular dystrophy (DMD)/BMD carriership, limb girdle muscular dystrophy or distal myopathy due to dysferlin or anoctamin 5 variants, sarcoglycanopathy, Pompe disease, McArdle disease, and others (Chapter 3, Box 3.22).

If confronted with an individual with a- or paucisymptomatic (myalgia, cramps, but no apparent muscle weakness) elevated CK without positive family history, one should recheck CK after 7 days and recommend the patient to reduce physical activities and refrain from alcohol.

If CK is still elevated, which is the case in ~30%, check whether this can be explained by a medical condition, substance abuse, or drug treatment (Chapter 3, Box 3.22). This is the case in more than 40% of the remaining cases and caused mostly by statins or thyroid, renal, or cardiac disease.

If all these causes are ruled out and CK is 1.5 times the upper limit of normal (this cut-off has been chosen by consensus), taking into account gender and race, then one should look for a neuromuscular cause (in approximately 10% of the cases). Some recommend performing EMG or muscle MRI first, and if these tests do not show abnormalities, the advice is to refrain from further evaluation and monitor the patient and CK. In this case, there is idiopathic hyperCKaemia. Others start genetic testing. Next-generation sequencing (NGS) can be very helpful in identifying the culprit gene. However, detection rate is approximately 50%. When gene panel analysis is negative, the following approach can be taken. Repeats (e.g., DM2) or large deletions/duplications (e.g., BMD, SMA) are currently not identified by NGS; proceed to whole exome screening and if this does not yield any results, consider performing whole genome screening. If a causative gene is not found, re-evaluate the phenotype (EMG, muscle MRI, ischaemic forearm test, muscle biopsy, dried blood spot), and consider carrying out additional tests, such as Sanger fill-in, copy number variation (CNV) analysis, and repeat analysis. This should always be done in close collaboration with the geneticist and the lab.

Patients with asymptomatic hyperCKaemia may be at risk for malignant hyperthermia (MH). If a (likely) pathogenic *RYR1* variant is found as explanation for hyperCKaemia, in vitro contracture test (IVCT) is recommended. Since IVCT is an invasive test, it seems that as yet there is not sufficient evidence to recommend this in every case with asymptomatic unexplained hyperCKaemia. Consequently, when patients with unexplained hyperCKaemia undergo anaesthesia, substances that may trigger MH (inhalational anesthetics and depolarizing muscle relaxants) should be avoided as a precautionary measure.

Suggested Reading

Brewster LM, Mairuhu G, Sturk A, van Montfrans GA. Distribution of creatine kinase in the general population: implications for statin therapy. *Am Heart J* 2007;154(4):655–661. doi: 10.1016/j.ahj.2007.06.008. PMID: 17892987.

Janssens L, De Puydt J, Milazzo M, et al. Risk of malignant hyperthermia in patients carrying a variant in the skeletal muscle ryanodine receptor 1 gene. *Neuromuscul Disord* 2022;32(11-12):864–869. doi: 10.1016/j.nmd.2022.10.003. Epub 2022 Oct 19. PMID: 36283893.

Lilleng H, Johnsen SH, Wilsgaard T, Bekkelund SI. Are the currently used reference intervals for creatine kinase (CK) reflecting the general population? The

Tromsø Study. *Clin Chem Lab Med* 2011;50(5):879–884. doi: 10.1515/CCLM.2011.776. PMID: 22070220.

Kley RA, Schmidt-Wilcke T, Vorgerd M. Differential diagnosis of hyperckemia. *Neurol Int Open* 2018;2: E72–E83.

Rubegni A, Malandrini A, Dosi C, et al. Next-generation sequencing approach to hyperCKemia: a 2-year cohort study. *Neurol Genet* 2019;5(5):e352. doi: 10.1212/NXG.0000000000000352. PMID: 31517061; PMCID: PMC6705647.

CASE 66  Exertional Rhabdomyolysis

Clinical History

A 45-year-old man was referred by the internist because of a second episode of rhabdomyolysis. Motor milestones had been normal, and he had always been good at sports, although he was used to having stiff calves after skiing. At the age of 39 years he once experienced a sensation of 'barbed wire' in his upper legs, evolving in quite severe myalgia building up over days. This complaint dissolved in the course of three weeks. CK activity in this period increased to 23,094 U/L and normalized completely. There was no history of dark urine. In the absence of a metabolic cause or a history of the use of drugs, this was interpreted as having been caused by a viral infection. In the preceding months, he had been cycling fanatically daily, up to exhaustion. After this episode he had cut down on his sporting activities, but recently he had taken up mountain biking. One day, he experienced the same sensations as six years earlier, albeit less severe. CK values rose to 8926 and normalized in a couple of weeks. In between these attacks, he did not have any muscle-related complaints such as cramps or myalgia. He had noticed for a long time, however, that he had firm calves, just as his deceased father and his eldest daughter. No one in the family had had muscle complaints similar to the patient's. He never had had surgery. His parents were not consanguineous.

Examination

Firm calves (Fig. 66.1) were noted. There was no weakness and no joint contractures.

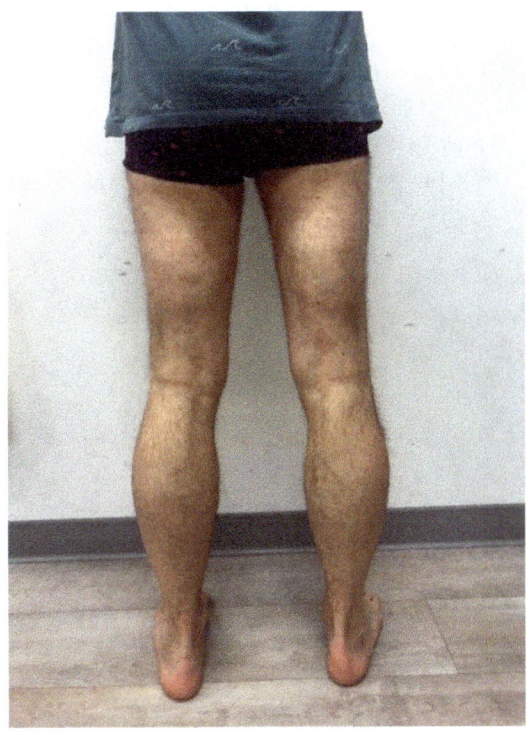

Figure 66.1 Firm calves in the described patient.

Diagnostic Considerations

Repeated attacks of rhabdomyolysis provoked by physical activity is highly suggestive of a neuromuscular cause. *RYR1* is a relatively frequent causative gene in exertional rhabdomyolysis. This diagnosis seemed to be corroborated by the family history, suggesting muscle hypertrophy in an autosomal dominant inheritance pattern (male-to-male transmission), but calf appearances vary widely in the general population. The normal CK in between attacks argued against a diagnosis of muscular dystrophy or McArdle disease. The absence of attacks during childhood argued against Lipin-1 deficiency. We decided to first perform investigations aimed at a CPT2 deficiency or another fatty oxidation disorder, as a positive result would allow for a targeted genetic analysis. If negative, we planned to request either a single-gene (*RYR1*) analysis or a multi-gene panel analysis. A single-gene test would have the disadvantage of necessitating further DNA analyses if negative. Genetic analysis using a large gene panel containing hundreds of genes would implicate a fair chance of finding a variant of unknown significance (VUS), and would still not capture a causative mitochondrial DNA defect.

Ancillary Investigations

CK was 187. Acylcarnitine profile was normal. A gene panel analysis disclosed heterozygosity for the probably pathogenic variant c.7300G>A p. (Gly2434Arg) in the *RYR1* gene. This variant is associated with an increased susceptibility to malignant hyperthermia.

Follow-Up

The patient was referred to a clinical geneticist. His eldest daughter, a sister, and her son were found to be affected with the mutation too. All family members received information and advice concerning rhabdomyolysis and the risk of anaesthetics. The patient resumed mountain biking, albeit 'with the brakes on'.

General Remarks and Suggested Reading

For more information on rhabdomyolysis, see **Case 53** (McArdle disease) and **Case 54** (CPT2 deficiency).

For more information on malignant hyperthermia, see **Case 56** (*RYR1*-related disease) and Chapter 8 (Management).

Video legends

Supplementary videos are available at www.cambridge.org/neuromuscular

Part I: Evaluation and Treatment of Patients with a Neuromuscular Disorder

Numbers	Title	Remarks
Video 1	EMG: Fibrillations and Positive Sharp Waves.	Fibrillations (amplitude 20–200 µV; duration 1–5 ms, frequency 0.5–15 Hz), positive sharp waves (amplitude 20–200 µV; duration 10–30 ms, frequency 0.5–15 Hz) and their combined presence in needle myography are shown (50 µV/division). In fact, positive sharp waves are the same potentials as fibrillations, with only their stop at the needle giving rise to a different morphology. They are produced by structurally detached muscle fibres (e.g., denervation, inflammation, and degeneration) and subsequent membrane instability. Their sound has a unique 'rain on the roof' pitch and, in contrast to motor unit potentials, their frequency is highly regular with linear change.
Video 2	EMG: Large and Polyphasic MUPs with Long Duration	Large polyphasic motor unit potentials (MUPs; often > 2000 µV amplitude, > 4 phases/turns) with long duration (> 15 ms) and giant potentials (> 10 mV amplitude) are shown, upon volitional contraction. Sprouting of nearby axons to previously detached muscle fibres (i.e., re-innervation) will give rise to fibre connections with different degrees of maturation in the parent motor unit. Consequently, action potential propagation is variable and underlies the polyphasic features and long duration of these altered MUPs. The size of the motor unit also increases, resulting in the enlarged MUPs. Their sound has a dull crackling pitch and, in line with normal MUPs, frequency is pseudo-regular (off-beat). These abnormal MUPs may have satellite potentials, can be unstable, and are often seen with reduced recruitment.
Video 3	EMG: Small Polyphasic MUPs with Short Duration.	Small polyphasic motor unit potentials (MUPs; typically < 500 µV amplitude, > 4 phases/turns) with short duration (< 6 ms) are shown. These are common in myopathies, with enhanced recruitment. However, they can also be seen early in the re-innervation process as well as in myasthenic syndromes. Inflammation, fibre degradation, and denervation will cause detached muscle fibres. Sprouting of nearby axons to such separated muscle fibres will give rise to fibre connections with different degrees of maturation in the parent motor unit. Furthermore, a smaller pool with increased heterogeneity of muscle fibre diameters is seen as some muscle fibres are lost and others regenerate. Consequently, the action potential propagation is variable, resulting in the polyphasic and short duration of these altered MUPs. Their sound has a sharp crackling pitch, and, in line with normal MUPs, frequency is pseudo-regular (off-beat).
Video 4	EMG: Complex Repetitive Discharges.	Complex repetitive discharges (CRDs) have an abrupt onset and termination, with moderate decay in between, and high frequency (5–100 Hz). CRDs are the result of depolarization of a single muscle fibre, followed by ephaptic transmission to adjacent denervated motor fibres and ultimately a self-propagating circuit in a muscle fascicle. CRDs should not be confused with short runs of positive sharp waves or myotonic discharges. Their sound is regular without significant change, often compared with the engine of a petrol motor bike.

Video legends

(cont.)

Numbers	Title	Remarks
Video 5	EMG: Myotonic Discharges.	Myotonic discharges have a unique waxing and waning pattern (firing rate 20–150 Hz, 20–300 μV), with a positive wave or brief spike morphology. Myotonic discharges are the result of an abnormally low depolarizing threshold of muscle fibres, and further perpetuation by cumulative after-depolarization. Hence, the cross-over of individual myotonic discharges underlies the waxing and waning pattern. Myotonic discharges should not be confused with short runs of positive sharp waves (sometimes referred to as 'pseudo-myotonia') or CRDs. Their sound is regular with exponential change, often referred to as 'dive bomber' or likened to a short thrust on the throttle of a motor engine.
Video 6	Ultrasound: Fasciculations	Fasciculations are focal areas of abrupt and irregular movements within the muscle (ultrasound). They have short duration and variable occurrence (one or multiple sites, low and high intensity). These should be discerned from muscle displacement by a pulsating artery (regular frequency), muscle contraction (larger part or all of muscle seen moving, often gradually), or probe movement (movement of the whole image).
Video 7	Example of Ultrasound Protocol for Dysimmune Neuropathies.	A diverse set of ultrasound protocols has been published to evaluate a range of different neuropathies. A practical protocol, evaluating median nerves and brachial plexus bilaterally, could be considered in suspected dysimmune neuropathies. Screening for potential changes in nerve size from wrist to axilla (median nerves), extraforaminal to supraclavicular (brachial plexus), and measuring nerve size at predetermined sites can be done relatively quickly (± 15 min). Use of appropriate reference values, interpretation within the appropriate clinical context, and careful consideration of potential imaging mimics are essential for accurate interpretation.

Part II: Neuromuscular Cases

Numbers	Title	Remarks
Video 1.1	Amyotrophic Lateral Sclerosis.	A patient with ALS showing florid fasciculation in his biceps brachii muscle.
Video 1.2	Amyotrophic Lateral Sclerosis	Patient with ALS – muscle atrophy, fasciculations, hyperreflexia in atrophic muscle, and extensor plantar response (Babinski reflex).
Video 2.1	Pseudobulbar Palsy	Patient with pseudobulbar palsy showing slow movements of an otherwise normal looking tongue. Brisk jaw jerk.
Video 2.2	Spastic Gait	Patient with myelopathy caused by cervical stenosis showing a spastic gait.
Video 5.1	Spinal and Bulbar Muscular Atrophy (Kennedy Disease)	Limb girdle walking pattern, tongue fasciculations, postural tremor.
Video 5.2	Spinal and Bulbar Muscular Atrophy (Kennedy Disease)	Perioral and tongue fasciculations, facial weakness visible when pouting the lips and showing the teeth.
Video 9.1	Miller–Fisher/GBS Overlap Syndrome	Ophthalmoplegia, areflexia, ataxia (and ptosis) compatible with Miller–Fisher syndrome (MFS). In addition, clear limb weakness that is compatible with GBS. Combination of these features is compatible with MFS/GBS overlap syndrome. Difficult walking due to limb muscle weakness and ataxia.

(cont.)

Numbers	Title	Remarks
Video 10.1	Chronic Inflammatory Demyelinating Polyneuropathy	Problems when rising from a chair (proximal limb muscle weakness) and walking with foot drop, due to distal weakness. Sensory loss and areflexia (not shown). Combination of both proximal and distal weakness (and clear features of demyelination with EMG examination) is compatible with diagnosis of typical CIDP.
Video 18.1	Peripheral Nerve Hyperexcitability: Morvan Syndrome	Peripheral nerve hyperexcitability – myokymia and fasciculations in leg muscles. Widespread and gross abnormal muscle movements (cramps, fasciculations, gross muscle twitches) especially in arms and legs, but also in all other parts of the body (only partially shown). In the presence of sleep disturbances and behavioural changes, and anti-Caspr2 and LGI1 antibodies: compatible with Morvan syndrome.
Video 27.1	Charcot–Marie–Tooth Disease	Steppage gait due to weakness of ankle dorsal flexors.
Video 31.1	Myasthenia Gravis	Provocation of asymmetric ptosis when looking upwards.
Video 35.1	Congenital Myasthenic Syndromes: Dok7, Before Treatment	Seven-year-old girl with Dok7-related CMS performing a 10-meter walk–run test. Note the inability to increase speed, and the endorotation of the right leg.
Video 35.2	Congenital Myasthenic Syndromes: Dok7, After Treatment.	One year after treatment with salbutamol. She is now able to run symmetrically, i.e., clear the floor with both feet. There is no longer any endorotation of the right leg.
Video 37.1	Becker Muscular Dystrophy	Gowers sign in a patient with Becker muscular dystrophy when getting up from a chair.
Video 39.1	Myotonic Dystrophy Type I	Action myotonia, percussion myotonia, foot drop, and steppage gait.
Video 39.2	Action Myotonia.	
Video 39.3	Percussion Myotonia.	
Video 41.1	Calpainopathy: Limb Girdle Muscular Dystrophy Type R1	Walking pattern in the described patient showing lumbar hyperlordosis and waddling gait.
Video 46.1	Caveolinopathy: Rippling Muscle Disease	Rippling muscle.
Video 52.1	Pompe Disease	Limb girdle weakness, and weakness of the muscles of the lower back and abdominal wall resulting in hyperlordosis and prominent abdominal wall extension. When walking, the patient bends backwards to remain stable.
Video 52.2	Pompe Disease	Proximal muscle weakness resulting in Gowers sign when rising from a chair.
Video 61.1	Anti-SRP-Positive Immune-Mediated Necrotizing Myopathy	Irreversible weakness ('damage') of hip anteflexors and hip abductors manifesting in a pronounced waddling gait in a 67-year-old woman with a 23-year history of SRP-pos IMNM.
Video 62.1	Inclusion Body Myositis	A 72-year-old woman with a 20-year history of IBM. Severe distal weakness of the arms with MRC 0 weakness of the deep finger flexors (flexing the distal phalanges). Facial weakness: firmly closing the eyes is incomplete, right more than left. Pouting the lips is weak. Whistling is not possible. Articulating consonants that require closing the lips is difficult, but there are no other features of dysarthria such as a nasal voice. Courtesy Dr Henk-Jan Westeneng.

Index

Locators in bold refer to tables; those in italic to figures; underline to videos

acetylcholine receptor (AChR)
 congenital myasthenic syndromes, 170
 neuromuscular junction disorders, 2–3
AChR-myasthenia gravis, 157–158, *160*
 clinical features, **157**
 clinical history/symptoms, 157, *158*
 compound muscle action potential, *159*
 diagnosis, 157, 158
 examination, 157
 follow-up, 157
 management, 158–161
 myasthenic crisis, 161
 prognosis, 158–161
acid alpha-glucosidase (GAA), **29–30**, 219
acid maltase *see* acid alpha-glucosidase
acute flaccid myelitis (AFM), 93
acute inflammatory demyelinating polyneuropathy (AIDP), 96
acute motor and sensory axonal neuropathy (AMSAN), 96
acute motor axonal neuropathy (AMAN), 96
adrenomyeloneuropathy, 78
AFM (acute flaccid myelitis), 93
AIDP (acute inflammatory demyelinating polyneuropathy), 96
alcohol-induced myopathies, 263, **264**, 265
alcoholic polyneuropathy, 130–131, **138**
 clinical history/symptoms, 130
 diagnosis, 130
 examination, 130
 follow-up, 130
 management, 131
 prognosis, 131
aldolase A deficiency (GSDX11, ALDOA), **33**
allodynia, **28**, 110, 132
alpha-dystroglycan, 191–192
ALS *see* amyotrophic lateral sclerosis
AMAN (acute motor axonal neuropathy), 96
amiodarone polyneuropathy, 137–139
 blue-grey discoloration of face/hands, *138*
 clinical history/symptoms, 137
 diagnosis, 137
 examination, 137
 follow-up, 137
AMSAN (acute motor and sensory axonal neuropathy), 96
amyloid myopathy, **49**, 249–250, 252
amyloidosis, 155, 155

amyotrophic lateral sclerosis (ALS), 1, 72–76, *73*
 clinical history/symptoms, 1, 71
 diagnosis, 1–2, 71–72, *73*
 differential diagnoses, **74–75**
 electrodiagnostic studies, **37**
 examination, 71
 follow-up, 72
 Gold Coast criteria for diagnosis, **74**
 management, 75–76
 multidisciplinary care, 76
 phenotypes, **72**
 spasticity management, 60
 videos, <u>272</u>
anaesthetic management, 60–63
Andersen–Tawil syndrome, 213, 215
ANO5 distal myopathy, 23–24
ANO5 gene, 202
anoctaminopathy, 203–205, *204*
anterior horn cell diseases, 1–2
antisense oligonucleotide mediated exon skipping, 174
antisense oligonucleotides (ASOs), 57
anti-synthetase syndrome (ASyS), **45**, 249
arachnodactyly, MTM1 myopathy, *238*, *239*
ASOs *see* antisense oligonucleotides
AsyS *see* anti-synthetase syndrome
ataxia, differential diagnoses, **26**
ATTR *see* transthyretin amyloidosis
ATTR-PN (transthyretin amyloidosis-polyneuropathy), 155, *156*
autonomic dysfunction, examination, 14
axial weakness
 differential diagnoses, **19–20**
 examination, 10
azathioprine, 160, 162, 248, **255**

Becker muscular dystrophy (BMD), 174, 177–179
 clinical history/symptoms, *176*, 176
 CT scan, *177*
 diagnosis, 176
 differential diagnoses, 176
 examination, 176
 follow-up, 176
 imaging, **45**
 incidence, 177
 muscle biopsy, *177*, 179
 phenotypical spectrum of dystrinopathies, *178*
 videos, <u>273</u>
Becker myotonia, 213, 215
behavioural problems, 7–8, 174
Beighton scale for hypermobility, **9**
bent spine (camptocormia), **19–20**

β enolase deficiency, **33**
Bethlem myopathy, 193–194
 clinical features, **194**
 clinical history/symptoms, 193
 CT scan, *195*
 diagnosis, 193
 elbow contractures, *193*
 examination, 193
 imaging, **45**
biopsy *see* muscle biopsy; nerve biopsy; skin biopsy
blue-grey skin discoloration, amiodarone polyneuropathy, 137, *138*
BMD *see* Becker muscular dystrophy
Borrelia burgdorferi see Lyme radiculopathy/Lyme disease
bortezomib, 107, **138**
botulism, **29–30**, 86
brachial plexus neuropathy *see* neuralgic amyotrophy
breathing problems *see* respiratory muscle weakness
Brody disease, 9, **32–34**, 228
Brown–Violetta–Van Laere syndrome, **16**, 18
bulbar muscles; *see also* spinal and bulbar muscular atrophy
 DM1, **184**
 examination, 9–10
 MG, 17
 postpolio syndrome, 92

CACNA1S gene, 213
 exertional rhabdomyolysis, *269*, 269
calpain-related limb girdle muscular dystrophy, 189–190, **190**
calpainopathy, 189–190, **190**, <u>273</u>
camptocormia (bent spine), **19–20**
cannabis-derived products, neuropathic pain, 60
CANOMAD syndrome (chronic ataxic neuropathy, external ophthalmoplegia, M-protein agglutination, disialosyl antibodies), **16**
carbohydrate metabolic myopathies, 224; *see also* McArdle disease; Pompe disease
cardiac function, **30–31**
 alcohol use, 265
 amyloidosis, 155, *156*
 Andersen–Tawil syndrome, 213, 215
 BMD, **178**, 179
 desminopathy, 211
 diagnosis, 6
 DM, 249

274

DM1, 184
DM2, 185, **186**, 186
drug-induced myopathies, 263–264
drug-induced polyneuropathies, 137
EDMD, **199**, 199–200
management, 59
MFMs, 210, **211**
myopathies, 4, **208**
OPMD, 197
PMDs, **232**
Pompe disease, **221**
pregnancy, 63
carnitine palmitoyltransferase (CPT) deficiency, **33–34**
clinical history/symptoms, 227
diagnosis, 227–228
follow-up, 228
types, 228–229
cataract, 6–7, **32–34**, 53, 185
CAV3 gene, 201
caveolinopathy, **123**, 201
clinical features, **201**
clinical history/symptoms, 200
diagnosis, 201
examination, 200–201
follow-up, 201
videos, 273
central core disease, **19–20**, **32**, 235, *236*, **236**, 236
central nervous system involvement, 7–8, 10, **22–23**, 123, 231, 234–235
cerebrospinal fluid, 1–2, 93, 94
cervical spondylotic myelopathy, 74–75
cervical stenosis, 78, *152*
channelopathies *see* skeletal muscle channelopathies
Charcot arthropathy, **153**
Charcot deformities, *151*
Charcot–Marie–Tooth disease (CMT), **64**, **273**
Charcot–Marie–Tooth disease type 1A, 144–148
classificatory features, **145–146**
clinical features, **146**
clinical history/symptoms, 144
diagnosis, 144
differential diagnoses, 145–146
examination, 144
follow-up, 144
management, 147
muscle atrophy, *147*
Charcot–Marie–Tooth disease type 2, **145–146**, 145–146
Charcot–Marie–Tooth disease (CMT) types 2A/2B, 150–151
clinical history/symptoms, *149*, 149
diagnosis, 150
examination, 149–150
follow-up, 150
RAS-associated protein gene, *150*, 150–151
chemotherapy-induced peripheral neuropathy (CIPN), **138**, 138
chloride channelopathy, 212
chloroquine (CQ), drug-induced myopathies, 263–264
CHRNE gene, 170
chronic fatigue syndrome, 165–166

chronic idiopathic axonal polyneuropathy (CIAP), 134
clinical features, **134**
clinical history/symptoms, 131–132
diagnosis, 132
differential diagnoses, **133**
examination, 132
follow-up, 132
risk factors, *134*
chronic inflammatory demyelinating polyneuropathy (CIDP), 108
clinical history/symptoms, 97
diagnosis, 97–98
diagnostic criteria, **97**
differential diagnoses, 43, **98**
distribution of symptoms in variants, *99*
examination, 97
follow-up, 98
imaging, 42–43, *44*
management, 98–99
prognosis, 98–99
videos, 273
chronic polyneuropathy, 132–134; *see also above*
differential diagnoses, **133**
prevalence, *133*
risk factors, *134*
chronic progressive external ophthalmoplegia (CPEO), 230, **232**, *233*
clinical history/symptoms, 230, *233*
clinical features, **232**
differential diagnoses, 230
examination, 230
follow-up, 230
management, 233
CIAP *see* chronic idiopathic axonal polyneuropathy
CIDP *see* chronic inflammatory demyelinating polyneuropathy
CIP/CIM *see* critical illness polyneuropathy/myopathy
CIPN *see* chemotherapy-induced peripheral neuropathy
cisplatin, **24–25**, *26*
CK *see* creatine kinase
claw hand
CMT, *144*, 144, **145–146**
leprosy, *142*, 142
CMS *see* congenital myasthenic syndromes
CMT *see* Charcot–Marie–Tooth disease
CNV analysis *see* copy number variant analysis
coasting effect, **24–25**, 139
Coats syndrome, 181
coenzyme Q 10,
collagen VI-related myopathies; *see also* Bethlem myopathy; Ullrich congenital muscular dystrophy
clinical features, **194**
imaging, 45
complex repetitive discharges (CRDs), EMG, **272**
congenital cranial dysinnervation disorders (CCDDs), **16**
congenital fibrosis of the extraocular muscles (CFEOM), **16**

congenital myasthenic syndromes (CMS), 3, 170; *see also* Dok7 myasthenic syndrome
diagnosis, 171
genes involved, *171*
management, 171–172
videos, 273
congenital myopathies, imaging, 45; *see also* nemaline myopathy
congenital ptosis, **16**
contractures *see* elbow contractures; muscle contractures
copper deficiency myelopathy, 78
copy number variant (CNV) analysis, 54; *see also* genetic testing
corticosteroids
drug-induced myopathies, **264**, 265
immunotherapy, 57–58
vasculitic neuropathy, 109–110
counselling, 65
FSHD, 182
OPMD, 197
spinal muscular atrophy, 86
CPEO *see* chronic progressive external ophthalmoplegia
CPT 2, *see* carnitine palmitoyltransferase
cramp, **178**
differential diagnoses, **27**
examination, 8
management, 60
cramp-fasciculation syndrome, **123**, 124
creatine kinase (CK), 268; *see also* hyperCKaemia
Bethlem myopathy, 194
BMD, 179
IIMs, 249
JDM, 244
McArdle disease, 224
myopathies, 40–41
non-dystrophic myotonic syndromes, 215
critical illness polyneuropathy (CIP)/myopathy (CIM), 136
clinical features, **136**
clinical history/symptoms, 135
diagnosis, 135
examination, 135
follow-up, 136
ICU-acquired weakness, 136
ventilator weaning, 136–137
CT scanning (computed tomography)
Bethlem myopathy, *195*
BMD, *177*
LGMD, *188*, 191
MG, 157
cyanocobalamin deficiency, 78
cytochrome b deficiency (Complex III), **33–34**
cytochrome-C-oxidase deficiency, **33–34**
cytostatic medication, drug-induced polyneuropathies, **138**, 138

Danon disease, **30–31**, **32**
dapsone, **138**, 143
DCM (dilated cardiomyopathy), **178**, 179
deafness, 16, 145–146
deep finger flexor muscles, 74–75

Index

Dejerine–Sottas phenotype, 146
dementia, frontotemporal
  ALS, 7, 53, *73*
  VCP distal myopathy, **19–20, 208**
demyelination
  CMT type 2, 145–146
  drug-induced polyneuropathies, 137, **138**
  GBS, 96
  neuropathies, *38*
dermatomyositis (DM), 251
  clinical features, 249
  clinical history/symptoms, *247*, 247, *250*, *251*
  dermatomyositis-specific autoantibodies, **250**
  diagnosis, 247
  differential diagnoses, 249–250
  examination, 247
  follow-up, 247–248
  imaging, 45
  muscle biopsy, 249–250
  short tau inversion recovery data, *248*
  skin abnormalities, **250**
dermatomyositis-specific autoantibodies (DMSAs), **250**
DES gene, 209
desminopathy, 211
diabetic neuropathy, 128–129
  classificatory features, **129**
  clinical history/symptoms, 127
  diagnosis, 127–128
  examination, 127
  follow-up, 128
  management, 129
  nerve injury patterns, *128*
diaphragm weakness, 87, 126, 137, **145–146**, 164, **192**
dilated cardiomyopathy (DCM), **178**, 179
distal anoctaminopathy, 202–203
distal filaminopathy, **204**
distal myopathies, **22–23**, 203, **205**; *see also* GNE myopathy
  clinical history/symptoms, 202, *202*, *204*
  diagnosis, 202–203
  differential diagnoses, **23–24**, 202–203
  examination, 202
  follow-up, 203
  short tau inversion recovery data, *203*
  showing rimmed vacuoles in muscle biopsy, **208**
distal myopathy with myotilin defect, **204**
distal myopathy with rimmed vacuoles *see* GNE myopathy
DM *see* myotonic dystrophy
DMD gene variants, 174, *175*, **178**; *see also* Becker muscular dystrophy; Duchenne muscular dystrophy
DMRV (distal myopathy with rimmed vacuoles) *see* GNE myopathy
DMSAs (dermatomyositis-specific autoantibodies), **250**
DNA testing *see* genetic testing
DNAJB6 gene, **21–22, 23–24**
Dok7 myasthenic syndrome, 170

clinical features, 170–171
clinical history/symptoms, 168–169
diagnosis, 169
examination, 169
follow-up, 169–170
management, 171–172
muscle biopsy, 169
muscle ultrasound, *170*
dorsal root ganglia (DRG), 114–115, **115**
dropped head, differential diagnoses, **19–20**
drug-induced myasthenia gravis
  clinical history/symptoms, 163
  diagnosis, 164
  drugs to avoid or use with caution, **165**
  examination, 163–164
  follow-up, 164
  management, 165
drug-induced myopathies, 263, **264**, 265; *see also* hydroxychloroquine myopathy
  alcohol, 263, **264**, 265
  clinical history/symptoms, 262
  diagnosis, 263
  examination, 263
  follow-up, 263
  hydroxychloroquine, 263–264, **264**
  muscle biopsy, *263*
  statins, 263, **264**, 264–265
  steroids, **264**, 265
  vitamin D deficiency, 263, **264**, 266
drug-induced polyneuropathies, 137–139
  clinical history/symptoms, 137
  cytostatic drugs, **138**, 138
  diagnosis, 137
  examination, 137
  toxins and drugs which can cause, **138**
Duane syndrome, **16**
Duchenne muscular dystrophy (DMD), 174–175
  clinical history/symptoms, *173*, 173
  comorbidities, 174
  diagnosis, 173
  DMD gene variants, 174, *175*
  examination, 173
  follow-up, 173–174
  imaging, 45
  phenotypical spectrum of dystrinopathies, **178**
dysautonomia, differential diagnoses, **26**
DYSF gene, 202, 203
dysferlinopathy, 203, *204*, 205
dysimmune neuropathies, **26–27**, *38*, **43**, **272**
dysphagia, management, 59–60
dystroglycanopathies, 191–192
dystrophin–glycoprotein complex (DGC), *190*

EDMD *see* Emery–Dreifuss muscular dystrophy
elbow contractures, Bethlem myopathy, *193*
electrodiagnostic studies, 35, *36*, *39*
  ALS, **37**
  IgM anti-MAG polyneuropathy, 103
  motor neuron diseases, 35

myopathies, 40–41
neuromuscular junction disorders, 38, *40*
neuropathies, 35, *38*, *39*
PPS, 92
videos, **271–272**
emerinopathies, imaging, **45**
emerins (nuclear envelope proteins), 200
Emery–Dreifuss muscular dystrophy (EDMD), 199–200
  clinical features, **199**
  clinical history/symptoms, 198
  diagnosis, 198–199
  examination, 198
  follow-up, 199
  MRI scan, *199*
  phenotypes, 200
EMG (electromyography) *see* electrodiagnostic studies
end-of-life care *see* palliative care
endocrine myopathy, 261–262
  clinical history/symptoms, 260
  diagnosis, 260–261
  differential diagnoses, 260
  examination, 260
  follow-up, 261
  muscle biopsy, *261*
eosinophilic granulomatosis with polyangitis (EGPA), 109
epimerase-kinase enzyme, 207; *see also* GNE myopathy
Erasmus Polyneuropathy Symptom Score (E-PSS), 132
ERM *see* exertional rhabdomyolysis
EURO-NMD-ERN recommendations, immunohistochemical stains, **49**
European Federation of Neurological Societies/Peripheral Nerve Society (EFNS/PNS), MMN diagnostic criteria, **119**
European Malignant Hyperthermia (MH) Group, 237
exertional rhabdomyolysis (ERM)
  clinical history/symptoms, *269*, 269
  diagnosis, 269–270
  examination, 269
  follow-up, 270
  RYR1 myopathy, 237
external ophthalmoplegia, 9, **16**

facial weakness
  differential diagnoses, **17**
  examination, 9
facioscapulohumeral muscular dystrophy (FSHD), 181–182
  clinical features, **181**
  clinical history/symptoms, 180
  diagnosis, 180
  examination, 180
  follow-up, 180
  imaging, **45**
  phenotypes, **181**
  pregnancy and obstetrics, **64**
family history
  genetic testing, 53
  history taking, 6–7
fasciculations
  differential diagnoses, **27**
  examination, 8

ultrasound, 272
fatigability/fatigue
   examination, 11–13
   management, 58
   SMA type 3, 90
   tests, **13**
fatty acid metabolism disorders, 33–34
fatty acid oxidation disorders (FAODs), 228, *229*
Fazio–Londe syndrome, **18**
fibreoptic evaluation of swallowing (FEES), 10
FKRP gene *see* limb girdle muscular dystrophy R9
flail arm syndrome, 72, *81*, 83
forced vital capacity, 10, 71, 72, 80, 96, 164, 207, 211
Friedreich ataxia, **28–29**
frontotemporal dementia *see* dementia
FSHD *see* facioscapulohumeral muscular dystrophy
functional neurological symptom disorder (FND), 14

GAA (acid alpha-glucosidase), 219
ganglionopathies, 114–115; *see also* paraneoplastic sensory neuronopathy
gastrointestinal involvement, management, 59–60
GBS *see* Guillain–Barré syndrome
gene–phenotype associations, 55
genetic(s)
   differential diagnoses, 146
   distal myopathies, 203
   DM2, 185–186
   EDMD, 200
   FSHD, 181
   MTM1 myopathy, 240
   myofibrillar myopathies, 210–211
   OPMD, 196–197
   peripheral neuropathies, 2
   RYR1 myopathy, 237
   SMA type 1, 86, 87
   SMA type 3, 88–90
genetic counselling *see* counselling
genetic testing, 52, *52*
   consequences of genetic diagnosis, 53
   family history, 53
   first-line tests, 53–54
   interpretation of results, 55–56
   mitochondrial DNA, 54
   NGS panels, 53–54
   second-line tests, 54
   structural variations, 54
genetic treatments, 57
genetic variants, significance of, 55–56
genome aggregation database (gnomAD), 55
Gestalt approaches, ix, 47
glutaric aciduria type I, **33–34**
glycogen metabolism disorders, 33
glycogen storage diseases *see* McArdle disease; Pompe disease
GNE myopathy, 207–209
   clinical features, **208**
   clinical history/symptoms, 206, *207*
   diagnosis, 206–207
   examination, 206

follow-up, 207
MRI scan, *207*
pregnancy and obstetrics, **64**
rimmed vacuoles in muscle biopsy, 207–208, **208**
Gottron papules, DM, *247*, 251
Gowers sign
   DMD, *173*
   videos, 273
Graves disease, **213**, 214, 262
GSDs (glycogen storage diseases) *see* McArdle disease; Pompe disease
Guillain–Barré syndrome (GBS), 94–96
   clinical history/symptoms, 94
   diagnosis, 94
   diagnostic criteria, **95**
   examination, 94
   follow-up, 94
   frequency of disease, *95*
   imaging, 43
   immunotherapy, 57
   management, 96
   MFS-GBS overlap syndrome, 96, 272
   prognosis, 96

Hashimoto thyroiditis, 261, 262
heart *see* cardiac function
hereditary inclusion body myopathy *see* GNE myopathy
hereditary motor neuropathies (HMN), 1
   diagnosis, 1–2
   therapies, 2
hereditary neuralgic amyotrophy (HNA), 126–127
hereditary neuropathy with liability to pressure palsies (HNPP), **145–146**, 147–148
hereditary sensory and autonomic neuropathies (HSAN), **145–146**, 145
hereditary sensory and autonomic neuropathy type 4, *150*, 152–153, *153*
   Charcot arthropathy, **153**
   clinical features, 152
   clinical history/symptoms, *151*, 151
   diagnosis, 151–152
   examination, 151
   follow-up, 152
   MRI scan, *152*
hereditary spastic paraplegia (HSP), **28–29**, 78, *153*
hereditary transthyretin amyloidosis-polyneuropathy (ATTRv-PN), 155, **156**; *see also* transthyretin amyloidosis
Hirayama disease, **22–23**, 74–75, 83
histochemical stains, muscle biopsy, 49
HMN *see* hereditary motor neuropathies
HNA (hereditary neuralgic amyotrophy), 126–127
HSAN *see* hereditary sensory and autonomic neuropathies
hydroxychloroquine, drug-induced myopathies, 263–264, **264**
hyperCKaemia (elevated creatine kinase), 268
   clinical history/symptoms, 266–267

diagnosis, 267
differential diagnoses, 32, 267
drug-induced myopathies, 264
examination, 267
follow-up, 267
MRI scan, *267*
hyperkalaemic periodic paralysis, **213**
hypermobility/hyperlaxity
   Beighton scale for hypermobility, **9**
   differential diagnoses, 28–29
   examination, 9
hyperthyroid myopathy, 262
hypokalaemic periodic paralysis (HypoPP), **213**
   clinical history/symptoms, 216
   diagnosis, 216
   examination, 216
   follow-up, 217
   short tau inversion recovery data, *217*
hypothyroid myopathy, 261–262
hypotonia
   collagen-related myopathies, **194**
   DM1, **184**
   nemaline myopathy, 241–242
   neonatal, **29–146**, 238–239
   Pompe disease, **221**
   RYR1 myopathy, 234–235
   SMA1, 85, *86*
   X-linked myotubular myopathy, 238

IBM *see* inclusion body myositis
ICI *see* immune checkpoint inhibitor
idiopathic brachial plexus neuropathy *see* neuralgic amyotrophy
idiopathic inflammatory myopathies (IIMs), 248–250
   management, 250–251
   types, 248
IENFD (intra-epidermal nerve fibre density), *112*
IgM anti-MAG polyneuropathy/IgM MGUS associated neuropathies, 101
   associated conditions, **102**
   clinical features, 101–103, **103**
   clinical history/symptoms, 99
   diagnosis, 100–101
   examination, 99–100
   follow-up, 101
   management, 103
   nerve motor conduction studies, *100*
   prevalence, 101
IIMs *see* idiopathic inflammatory myopathies
imaging, 42; *see also specific imaging modalities*
   motor neuron diseases, 42
   myopathies, 44–46, **45**
   neuropathies, 42, *43*, 44
   POEMS syndrome, 105
immune checkpoint inhibitor (ICI)-related myasthenia gravis, 164
   clinical history/symptoms, 163
   diagnosis, 164
   examination, 163–164
   follow-up, 164
   management, 165
immune-mediated necrotizing myopathy (IMNM), 255–256, 265

Index

immune-mediated necrotizing myopathy (IMNM), (cont.)
 clinical features, 249
 clinical history/symptoms, 252
 diagnosis, 252–253
 examination, 252
 follow-up, 253–254, *254*
 imaging, **45**
 in juveniles, 246
 management, *255*
 MRI scan, *254*
 muscle biopsy, *253*
 statins, *254*
 videos, **273**
immunohistochemical stains, ERN-EURO-NMD recommendations, 49
immunotherapy, management of neuromuscular disorders, 57–58
inclusion body myositis (IBM), **208**, 248, 257–259
 clinical features, **249**, 257
 clinical history/symptoms, 256–257, *258–259*
 diagnosis, 257, 259–260
 examination, 257
 follow-up, 257
 imaging, **45**
 management, 260
 muscle atrophy, *258–259*
 muscle biopsy, *258*
 videos, **273**
infantile-onset Pompe disease (IOPD), **221**, 223; *see also* paediatrics
intensive care unit (ICU)-acquired weakness, 136–137; *see also* critical illness polyneuropathy/myopathy
intra-epidermal nerve fibre density (IENFD), *112*
Isaac syndrome, 37–38, **123**, *124*

joint contractures
 differential diagnoses, **28–29**
 examination, 9
juvenile dermatomyositis (JDM), 244–245
 clinical history/symptoms, 243, *244*
 diagnosis, 243–244, 245–246
 examination, 243
 follow-up, 244
 management, 246
 MRI scan, *245*
 muscle biopsy, *244*, 245
juvenile immune-mediated necrotizing myopathy (IMNM), 246

KCNJ2 gene, **213**, 215
Kearns–Sayre syndrome (KSS), **232**
Kennedy disease *see* spinal and bulbar muscular atrophy

lactate dehydrogenase A deficiency (GSDXI, LDHA), **33**
LAMB2 gene, 170
Lambert–Eaton myasthenic syndrome (LEMS), 3, 166–168
 clinical history/symptoms, 165–166, *167*

comparison with myasthenia gravis, **167**
 development of symptoms, *167*
 diagnosis, 166
 electrodiagnostic studies, 38, *40*
 examination, 166
 follow-up, 166
 management, 168
laminopathies, imaging, **45**
lamins (nuclear envelope proteins), 200
Lasègue sign, Lyme radiculopathy, 141
late-onset Pompe disease (LOPD), 219–222, **221**
LEMS *see* Lambert–Eaton myasthenic syndrome
leprosy (*Mycobacterium leprae*), 143
 clinical history/symptoms, *142*, 142
 diagnosis, 142–143
 differential diagnoses, 142
 examination, 142
 follow-up, 143
 skin biopsy, *143*
limb girdle muscular dystrophies (LGMDs), 188–189
 clinical history/symptoms, 187
 CT scan, *188*
 diagnosis, 187
 dystrophin–glycoprotein complex (DGC, *190*
 examination, 187
 follow-up, 188
 imaging, **45**
 pregnancy and obstetrics, **64**
 scapula winging, *187*
 subtypes, **188**, **189**, **203**; *see also below*
 videos, **272**
limb girdle muscular dystrophy R1, 189–190, **190**
limb girdle muscular dystrophy R9, 192
 clinical features, **192**
 clinical history/symptoms, 191
 diagnosis, 191
 differential diagnoses, 191
 examination, 191
 follow-up, 191
limbic encephalitis, **123**
LGMDs *see* limb girdle muscular dystrophies
LOPD (late-onset Pompe disease), 219–222, **221**
LPIN1 deficiency, **33–34**
lung weakness *see* respiratory muscle weakness
Lyme radiculopathy/Lyme disease, 141
 clinical features in children, **141**
 clinical history/symptoms, 139, *140*
 diagnosis, 140–141
 examination, 139–140
 follow-up, 141
 MRI scan, *140*

malignant hyperthermia, **213**, 235–237, 268, 270
 anaesthetic use, 60–62
 exertional rhabdomyolysis, 270
 RYR1 myopathy, **236**, 237
Malignant Hyperthermia (MH) Group, 237

man-in-the-barrel *see* flail arm syndrome
management of neuromuscular disorders, 57; *see also under specific conditions*
 anaesthetics, 60–63
 cardiac involvement, 59
 care transitions throughout life course, 65–66
 gastrointestinal involvement, 59–60
 genetic counselling, 65
 genetic treatments, 57
 immunotherapy, 57–58
 multidisciplinary care, 58–59
 pain management, 60, *61*
 POEMS syndrome, 107
 pregnancy and obstetrics, 63–65, **64**
 rehabilitation and palliative care, 58
 respiratory muscle weakness, 59
 surgery, 60–63
 telemedicine, 66
MC (myotonia congenita), **213**, 215
McArdle disease, 225
 clinical features, **225**
 clinical history/symptoms, 224
 diagnosis, 224–225
 follow-up, 225
 muscle biopsy, *224*
 rhabdomyolysis, **225**, 225–226
McLeod syndrome, **32**
Marcus Gunn ptosis, **16**
Marinesco–Sjögren syndrome, **33–34**
Medical Research Council scale for assessment of muscle strength, **11**
MELAS (mitochondrial encephalomyopathy with lactic acidosis and stroke-like episodes), **232**
MEMSA *see* myoclonic epilepsy, myopathy, sensory ataxia
MERRF *see* myoclonus epilepsy with ragged red fibres
MFMs *see* myofibrillar myopathies
MFN2 gene, *149*
MFS *see* Miller–Fisher syndrome
MG *see* myasthenia gravis
MGUS (monoclonal gammopathy of undetermined significance) polyneuropathy *see* IgM anti-MAG polyneuropathy
microscopic polyangiitis (MPA), 109
Miller–Fisher syndrome (MFS), 96
 MFS-GBS overlap syndrome, 96, **272**
mitochondrial DNA (mtDNA) testing, 54
mitochondrial encephalomyopathy with lactic acidosis and stroke-like episodes (MELAS), **232**
mitochondrial myopathies, 230, **232**; *see also* primary mitochondrial disorders
mitochondrial neurogastrointestinal encephalomyopathy (MNGIE), **232**
mitochondrial trifunctional protein (MTP) deficiency/ LCHAD deficiency, **33–34**
Miyoshi myopathy, 202–203, **204**, *205*

Index

MLPA (multiplex ligation-dependent probe amplification), 54
MMN *see* multifocal motor neuropathy
modified Erasmus GBS Respiratory Insufficiency Score (mEGRIS), 94, 96
Moebius syndrome, 16, 17
monoclonal gammopathy of undetermined significance (MGUS) *see* IgM anti-MAG polyneuropathy
Morvan syndrome, 123, 124
   clinical history/symptoms, 122
   diagnosis, 122–123
   electrodiagnostic studies, 37–38
   examination, 122
   follow-up, 123
   videos, **273**
motor neuron diseases, 1; *see also* amyotrophic lateral sclerosis; primary lateral sclerosis; progressive muscular atrophy
   differential diagnoses, 35
   electrodiagnostic studies, 35
   imaging, 42, **45**
MR (magnetic resonance) imaging, 42
   EDMD, *199*
   GNE myopathy, *207*
   HSAN, *152*
   hyperCKaemia, *267*
   IMNM, *254*
   JDM, 245
   Lyme radiculopathy, *140*
   MMN, *121*
   segmental SMA, *83*
MTM 1 myopathy, *see* X-linked myotubular myopathy
multidisciplinary care, 58–59
multifocal motor neuropathy (MMN), *118*, 120–122
   clinical history/symptoms, 118
   diagnosis, 118–119, *120*
   diagnostic criteria, 119
   differential diagnoses, **120**
   examination, 118
   follow-up, 120
   imaging, 42, *44*
   immunotherapy, 57
   MRI scan, *121*
multi/minicore myopathy, 16
multiminicore disease, 19–20
multiple acyl-coenzyme A dehydrogenase deficiency (MADD), 33–34
multiplex ligation-dependent probe amplification (MLPA), 54
muscle(s), action and innervation, 11, 12
muscle biopsy, 47, 48
   BMD, *177*, *179*
   DM, 249–250
   Dok7 myasthenic syndrome, *169*
   drug-induced myopathies, *263*
   endocrine myopathy, *261*
   IBM, *258*
   IMNM, *253*
   JDM, *244*, 245
   McArdle disease, *224*
   MFM, *210*
   MTM1 myopathy, *239*
   normal muscle tissue, *48*
   rimmed vacuoles, 207–208, **208**
   RYR1 myopathy, *235*
   stains, *47*, **49**
   techniques and tissue preparation, 48
muscle chloride channelopathy, 212
muscle contractures
   differential diagnoses, 27
   examination, 9
muscle glycolysis disorders, 224; *see also* McArdle disease
muscle hypertrophy, differential diagnoses, 28
muscle ultrasound (MUS), 42
muscular dystrophies, *190*; *see also* Becker muscular dystrophy; Duchenne muscular dystrophy; Emery–Dreifuss muscular dystrophy; limb girdle muscular dystrophies
MuSK-myasthenia gravis, 162–163
   clinical features, **162**
   clinical history/symptoms, 161
   diagnosis, 162
   examination, 161–162
   follow-up, 162
   management, 163
   tongue abnormalities, *162*
myalgia and cramps syndrome, 178
myasthenia gravis (MG), 2–3; *see also* AChR-myasthenia gravis; drug-induced myasthenia gravis; immune checkpoint inhibitor-related myasthenia gravis; MuSK-myasthenia gravis
   comparison with LEMS, **167**
   electrodiagnostic studies, 38, *40*
   examination, 11–13
   fatigability tests, 13
   pregnancy and obstetrics, **64**
   videos, **273**
myasthenic crisis, 161
Mycobacterium leprae see leprosy
myoclonic epilepsy, myopathy, sensory ataxia (MEMSA), **232**
myoclonus epilepsy with ragged red fibres (MERRF), **232**, *233*
myofibrillar myopathies (MFMs), **208**, 210–211
   clinical features, **211**
   clinical history/symptoms, 209
   diagnosis, 209
   examination, 209
   follow-up, 209–210
   muscle biopsy, *210*
myokymia
   differential diagnoses, 27
   examination, 8
myosin myopathy (MyHC IIa), 16
myositis *see* idiopathic inflammatory myopathies; immune-mediated necrotizing myopathy
myositis-associated antibodies (MAAs), 245
myotonia
   differential diagnoses, 27
   examination, 8–9
myotonia congenita (MC), **213**, 214, 215
myotonic discharges, EMG, **271–272**
myotonic dystrophies; *see also below*
   imaging, 45
   videos, **273**
myotonic dystrophy type 1 (DM1), 183–185
   clinical features, **184**, **186**
   clinical history/symptoms, 182, *183*
   diagnosis, 182–183
   examination, 182
   facial appearance, *183*
   follow-up, 183
   management, **184**
myotonic dystrophy type 2 (DM2), 185–186
   clinical features, **186**, 186
   clinical history/symptoms, 185
   diagnosis, 185
   examination, 185
   follow-up, 185
   phenotypes, 186
myotubular myopathy *see* X-linked myotubular myopathy

NA *see* neuralgic amyotrophy
NARP (neuropathy, (episodic) ataxia and retinitis pigmentosa), **232**
NEB gene, 241
nemaline myopathy, 241–243
   clinical features, **242**
   clinical history/symptoms, 240
   diagnosis, 241
   differential diagnoses, 241
   examination, 241
   follow-up, 241
   rods in muscle fibres, *241*, 242
   TPM2 gene, 242
neonatal hypotonia, differential diagnoses, 29–30
neonatal myasthenia gravis, 16, 17
neostigmine test, 13
nerve biopsy, 48–50
   IgM anti-MAG polyneuropathy, 103
   vasculitic neuropathy, *108*, 108, 109
nerve motor conduction studies, IgM anti-MAG polyneuropathy, *100*
nerve pain, management, 60
nerve ultrasound (NUS), 42
neuralgic amyotrophy (NA), 19, 125–126
   clinical features, **126**
   clinical history/symptoms, 124–125, *125*
   diagnosis, 125
   examination, 125
   hereditary, 126–127
   management, 126
   prognosis, 126
neurofilament light chain, 79
neuromuscular junction disorders, 2–3; *see also* myasthenia gravis
   electrodiagnostic studies, 38, *40*
   therapies, 3
neuronopathies, 2, 25, 26, 37; *see also* sensory neuronopathies
neuropathic hereditary transthyretin (TTR) amyloidosis, 155, **156**
neuropathic pain, 2
neuropathy, (episodic) ataxia and retinitis pigmentosa (NARP), **232**

279

Index

neutral lipid storage disease, 30–31, **32**
next-generation sequencing (NGS) panels, 53–54; *see also* genetic testing
Nonaka myopathy *see* GNE myopathy
nondystrophic myotonias, 212, **214**, 215
nuclear envelope proteins, 200
nutritional deficiencies, myopathies, 263

obstetrics, management, 63–65, **64**
oculopharyngeal muscular dystrophy (OPMD), 196–197, **208**
    clinical features, **197**
    clinical history/symptoms, 196
    diagnosis, 196
    examination, 196
    management, 197
oculopharyngodistal myopathy, **16**, 18
ophthalmoplegia, external, 9, **16**
overlap-myositis, clinical features, 249

PABPN1 gene, 196–197
paediatrics; *see also* juvenile dermatomyositis
    care transitions throughout life course, 65–66
    examination, 7–14
    immune-mediated necrotizing myopathy, 246
    Lyme radiculopathy, **141**
    Pompe disease, **221**, 223
pain
    differential diagnoses, **28**
    management, 60
    treatment algorithm, *61*
palliative care, 58
    ALS, 76
    SMA type 1, 87
PAN *see* polyarteritis nodosa
paramyotonia congenita, **213**
paraneoplastic sensory neuronopathy, 115
    antibodies associated with cancer in, **116**
    clinical history/symptoms, 114
    diagnostic criteria, **115**
    examination, 114
    follow-up, 114
    ganglionopathies, 114
Parsonage–Turner syndrome. *see* neuralgic amyotrophy
percussion-induced muscle mounding (PIMMs), caveolinopathy, 201
percussion-induced rapid contractions (PIRCs), caveolinopathy, 201
peripheral nerve hyperexcitability syndromes, **123**, *123*. *see also* Isaac syndrome; limbic encephalitis; Morvan syndrome; rippling muscle disease; stiff person syndrome
    electrodiagnostic studies, 37–38
    spectrum of disorders, *124*
    videos, **272**–**273**
PET (positron emission tomography), POEMS syndrome, *105*
PGT (pre-implantation genetic testing), 65
    phosphatidic acid phosphatase deficiency, 33–34

phosphofructokinase deficiency (Tarui disease/GSDVII), 33
phosphoglycerate kinase deficiency (PGK1), 33
phosphoglycerate mutase deficiency (GSDX), 33
Pierson syndrome, 170
Plexopathy, electrodiagnostic studies, 37
PLS *see* primary lateral sclerosis
PMA *see* progressive muscular atrophy
PMDs *see* primary mitochondrial disorders
PMP-22 gene,
    CMT, 144, 146–147
    HNPP, **145**–**146**, 147–148
POEMS *see* polyneuropathy, organomegaly, endocrine manifestations, monoclonal protein, and skin changes
polio-like syndrome, West Nile virus, 93
poliomyelitis anterior acuta, 1, 91; *see also* postpolio syndrome
polyarteritis nodosa (PAN), 109
polyneuropathies, 2; *see also* chronic polyneuropathy
    demyelinating features, 38
    electrodiagnostic studies, 37, *38*, *39*
    risk factors, *134*
polyneuropathy, organomegaly, endocrine manifestations, monoclonal protein, and skin changes (POEMS), 105–107
    clinical history/symptoms, 104, *106*
    diagnosis, 104–105
    diagnostic criteria, **106**
    examination, 104
    follow-up, 105
    management, 107
    muscle atrophy and skin discolouration, *104*, 105
    PET imaging, *105*
    prognosis, 107
polyradiculopathy, electrodiagnostic studies, 37
Pompe disease, 219–222
    clinical features, **221**
    clinical history/symptoms, 218, *218*, *221*
    diagnosis, 218–219
    examination, 218
    follow-up, 219
    imaging, 45
    management, 223
    muscle weakness distribution, *220*
    pregnancy and obstetrics, **64**
    respiratory muscle weakness, *222*
    videos, **273**
postpolio syndrome (PPS), 92–93, *92*
    clinical history/symptoms, 91
    diagnosis, 1–2, 91
    diagnostic criteria, **93**
    examination, 91
    follow-up, 91
postural tremor, differential diagnoses, 27
PP (primary periodic paralyses), **213**, 215
PPS *see* postpolio syndrome
prednisolone/prednisone, 157, 160, 162

pregnancy, 63–65, **64**
pre-implantation genetic testing (PGT), 65
primary lateral sclerosis (PLS), 40–41, 79
    anterior horn cell diseases, 1
    clinical history/symptoms, 1, 77, 80
    diagnosis, 77
    diagnostic criteria, **77**, 79
    differential diagnoses, **78**
    examination, 77
    follow-up, 77
    frequency of disease, 79
    prognosis, 80
primary mitochondrial disorders (PMDs), 230–231
    clinical features, **231**, *233*
    with neuromuscular features, **232**
primary periodic paralyses (PP), **213**, 215
progressive muscular atrophy (PMA), 1, 80–81
    clinical history/symptoms, 1, 79
    diagnosis, 1–2, 80
    examination, 79–80
    flail arm syndrome, *81*
    follow-up, 80
    frequency of disease, 80
pseudobulbar palsy, <u>272</u>
ptosis, examination, 9
PURA gene, 170
pyroxidine deficiency, 138

quadriceps sparing myopathy *see* GNE myopathy

Rab7 gene, *150*, 150–151
ragged red fibres, mitochondrial myopathies, *233*; *see also* myoclonus epilepsy with ragged red fibres
RAPSN gene, 170
repetitive nerve stimulation (RNS), 171
respiratory muscle weakness
    differential diagnoses, **19**
    examination, 10
    JDM, 246
    management, 59
    Pompe disease, *222*
reversible infantile respiratory chain deficiency (RIRCD), **232**
rhabdomyolysis (RML), 270; *see also* exertional rhabdomyolysis
    CPT2 deficiency, 227–228
    differential diagnoses, **32**–**34**
    drug-induced myopathies, 263, 265
    McArdle disease, **225**, 225–226
    mitochondrial disorders, 232
    RYR1 myopathy, 237
riboflavin transporter deficiency (RTD), **16**, 18
riluzole, 76
rimmed vacuoles, muscle biopsy, 207–208, **208**; *see also* GNE myopathy
rippling muscles, 201
    caveolinopathy, 200–201
    differential diagnoses, **27**
    examination, 9

280

rippling muscle disease, 123; see also
  caveolinopathy
RIRCD (reversible infantile respiratory
  chain deficiency), 232
RML see rhabdomyolysis
RNS (repetitive nerve stimulation), 171
rods, in muscle fibres, 241, 242; see also
  nemaline myopathy
RYR1 gene, 269
RYR1 myopathy, 235–237
  clinical features, 236
  clinical history/symptoms, 234, 234
  diagnosis, 234–235
  examination, 234
  follow-up, 235
  muscle biopsy, 235
  types, 236, 236

SAAM (statin-associated autoimmune
  myopathy), 265
SANDO (sensory ataxic neuropathy,
  dysarthria, ophthalmoplegia), 232
sarcoid myopathy, 21–22, 249–250
sarcoglycanopathies, 30–31, 32–34, 59,
  227
SBMA see spinal and bulbar muscular
  atrophy
scapular winging
  differential diagnoses, 20
  examination, 10
  LGMD, 187
  Lyme radiculopathy, 140
  NA, 125
SCLC see small-cell lung cancer
SCN4A gene, 213
segmental muscular atrophy, 1, 82,
  83–84
  clinical history/symptoms, 82
  diagnosis, 1–2, 82
  differential diagnoses, 82
  examination, 82
  follow-up, 83
  MRI scan, 83
  therapies, 2
sensory ataxic neuropathy, dysarthria,
  ophthalmoplegia (SANDO), 232
sensory neuronopathies (SNN),
  114–115; see also paraneoplastic
  sensory neuronopathy
  antibodies associated with cancer in
    SNN, 116
  diagnostic criteria, 115
serum creatine kinase see creatine kinase
SFN see small-fibre neuropathy
shawl sign, 247
single-fibre electromyography (SfEMG),
  38
skeletal muscle channelopathies, 213,
  214–215
  clinical history/symptoms, 212
  diagnosis, 212
  examination, 212
  follow-up, 214
  types, 213
skin abnormalities
  DM, 250
  examination, 8
skin biopsy, 50–51
  leprosy, 143

SFN, 111
skin discolouration, POEMS syndrome,
  104, 105
skin lesions, vasculitic neuropathy, 108
skin rash, JDM, 243, 244
SMA see spinal muscular atrophy
small-cell lung cancer (SCLC), 166–168,
  167
small-fibre neuropathy (SFN), 111–113
  associated conditions, 111
  causality, 113
  clinical history/symptoms, 110
  diagnosis, 110–111, 112–113
  differential diagnoses, 111–112
  examination, 110
  follow-up, 111
  grading, 112
  intra-epidermal nerve fibre density,
    112
  management, 113
  phenotypes, 113
  skin biopsy, 111
  symptoms suggesting, 110
small interfering ribonucleic acids
  (siRNAs), 57
small polyphasic motor unit potentials,
  EMG, **271–272**
SMPX distal myopathy, 208
sodium channel myotonia, 213
spastic paraplegia, differential diagnoses,
  78
spasticity of gait, **272**
spasticity, management, 60
spinal and bulbar muscular atrophy
  (SBMA), 1, 84–85, **85**
  clinical history/symptoms, 84, 85
  diagnosis, 1–2, 84
  examination, 84
  follow-up, 84
  videos, **272**
spinal muscular atrophy (SMA), 1; see
  also segmental muscular atrophy
  and see below
  diagnosis, 1–2
  genetic treatments, 57
  imaging, 45
  pregnancy and obstetrics, 64
  therapies, 2
spinal muscular atrophy (SMA) type 1,
  86, 87
  clinical history/symptoms, 85
  diagnosis, 86
  differential diagnoses, 86
  examination, 85–86
  follow-up, 86
  management, 87
spinal muscular atrophy (SMA) type 3,
  89–90
  classificatory features, 89
  clinical history/symptoms, 88
  diagnosis, 88–89
  examination, 88
  follow-up, 89
  management, 90
  phenotypes, 90
statin-associated autoimmune
  myopathy (SAAM), 265
statins, 254, 263, **264**, 264–265
steroids see corticosteroids

stiff person syndrome, **123**
stiffness, differential diagnoses, 28
STIR see short tau inversion recovery
surgical options, 60–63
swallowing difficulties, management,
  59–60

TANGO2-syndrome, 33–34
Tarui disease, 33
telemedicine, 66
tendon reflexes, 13–14
therapy see management of
  neuromuscular disorders
thiamine deficiency, alcoholic
  polyneuropathy, 131
thymidine kinase 2 deficiency, 33–34
thyroid-associated ophthalmopathy, 262
thyrotoxic hypokalaemic periodic
  paralysis (TPP), 213
tick bites, vasculitic neuropathy, 108; see
  also Lyme disease/Lyme
  radiculopathy
time course of disease, history taking, 5
tongue abnormalities
  differential diagnoses, 28
  examination, 10
  MuSK-myasthenia gravis, 162
TPM2 gene, 242
TPP (thyrotoxic hypokalaemic periodic
  paralysis), 213
transthyretin amyloidosis (TTR), 155,
  155
  clinical history/symptoms, 154
  diagnosis, 154
  differential diagnoses, 154
  examination, 154
  follow-up, 154–155
  genetic treatments, 57
  neuropathic type, 155, **156**
transthyretin familial amyloid
  polyneuropathy see hereditary
  transthyretin amyloidosis-
  polyneuropathy
transthyretin (TTR) transport protein,
  155
treatments see management of
  neuromuscular disorders
tremor, differential diagnoses, 27
Trendelenburg sign
  Lyme radiculopathy, 140
  Pompe disease, 218
TTR amyloidosis see transthyretin
  amyloidosis
TTR (transthyretin) transport protein,
  155

Ullrich congenital muscular dystrophy
  (UCMD), 45, **194**, 194, 195
ultrasound (US), 42; see also muscle
  ultrasound; nerve ultrasound
  Dok7 myasthenic syndrome, 170
  videos, **272**

vaccine-derived poliovirus (VDPV), 93
Valsalva manoeuvre, 14
vascular endothelial growth factor
  (VEGF), 105
vasculitic neuropathy, 109–110
  classificatory features, **109**

Index

vasculitic neuropathy (cont.)
  clinical history/symptoms, 107, *108*, **109**
  diagnosis, 108, 109
  examination, 107–108
  follow-up, 108–109
  management, 109–110
  nerve biopsy, *108*, 108
VCP distal myopathy, **208**
ventilator weaning, ICU-acquired weakness, 136–137
very long-chain acyl-CoA dehydrogenase deficiency (VLCAD), **33–34**, 229
video fluoroscopic swallow studies (VFSS), 10
videos
  case studies, 272–273
  EMG, 271–272
  ultrasound, 272

vitamin B1 deficiency, alcoholic polyneuropathy, 131
vitamin B6 deficiency, 138
vitamin B12 deficiency, **78**
vitamin D deficiency, 263, **264**, 266
voltage-gated calcium channels, 3

Wartenberg migrant sensory neuropathy, 117–118
  clinical features, **117**
  clinical history/symptoms, 116–117
  diagnosis, 117
  examination, 117
  follow-up, 117
Welander distal myopathy, **208**
West Nile virus (WNV), 93; *see also* postpolio syndrome
Western blot analysis, *177*
whole exome-sequencing (WES), 53

winging, scapula *see* scapula winging
X-linked dilated cardiomyopathy (DCM), **178**, 179
X-linked muscular dystrophy *see* Emery–Dreifuss muscular dystrophy
X-linked myotubular myopathy (MTM1), 239–240
  arachnodactyly, *238*
  clinical history/symptoms, 238, **239**
  diagnosis, 238–239
  examination, 238
  follow-up, 239
  muscle biopsy, *239*
X-linked recessive diseases. *see* Becker muscular dystrophy; Duchenne muscular dystrophy

For EU product safety concerns, contact us at Calle de José Abascal, 56–1º, 28003 Madrid, Spain or eugpsr@cambridge.org.